BLEED

BLEED

DESTROYING MYTHS AND MISOGYNY IN ENDOMETRIOSIS CARE

TRACEY LINDEMAN

Published by ECW Press
665 Gerrard Street East
Toronto, Ontario, Canada M4M 1Y2
416-694-3348 / info@ecwpress.com

Editor for the Press: Jennifer Knoch
Cover design: Tree Abraham
Author photo: Ben Cruz

LIBRARY AND ARCHIVES CANADA CATALOGUING IN
PUBLICATION

Title: Bleed : destroying myths and misogyny in
endometriosis care / Tracey Lindeman.

Names: Lindeman, Tracey, author.

Identifiers: Canadiana (print) 20220429065 | Canadiana
(ebook) 20220429170

ISBN 978-1-77041-653-6 (softcover)
ISBN 978-1-77852-146-1 (Kindle)
ISBN 978-1-77852-145-4 (PDF)
ISBN 978-1-77852-144-7 (ePub)

Subjects: LCSH: Endometriosis—Treatment. | LCSH:
Endometriosis—Patients—Care. | LCSH: Discrimination
in medical care.

Classification: LCC RG483.E53 L56 2023 | DDC
618.1/42—dc23

This book is funded in part by the Government of Canada. *Ce livre est financé en partie par le gouvernement du Canada.* We
acknowledge the funding support of the Government of Ontario through Ontario Creates. Creation of this work was funded
in part by an Ontario Arts Council grant.

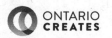

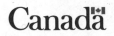

PRINTED AND BOUND IN CANADA

PRINTING: FRIESENS   5   4   3   2

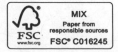

For all of us.

CONTENTS

PROLOGUE
anger can be power

Have you ever been told the pain you feel is imaginary? That the mental anguish you experience from being trapped in a cycle of feeling bad, then feeling bad about feeling bad, could be solved with a better attitude and a brisk walk? Or, have you tried yoga? Meditation? Eating probiotic yogurt? Drinking unicorn blood on a full moon? Perhaps you just need to get off your phone, get out into nature, get into woodworking, go on a vision quest, maybe learn to crochet or take up archery or create YouTube makeup tutorials. I hear Kegels help. Get that pelvic floor into fighting shape!

When you have an invisible disease like endometriosis, you hear versions of this *all the time*. Your friends will tell you they get cramps too. Your partner will tell you to relax. Your doctor will suggest hormonal birth control to tame the pain and the bleeding, and then antidepressants to control the depressive side effects of the birth control, and then when your libido is sufficiently annihilated by the antidepressants, they will simply shrug and ask, "Have you tried losing weight?"

This is death by a million papercuts, little barbs of misogyny meant to undermine your suffering and shut you up. No one wants to hear about the feeling of daggers being plunged into your abdomen and twisted around. No one wants to know how sad, how lonely, how angry you are—not only about being sick, but about how your doctors won't do more than the barest of minimums to help you be a little less sick. You are an island.

There are, according to the World Health Organization, 190 million islands on this planet: people with endometriosis. The real figure is probably double that; about 10 percent of people assigned female at birth are said to experience the disease,[1] and there are about four billion of us in the world.[2] Some people don't know they have it. Others *know* they have it but haven't persuaded the right people to give them a diagnosis. In North America, and much of the Westernized world, people spend an average of seven to ten years trying to get properly diagnosed.[3] Not seven to ten years from the onset of symptoms, but seven to ten years of actively and persistently lobbying doctors to try and figure out what's wrong with them. As such, the average age at diagnosis is somewhere around twenty-eight.[4]

So, what exactly is endometriosis?

In the simplest of terms, it's a disease defined by the growth of endometrial-like tissue outside of the uterus.[5] These growths—called endometriomas, lesions and adhesions—attach to ovaries, fallopian tubes and the exterior of the uterus, as well as the bowel and sometimes as far away as the kidneys, diaphragm, lungs and in rare cases, the brain.[6] For some people, it's as if a bottle of glue was poured into their abdomen; as the glue hardens, organs become stuck together. In an overwhelming majority of cases, the disease is marked by chronic pain and inflammation, infertility and long, heavy menstrual periods. Migraines, digestion problems and sexual dysfunction (including painful orgasms!) are also common. Endometriosis can occur in anyone born with a uterus, and in a microscopic handful of people born without one.[7] There is no cure. Worse, there's not even scientific consensus on how it's caused or how it operates. That said, some researchers suspect the disease has genetic and epigenetic foundations (the latter meaning changes in gene functioning and expression that don't change our DNA sequence[8]), with strong links to hormonal and autoimmune functioning.[9]

All this, and still endometriosis is overwhelmingly treated like a bad period—by the people in our lives, by the medical system that's meant to treat us and by those who create the policies and laws that shape and perpetuate this misunderstanding. This isn't a coincidence. It is *systemic* disregard for our lives.

Endometriosis was first described in literature nearly four thousand years ago and was officially named in the mid-1920s.[10, 11] Birth control was first approved for the treatment of endometriosis in 1957—and, well, not much has happened since then when it comes to new treatments. We're told to take birth control and hope for the best. Or maybe get pregnant? *I hEaR iT's a CuRe.*

This inertia exists at the same time that mere fractions of per-capita pennies are going to publicly funded endometriosis research, if a nation funds research on endo at all. Instead, the pharmaceutical industry has become both the biggest funder and the biggest profiteer of endo research. Drugmakers are collectively raking in billions off the backs of desperate endometriosis patients, and too many physicians are allowing it to happen. Some are even enthusiastically enabling it by accepting consulting fees, travel, drinks and dinner from drug companies—a widespread practice that has proven to influence the prescribing practices of doctors.[12] Meanwhile, surgical experts and patient advocates are left to piss in the wind, trying to get medical colleges to recognize excision—not drugs—as the real gold standard of care.

Endometriosis isn't the only disease that yields so much systemic mistreatment. Another tenth of people assigned female at birth have polycystic ovarian syndrome (PCOS),[13] a hormonal disorder that often causes pain and infertility. A quarter of us have pelvic floor disorders.[14] One in three experience pain during penetrative sex.[15] Did you know sex isn't supposed to *hurt*? (Unless, of course, you want it to.)

There are so many of us, and yet patients feel alone, each of us toiling away in our own bubbles while trying to understand why no one seems to care.

Even those who develop fatal diseases get alienated when those diseases are coded female. Cervical cancer is becoming increasingly common, killing 342,000 globally in 2020 alone.[16] Mortality is highest in places with high poverty rates and insufficient screening for human papillomavirus (HPV), the viral infection known to cause cervical cancer that is most commonly transmitted through sex acts. Those locales include sub-Saharan Africa, Eastern Europe and central Asia.[17] Americans living in high-poverty areas are twice as likely to die from cervical cancer than those in low-poverty areas.[18] Even as a place where Pap smears and HPV vaccines have been routinized,[19] the U.S. is home to massive health inequities that worsen outcomes for a lot of people. For instance, white patients with cervical cancer have a five-year survival rate of 71 percent, while Black patients have a 58 percent rate.[20] Rural Black cervical cancer patients have even slimmer chances of surviving.[21]

Do the dismal math on all this, and it becomes clear we are being given care by a system that fundamentally does not care about us. That's not to say there aren't some very nice, responsible, ethical doctors out there—there are. But they are operating within a system that is rotten to the core, and having good actors in a bad system is not good enough.

Unfortunately, we can't dismantle systems merely by knowing how they work. Instead, we learn to circumvent them. So many people who've been through the medical wringer know this to be true: that systemic reform is a dream, and that making do is the reality. That's why we do our own research and become internet scientists trying to make sense of academic journalese on endometriosis. As we search, we discover there's a community out there—online groups and pages and endo influencers and hashtags turning upwards of 400 million lonely islands into archipelagos, united in our grief and frustration, learning from each other what we haven't been taught by the medical system. This information is critical, and the method of delivery can reach populations who've been traditionally excluded from healthcare systems and movements. But there is also a lot of misinformation, hyperbole and clickbait, and those thrive in the absence of effective, empathetic patient-doctor communication.

This isn't only a physical disease. It's also a psychologically opportunistic one that preys on what makes us insecure, different and disadvantaged—all of which are consequences of systemic and cultural forces pushing us to our limits. In this way, it's also a social disease.

In *BLEED*, I've attempted to weave together the histories and modern realities of female subjugation, hysteria and power imbalances in healthcare to show how the system came to be. There are no self-help tricks here. We have for too long carried the burden of helping ourselves because no one else will. Consider this an evidence file, proof that amid all the stories people love to hear about bootstrapping personal triumph over chronic illness, we are in reality set up to fail.

◆

Endometriosis is a disease almost exclusively affecting people assigned female at birth, including cisgender, non-binary and trans people. Cis women—people whose gender corresponds to their sex at birth—are the vast majority of sufferers when it comes to numbers. Proportionally, though, some early research suggests trans men have a higher incidence rate of endo than cis women,[22] and that gender-affirming care—including hormone replacement therapy—can affect the social and physical experience of the disease.[23]

Despite its cross-gender spectrum, endo is still largely considered to be a "women's disease," painted into a neglected, mistreated corner by the misogyny—and homophobia, and transphobia—rampant in medicine, and in larger society. That gets further compounded by layers of racism, classism, ableism, ageism and the stigmatization of fatness and mental illness. Gender norms are entrenched in the language and beliefs around endometriosis, and we haven't yet figured out how to talk about the disease in an infallibly inclusive way. In fact, some cis patients assert ownership of endo by excluding trans and non-binary people from communities and conversations—as if inclusion demands giving up the *meaning* of their suffering.

I get it: endometriosis feels patently female to cis women, from the places in our bodies where we feel pain, to the paternalism and patriarchal oppression we face when trying to access care. It is a disease associated with menstruation—a supposed beacon of femininity and womanhood. When we get our periods, we're taught that pain is intrinsic to the female experience and therefore doesn't matter. We know this to be true because the men and boys around us don't seem to face the same doubt and dismissal. Our periods become symbols of our alienation and oppression, and our communities are venues for resistance—of which some are extremely protective. What those people don't consider is that many young trans and non-binary people receive the same misogynistic messaging about suffering and self-worth—except, for them, it comes with the aggravated assault of healthcare that doesn't know how to manage menstruation, endo or other pelvic diseases *without* the systemic hatred of women. This is how so many trans and non-binary patients end up being treated as "woman-adjacent"—a reality that can cause people profound harm.

With the view of gender as a binary, we've been tricked into the idea that women only exist as antonyms to men. This is why so much of female suffering is measured against the backdrop of male privilege. I've heard many people say, "If cis men got endometriosis, it would already be cured." That may be true. We've certainly taken male sexual dysfunction seriously—Viagra has been on the market so long its patent expired.[24] And if there were any chronic pain conditions that exclusively affected cis men, we would probably take those more seriously too. Overall, though, the man-versus-woman argument is so tired. It presupposes that the only pain of consequence is that of cis men, when really no one should have to live a life of suffering. And, by playing into a gender binary, we also play into a series of binaries that falsely portray women as a monolith that is only treated differently in comparison to men, when in truth each of us faces disparities in care based on who we are and what we look like. This is precisely why being willfully exclusionary harms us more than it helps us. Owning endometriosis is not a privilege. Four millennia of awful medical care would suggest that designating endo a "women's disease" has never helped *anyone* get better treatment. Instead, it's like being in a boat with a hole in it: the more people we have bailing us out, the greater the chance that we all survive. To that end, *BLEED* includes some best practices laid out in the Trans Journalists Association style guide.[25] Instead of using "women" as shorthand to refer to sufferers, I use "endo patients" and other similarly inclusive terms. I also use "female/male" and "women/men" when contextually appropriate, and sometimes I use "assigned female at birth," shortened to AFAB. When I say "we" and "us," I am talking about all endo patients unless otherwise specified. Similarly, when I say "women" without a qualifier, I mean *all* women. Even with these guardrails, though, my execution of inclusion may not be flawless—and so I humbly ask for grace.

◆

In 1962, Dr. Robert W. Kistner—an endometriosis specialist who helped write the playbook on using hormonal birth control as an endo "cure"—wrote:

> Endometriosis has been noted with increasing frequency during the past two decades; several reports have indicated that it is found in 5–15 percent of pelvic

operations. It is not frequent in the Negro and seems to be found most often among women of the higher socio-economic groups. The median age is about 37 years, but about 15 percent of patients are under 30. It has been suggested that a specific body-type and psychic demeanor are frequently found: meso-morphic but underweight, overanxious, intelligent, egocentric and perfectionist. These characteristics represent a personality pattern in which marriage and childbearing are likely to be deferred and, therefore, predispose the woman to prolonged periods of uninterrupted ovulation.[26]

This passage is more than sixty years old, and yet the myths within it are relevant to the modern experience. Our genders, ethnicities, socioeconomic statuses and classes, body sizes, disabilities and sexualities are used and abused to give us privileges and to discriminate against us. On top of that, actual physical symptoms of diseases like endometriosis vary in severity, meaning people's quality of life is unevenly affected. Hence, there is no single experience of the disease. We all face different barriers, which create strains of personalized oppression that influence our experiences. What I've faced as a straight, white cis woman is just one version of the truth. To better represent our plural reality, *BLEED* includes the voices of people with different privileges and disadvantages to illustrate that there is no consistency in baseline medical care. Rather, it's meted out like Halloween candy based on how much we like someone's costume.

Some may wonder why we put up with all this nonsense. To that I answer, Do we really have a choice? We either live with it, or stop living. Whenever we try to exercise choices about our own bodies, we are penalized by discrimination. Abortion? Don't be so promiscuous. Gender transition? You might change your mind. Having a child?

Excellent! Unless, of course, you are too young, too old, too fat, too poor, too disabled, too Black or brown. *Not* having a child? Well then, you're just selfish.

Judgment of women who choose to be child-free is near to my heart, because I count myself among their ranks. I'm not talking about those who have difficulty conceiving, but women who could theoretically conceive if they wanted to and who choose not to. We all have different motivations for making this choice, but whatever our reasoning, the result is usually the same: we get put dead last for endometriosis care because our plight is about pain, not reproduction.

Challenges to bodily autonomy are outcroppings of white supremacist, paternalistic, patriarchal systems that are fueled by discrimination and the belief that women cannot be trusted to make decisions—especially not about sterilization—even if those decisions impact no one but them. The more discrimination we endure, the more we are told our bodies do not truly belong to us. The experience of gynecological illness follows suit: *I went to the doctor's office because it feels like my abdomen is full of tiny knives, and all I got was this lousy birth control script.* There is nothing wrong with you, we are told. Take two Advil and don't call me in the morning. This lack of concern has psychological effects, from internalized sexism to rumination to suicidality.

It's easy to understand why some people turn away from the system entirely.

◆

My endometriosis story begins at the age of eleven, when my period came crashing into my life. By fourteen, I was on the pill and taking prescription-strength naproxen to try to control it. I missed hundreds of days of school because of pain, bleeding and anxiety. But then I learned to cope by being a high-functioning person. I didn't have time to be unwell. I went to university, where I worked seventy hours a week on top of being a full-time student. More than fifteen years later, I'm still unpacking my relationship between productivity and denial.

I spent a decade asking, pleading, crying for a total hysterectomy to help me manage extreme pain—both the physical experience and the psychological anguish of facing a life sentence of agony. I never wanted kids so the hysterectomy felt like common sense to me, yet the mere specter of change-your-mindism was enough to make my doctors back away and deny the operation.

I lived my medical struggle relatively quietly until recently. As a Serious Journalist writing about Serious Stuff, I had to ask myself how much I wanted people to know about my body. I felt weak for letting the pain reverberate throughout my life. For the longest time, it felt like if I opened the door and finally talked about it, my health problems would grow to define me. Worse, they could change how people see me. I could look crazy for taking on a system that society views as an altruistic force constructed for the good of mankind.[27]

But as a Serious Journalist, I also couldn't ignore the bigger story here: endometriosis care is systemically flawed. Even with a few good actors, the system is rife with power-trippers and gaslighters who lean on misogyny—consciously or otherwise—to deny us help and hope. I came to realize the only ones who benefited from my continued silence were the ones who silenced me in the first place by telling me what I felt wasn't real, that it was all in my head. And so the past few years have been a series of public coming-outs: coming out about endometriosis, coming out about a lifelong struggle with depression and anxiety, coming out about my anger.

It has been revelatory. Not only am I learning just how profoundly all this has shaped me, but I am also learning that I am not alone. I am fighting for myself and for others, so that together we can fight the machine that oppresses us.

I have to admit that I was always a bit of an anti-authoritarian. Within the library's CD collection I found punk rock, two big middle fingers pointed at everything I hated about this world. It framed my desire to fight for what I thought was right: a community that genuinely cares about the well-being of the people in it. I would flip open the inserts and pore over the lyrics, examining the musical missives about finding solidarity and fighting systems. I found enormous meaning in those liner notes. When I think about everything I've been through, a particular lyric comes to mind. It's from the Clash song "Clampdown," off their 1979 *London Calling* album. Over a quick, punchy drum pattern just before the second verse kicks in, Joe Strummer and Mick Jones sing in unison: "Let fury have the hour / Anger can be power / Do you know that you can use it?"

That phrase has been flipping over in my mind for the past couple of years: *anger can be power*.

So often we are told to lie back and take it. We must accept the things we cannot change, lest our anger consume us. But why *not* be consumed? There is a certain utility in consumption. When focused, anger can be a catalyst and an engine for change. The systems that oppress us benefit from our silence and compliance, and they make us complicit in our own abuse by forcing us to engage on their terms.

Throughout *BLEED*, I've woven the history of our oppression and how the medical system—both as itself and as a proxy for society at large—benefits when it transforms us into helpless sufferers. To break the system, we first need to understand the forces shaping it. We need to demand change. We need to be angry.

It seems to me the world has been afraid of female anger for a very long time and has invested incredible amounts of money and energy to coax us out of using it. "Everything can be used / except what is wasteful / (you will need / to remember this when you are accused of destruction)," said the self-described Black, lesbian, mother, warrior and poet Audre Lorde in a keynote address at the 1981 National

Women's Studies Association Conference.[28] "Every woman has a well-stocked arsenal of anger potentially useful against those oppressions, personal and institutional, which brought that anger into being. Focused with precision it can become a powerful source of energy serving progress and change. And when I speak of change, I do not mean a simple switch of positions or a temporary lessening of tensions, nor the ability to smile or feel good. I am speaking of a basic and radical alteration in those assumptions underlining our lives."

BLEED is heavy and deals with a lot of things we don't often say out loud. It's difficult, but I promise you it's worth it. We deserve to be heard and to tell our stories without feeling like we have to protect other people from the truth. As sufferers of sick bodies and sick systems, it is easy to find ourselves in the high seas of hopelessness. Sometimes it takes everything we have just to keep our heads above water. But if this book makes you angry, I urge you to hold onto that feeling. Anger is a power plant that can generate energy that spurs us to action. You can use it to make a difference—if not for yourself, then for someone else. This is my difference.

1. WHAT DO I GET?

navigating the healthcare minefield

The day before my appointment with the surgeon, I asked my boyfriend to write a letter attesting to our plans to never, ever procreate.

Stunned, he squinted at me in a mix of confusion and incredulity. He knew me as a strong-willed woman, a take-no-shit kind of person. Why would I need his permission to do something to my own body?

But he'd never seen me in a doctor's office. Within those confines, I instantly transformed into an anxious mess. He didn't know about my little black pocket notebook, the one I'd recently purchased so I could jot down all my medical talking points and requests. He'd never seen me dissociate by reading from it during doctors' appointments, or by taking copious notes in the sloppy cursive I'd honed over a few million lines of interview notes. He couldn't fathom just how awful my medical care had been, nor how it conspired with visceral memories of childhood abandonment and violence to produce a form of complex post-traumatic stress that, in moments of vulnerability, often left me feeling powerless. He thought my preparedness was an exaggeration, but to me it was critical in case my mind went limp again under the mental strain of playing that tired game with doctors. You know the one, right? It's what happens when you want something they don't want to give you, so you find yourself negotiating, appealing, appeasing—trying to insist and argue while still deferring, so that you're not sent home with nothing. By then, I'd been asking for a hysterectomy for ten years, my fixation becoming more intense with each denial.

He opened a blank document and began typing: *I have watched Tracey suffer for many years—*

"I don't need you to tell him how you've watched me suffer. *I* can do that," I snapped, bristling with nervous energy as I stood behind him, watching him hunt and peck at his slim white keyboard.

"I don't know anything about this doctor," I huffed. "But I *know* how the system works, and I don't want to hear, 'Your husband might want kids.'"

He frowned at my impatience and looming presence. He was a prosaic writer and his long thin fingers typed *so* slowly. He fretted over his sentence transitions. Should this be a *hence* or a *however?* At my core I understood: he wanted to help me by getting this right. Still, each blink of the stalled cursor twisted my anxiety into more knots. My shoulders curled inward and the muscles surrounding my ribcage tightened, forcing my lungs to heave as I inhaled hard through my nose. My tongue spread itself firmly against the roof of my mouth. My jaw clenched. A high-pitched whine circled my brain, stuffing my ears with the sound of a million cicadas on a late summer's day. My gaze became unfocused and unblinking—that blank, hardened stare that could bore holes through the backs of people's skulls; the stare that washes over my face whenever I suddenly find myself in a situation I can no longer tolerate.

Ah yes, my old friend fight or flight. The feeling of having no options. It presses the gas pedal on my sympathetic nervous system, causing my brain to spin out like it's doing joyless donuts in a parking lot. But I'm spinning too fast, and I can't catch my thoughts. That's when the limpness takes over, muffling my circling thoughts with a thousand-pound duvet until all I can hear is the droning static of my synapses in overdrive. It's the sound of being unable to cope with even just one more speck of bullshit.

Although we'd been together for six years by then, my boyfriend could not possibly comprehend how important this letter was. It felt like my key to finally winning the game I'd been playing for more than half my life. Presented with this evidence, the surgeon could not possibly prioritize my supposed fertility over my pain. *See? It's not only my choice but also my male overseer's choice, therefore you have to do it.*

When I look back at that October day now, I realize this wasn't only a doctor's visit. This was a life-or-death moment, bookended on one side by metastasized desperation and on the other by an almost constant desire to be teleported off this planet. Over the past twenty-four years, I'd seen countless doctors about my extreme cramps and bleeding, and I'd only just received a diagnosis a couple weeks earlier. I was on the same pain medication I'd been prescribed as a fourteen-year-old, an anti-inflammatory that can cause stomach ulcers with overuse. So many medical professionals had told me that losing weight would solve my pain. When I lost weight but still felt pain, they told me to lose some more. Would I only have relief once I disappeared?

I have been so thoroughly traumatized by my medical experiences that even the thought of attending a doctor's appointment fills me with dread. So often the tears begin rolling down my cheeks before the doctor has even had a chance to sit down. At some point, seeing a doctor became like some kind of reverse exposure therapy, each visit making me more traumatized. For two decades, I oscillated between frustrated stoicism and pleading for help. I would go months and even years without bothering to see a doctor about my pain or the side effects of the medications they put me on. Every now and then, though, I'd pick the thread up again when I decided I'd had enough. People with chronic pain understand this intermittence as a way to juggle the demands of everyday life with the bigger picture, all while living in perpetual misery. But I could never shake the feeling that to doctors it looked suspicious—that my pain could not be as intense as I said it was because if it was, I'd be in their office every other week and in the ER every other month. Every doctor's visit left me feeling like I'd either complained too much or not enough, but never the right amount to get actual help. I'd been gaslit for so long that every new doctor felt like a new adversary, someone I had to fight. If this was the game, I didn't understand the rules of engagement.

I grew up and spent most of my life in Montreal—the Europe of North America, that mystical place where everyone is beautiful and speaks French and smokes cigarettes on sidewalk terrasses (patios) while sipping cappuccinos or red wine. The place where no buildings can be taller than the cross on the mountain and where Leonard Cohen haunted the Main, stopping in at Bagel Etc. for his eggs, bacon and allongé.[29]

That city is a part of my soul, even with its many frustrations. Among them is the inability to get a family doctor, the sometimes years-long wait times to see a specialist and the interminable waits in the ER. I remember a visit at the age of fourteen to an ER after two of my lower-back vertebrae slipped; the woman sitting across from me in the general waiting room bawled as she clung to her miscarried fetus that she'd scooped into a mason jar. After seven hours, they sent me home with oxycodone—a bottle of tiny green pills that disappeared into my mother's room, never to be seen again. Unlike other places where finding a doctor is more of a choose-your-own-adventure game, in Quebec you put yourself on a list and often wait years until you are assigned to a doctor. If and when you do get a family doctor, you hold onto them for dear life even if you hate their guts. You don't get a second option.

The services available to people without family doctors are a crapshoot, and I did not have a winning streak. As a teen, I was a ward of the walk-in state. No assigned doctor, no comprehensive file, just a fixture in a clinic waiting room, watching muted TVs while waiting to shuffle across the cheap industrial carpet into one of the exam rooms. It was there where I was first prescribed the birth control pill and naproxen, at age fourteen. That's pretty much all they could do for me, said the doctor on duty. If only I had a family doctor, I often thought; they would help me see the right people and get the right tests to figure out why I had such incredible pain.

Ten years later, I finally did get a family doctor. By then I'd tried several different brands of birth control pills to manage my period pain and bleeding, but each one was worse than the last. If they didn't cause spotting, they gave me acne, intense mood swings, and awful PMS, or made me feel straight-up depressed. The family doctor suspected it was endometriosis but said the treatment was the same whether or not I had an official diagnosis: birth control and pain-killers. Why tax an overburdened healthcare system looking for something we already know how to treat? she rationalized.

Exasperated and desperate, I tried to force her hand: at twenty-six, I stopped taking birth control because of the side effects. How about a hysterectomy instead? I implored. I had never wanted kids, I told the doctor, so why suffer? No, she replied—the menopause alone would grind my teeth into dust, break all my bones, destroy my life. But getting pregnant *could* help with the pain and bleeding, she continued, a lilt in her voice. Perhaps I shouldn't dismiss it out of hand.

By thirty-three, I wasn't any better off. In fact, I was worse. It had been seven years since I'd abandoned the pill, time that allowed my mental state to level out to some extent. The downside was that I was bearing the full brunt of my periods—wicked stretches of six, seven, eight days where I hated being alive. It was then when, a half-dozen internal pelvic ultrasounds and bucketfuls of naproxen later, I followed my partner to a new city. The move gave me both the opportunity and the daunting, exhausting task of sifting through a new-to-me pool of doctors.

I'd become fixated on getting a hysterectomy. I wanted my uterus, ovaries and fallopian tubes to be extracted for my motionless, anesthetized body. And I wanted what they found inside me to be awful, worse than anyone ever suspected, to finally prove once and for all that something was actually wrong with me. I wasn't a hysterical hypochondriac looking for drugs or attention. I was *sick*, and these people should be *ashamed* for making me keep a uterus I didn't even want, and which probably didn't even work anyway. I fantasized about shoving my results in the faces of all the doctors who had ever denied me. See? *See?*

◆

It was with all this wreckage that I stood behind my boyfriend, wishing he could understand the medical trauma, wishing he could read my mind, wishing he could instantly empathize and give me all the softness I craved.

But how could he? In modern times, straight cis men rarely face such rote institutional denial of their right to choose, especially when it comes to reproduction. Instead, they benefit from a culture where vasectomies are seen as a defense against gold diggers and unwanted children—a noble choice made for the benefit of society, really. In the U.S., the idea of male sterilization is so commodified that some men schedule their vasectomies to coincide with college basketball's March Madness—an opportunity to use medical leave from work to enjoy televised sports.[30] Some urologists call it Vas Madness, offering free pizza coupons and ice bags printed with team logos to patients who book their vasectomies during the basketball tournament.[31]

It's true that not all male sterilization has been voluntary. Although historically women have been the primary targets of government sterilization programs, sterilization was also used against some disabled men and men of color, particularly Black and Indigenous men.[32]

Today, some trans men and women are required to be sterilized in order to have the gender on their ID changed.[33] And most vasectomies are reversible in ways that female sterilization is not, which perhaps makes it an easier procedure to commodify. Still, the reality is that sterilized men are an unremarkable piece of the social landscape, as easy to ignore as a suburban stop sign. Women without children, however, are often treated like a car on fire on the side of the road, and everyone's welcome to come by to point and gawk. Your aunts at the family barbecue tease you, telling you you're getting a bit old. Your boss gives coworkers with less seniority but more offspring first dibs on summer vacation and flexible working arrangements. And so, so many people talk about "the clock": family, friends, doctors, co-workers, the guy at the corner store—they're all keeping tabs on your supposed hormonal timepiece. Can't you hear it tick-tick-ticking away your chance to give birth to the miracle of life?

Women without children are subjected to this kind of commentary at every turn. While I am sensitive to the heartbreak of infertility, there is an important distinction to make here: to be intentionally childless is called child-free, nomenclature to differentiate ourselves from the people who want kids but can't have them.[34] There are major disparities between how these two groups are treated, both medically and socially. A person desperate to get pregnant is more likely to be met with compassion and kindness than a person desperate to *never* get pregnant.[35] I saw it firsthand: as a reasonably able-bodied white cis woman, I had no socially acceptable excuse that qualified me to shun the reproductive imperative. Though I'd never had my fertility tested, I still had the *potential* to breed more members of the white race. Why wouldn't I jump at the opportunity?

Pronatalism underpins modern society, having built the pedestal upon which the uterus rests—a sacred, supreme vessel no one is allowed to touch except for breeding purposes. However, we need to acknowledge the inequalities in healthcare (and in society) that are created when we prioritize children and the idea of having them, because these conversations have direct and life-changing implications for the treatment of women. This acknowledgment is long overdue: the number of women choosing to be child-free is climbing, but we still live in a world with norms and systems built on the premise that most women will at some point become mothers. By making child-bearing the focal point of female healthcare, we become immune to caring about women's actual lives.

We can see this at work in a lot of different ways. One such way is how doctors can refuse to help patients get tubal ligations or hyster-ectomies by citing personal, religious or moral reasons. Like with abortion, their metaphorical "conscientious objector" card trumps a patient's needs. According to American College of Obstetricians and Gynecologists (ACOG) guidelines, these doctors should either prescribe another kind of birth control or refer patients elsewhere. But these guidelines aren't actual rules (provincial/state authorities set those), and they don't specify if a doctor should make an *effective* referral to a non-objecting practitioner.[36] In these gray zones, doctors consulting these guidelines may consider prescribing another form of birth control as good enough as far as their duty to their patient goes.

That's how objections usually go: no grand statement of conscience but rather cowardly stalling, demurring, running patients through the wringer a few more times. Allowing for conscientious objection on matters of female reproductive freedom—as most jurisdictions and medical associations do—cements the message that the medical system doesn't have to be accountable for its entrenched sexism.

The mental gymnastics used to justify denial of care are incred-ibly perplexing, especially when you consider one fundamental thing: doctors aren't forced to work with people of reproductive age. If a doctor goes into medicine knowing they have a problem with abor-tion or voluntary sterilization, why not choose a field outside of that realm from the start? They can easily choose to work in literally any other specialty, from geriatrics to oncology to orthopedics. There is no shortage of alternative careers for general practitioners and gynecologists with moral qualms about giving patients reproductive control over their own bodies. Yet here they are. They get the privilege of entering a field knowing they will deny certain types of care to certain types of people, and they get to do this because they know the system will always defend their interests. This is little more than an ego trip, a patriarchal power move aided and abetted by medical colleges and medical institutions that care more about doctors than the patients they serve. Worse, institutions along with medical colleges and boards enable this behavior by making the process of filing complaints against doctors difficult and intimidating, meaning that a lot of bad medicine goes undocumented.

These dynamics are paternalism and patriarchy at work. In gynecology in particular—a medical field defined by male power over women—there's nothing that forces doctors to respect the reproductive wishes of their patients. And sure, I guess we don't want to live in a world where anyone is forced to do anything they find objectionable. But at the same time, their use and abuse of this privilege *forces* patients to seek help elsewhere, often at personal financial cost. For instance, if a patient seeking an abortion doesn't have the resources or the ability to see another doctor—which is a huge problem for low-income people and those living in rural or remote communities—they might be inclined to take drastic measures, ranging from throwing themselves down the stairs to resorting to back-alley butchers.

To have to ask for permission to do something to your own adult body, and risk being denied, attacks the very heart of inalienable constitutional rights—yet so many of the world's societies wholeheartedly endorse this prejudice when it comes to people with uteruses. On voluntary sterilization, even some feminist and pro-choice circles treat the matter as separate from abortion, as if that issue is either less important or still too taboo to touch.

My point is, reproductive freedom isn't only about abortion and deciding whether to have a child, but also about deciding to *never* have children and allowing that to be a legitimate, uncontroversial option for people. Unfortunately, we're still a long way off from that ever happening. Instead, we are routinely denied choice and agency under the guise of the biological clock—the idea that every woman, when faced with increasing age and declining fertility, will one day wake up with babies on the brain.[37] As such, a not-insignificant number of medical professionals feel they have a responsibility to dissuade young female patients from making choices that will impact their future fertility, even when those patients enthusiastically insist they will never, ever want children. This gets even more complicated for people with diseases such as endometriosis. Our misery is wrapped up in the reproductive system, yet we are routinely barred from touching it. Instead, we are prescribed medications with whole-body side effects that are seen to preserve whatever fertility we might have, whether we want that fertility or not. This is treated as a sacrifice we should be willing to make to ensure we don't make choices we might regret. These ideas are outcroppings of the view that a woman defining the parameters of her own existence is unsafe for society.

Men? Oh, well, they're just making personal choices.

These bitches are burning down the empire.

◆

Kelly O'Shea, a thirty-three-year-old cis woman and epidemiologist in Chicago, knew from the age of five that she didn't want kids.[38] It was an easy decision for her to make.

Getting a doctor to remove her uterus, though? The opposite of easy, even with endometriosis. There were the nice doctors who demurred, telling her they'd "talk about this later." The most manipulative doctor made "sad puppy-dog noises" when O'Shea told them she didn't want kids, then demanded to know what would happen if she met a man who *did* want children. Surely, she would change her mind! Another doctor, who worked on the university campus where O'Shea was a student, denied that her back pain could be related to her period and insulted her for not knowing the difference, then went on to perform a rough, careless pelvic exam that O'Shea ultimately reported as an official Title IX sexual assault complaint.

It's no wonder that O'Shea's collection of negative medical encounters have given her hair-trigger anxiety about doctors. She just can't help but get stressed about medical appointments, even though she knows it never works in her favor. Instead, it made her easier to typecast as the crazy patient. She can almost hear doctors thinking, "You're obviously a hot mess, probably a hypochondriac who made up these problems." O'Shea was left with this feeling so often that she now goes into appointments with a retort loaded and ready to fire: "You don't know me. You just walked in the room. You've known that I existed for maybe two hours, when you looked at your schedule this morning."

The night before the appointment in which she was approved for a hysterectomy, O'Shea spent hours printing off scientific papers and highlighting passages. As if preparing for court, she briefed her husband and her mom, witnesses she'd recruited to testify to her lifelong wish to be child-free. She intended to make an airtight case for her hysterectomy. The next morning, with her stack of research papers tucked under her arm and her witnesses on standby, O'Shea sat in the waiting room steeling herself for the encounter. "I'm five feet tall. I'm small. I'm a little white girl," she tells me. "I don't look super intimidating. But I think it's always good to go in with an attitude of 'I'm not to be fucked with.'"

A lot of people don't understand why doctors make people like O'Shea and me so damned nervous. We're both reasonably privileged people, with our whiteness and university educations there to break our falls. As we conversed, though, we immediately found a kind of kinship: we both independently knew that without supporting evidence to rationalize our choices to be child-free, our cases would be thrown out. A 2019 research paper on child-free people trying to get voluntary sterilization notes that 52 percent of patients do research and prepare before an appointment; it also found that while men anticipated being approved for sterilization, women anticipated rejection.[39]

The accountability bar for treating endometriosis patients is already so low that a toddler could walk right into it. The disease is considered difficult, and the patients even more so—hardly an incentive to help. The bar is only as high as it is because of the idea that medicine should at least endeavor to "fix" defective women so they can procreate. But when a patient doesn't want kids, why bother? That puts child-free patients on an ice floe and sends them out to sea. The abysmal lengths to which some child-free people have to go to get care is downright disturbing. And yet my conversation with O'Shea is punctuated by emphatic "mmhmms" and knowing "ughs." We know so profoundly, so viscerally how we are so often perceived: we are the most useless of women.

And so I couldn't blame my partner for not being cursed with a uterus. I couldn't blame him for not understanding how his white girlfriend could have possibly experienced discrimination. Still, his inability to commiserate melted into everyone else's inability to commiserate, and it became an extension of the medical gaslighting I had endured for so long. Even on bad period days, he saw me working at my computer, a hot water bottle pressed to my abdomen and a plug-in heated cape draped over my back. If I could work, how could it possibly be as bad as I said it was?

As a good friend of mine always says, resilience is futile.

And so I shooed him away from the keyboard and took his seat. My fingers hurried across the keyboard, picking away at the words he wrote. Shift, option, arrow key, arrow key, backspace. Kill the transitions. Shorten the sentences. Get to the point. We are never having children.

2. OH BONDAGE, UP YOURS!

how the system got its power

Denise was in her early thirties when she first told a healthcare professional about her period pain.[40]

Desperate for relief, she'd stopped in over lunch at a Toronto pharmacy close to the office where she worked as a civil servant. Standing at the counter during the noon-hour rush, she told the pharmacist she'd already taken six Tylenol, two Aleve and one Advil that day. Those 1,600 milligrams of over-the-counter analgesics couldn't even touch her pain.

"Uh, it sounds like you need to talk to your doctor," he answered.

Her periods hadn't started off this terrible. From her first one at age fourteen until her mid-twenties, she'd barely had PMS or cramps, and she didn't bleed particularly heavily. Sure, there were the persistent migraines, but compared to the misery some friends seemed to endure, she figured she'd had it relatively easy.

Then it started. In her late twenties, the bleeding became heavier. A few years later, *wham!* The pain punched her right in the gut, sending her reeling. By the time she told her doctor, she'd already been playing painkiller roulette, hoping to find the right combination of off-the-shelf drugs that would let her get out of the bed in the morning and go to work. When she finally told her doctor that what she was doing wasn't cutting it, he replied, "That's excessive," then prescribed her five naproxen.

Chances are, if you have endometriosis, you've taken—and have been disappointed by—naproxen at some point in your life. It's a nonaddictive anti-inflammatory drug that somehow became the primary go-to pain reliever for people with endometriosis.[41] Some people know it as Aleve, which comes in 220-milligram tablets and can be bought at any pharmacy.[42] Prescription-grade naproxen typically comes in big, blue 550-milligram tablets, which can be taken twice a day, twelve hours apart; any more and you run a greater risk of burning a hole through your stomach. Unfortunately, that dosing schedule allows breakthrough endo pain to trickle in. (What a lot of doctors and pharmacists fail to mention is that you can take 500 milligrams of Tylenol at four-hour intervals between those twelve hours.[43])

Denise looked at the script. It was barely higher than what she'd already been taking. Why didn't her pain ever seem to matter?

She thought back to being thirteen. She hadn't gotten her period yet but was having sharp, stabbing pains in her abdomen. When she went to the doctor, he told her he didn't know what it was and sent her away. In actuality, she was in the throes of an appendicitis attack. She got a second opinion, and that doctor, a Filipino man, ordered emergency surgery. "You need to remove it, like, now," he told her. She did. A handful of months later, she got her first period.

She wonders whether the first doctor shrugged off her pain because she was Black—because now, a couple decades later, it was happening again. She grudgingly took the script to the pharmacy and accepted her allotment of five single naproxen tablets, using them alongside her over-the-counter cocktail. Then one day while hanging out with a few girlfriends, the conversation turned to cysts and fibroids, and how painful they were during menstruation. A lightbulb went off. That could explain her agony—maybe she had them too. She returned to her doctor to ask him that very question.

Impatiently, he asked her if she wanted to do a transvaginal ultrasound and shut down her request for a gynecologist referral. "He was mad. He said, 'You don't need to see a gynecologist,'" Denise says. "It was like he thought, 'What am I here for, then?'" Besides, she remembers him saying dismissively, she probably *did* have either cysts or fibroids, since a lot of Black women get them. And as her ultrasound results soon showed, she did in fact have them: one of each. Her doctor seemed nonplussed, telling her they were too small to merit intervention.

That was that. There was nothing more to be done. Denise continued filling her script for five naproxen a month.

◆

For most of my life, I thought I got poor medical treatment because of something I did. During appointments, my mounting doctor anxiety made me seem argumentative, irrational and/or mentally unstable. I mean, who cries while getting an ear infection checked out? These were involuntary reactions shaped by my awful track record with institutionalized medicine, shiny little flecks of trauma sprinkled on top of otherwise totally benign, routine encounters. Not being able to instantly overcome the trauma frustrated me so intensely; I knew it wasn't a good look, and yet I could not stop myself from breaking down. Surely, I thought, these were the reasons why my doctors didn't seem particularly concerned about what was happening to me. By tripping into the archetype of the hysterical woman, I had made it easy for them to write me off. Only when I learned to control myself, I reasoned, would I get the care I needed.

It was only in my thirties when I realized my medical mistreatment wasn't even about me. By then I'd heard countless stories from other endometriosis sufferers, as well as from people with autoimmune diseases,[44] PCOS and all kinds of other mysterious female-coded illnesses.[45] This was a group of people who felt as though they'd been thrown away by the medical system. Like them, I had also been unwittingly cast into a role for which I did not have the script. We each floundered around in our own bubble of turmoil, unaware of just how interconnected it all was.

When this dawned on me, I was flooded by two overwhelming emotions.

First, relief. I *wasn't* alone.

Then, anger. I wasn't *alone*. This was systemic.

♦

Symptomatically and systemically, endometriosis patients challenge institutional medicine in ways other diseases and patients do not. Because destroying misogyny is central to becoming empowered, endo patients pose a much greater threat to society's power structures than we may appreciate.

In Western medicine, there is a concept called the sick role, and it relates to how medical professionals—and larger society—expect sick people to behave. The theory was first introduced in 1951 by American sociologist and Harvard professor Talcott Parsons, who considered sickness both a biological problem and a sociological one.[46] A quarter century later, he wrote an updated definition of the sick role to be more inclusive of chronic illness and to more thoughtfully evaluate doctor-patient power dynamics.[47]

A quick note: Parsons used the role of the doctor as a representative for all healthcare personnel, and I'm doing the same throughout *BLEED*. After all, doctors are our main point of contact when seeking endometriosis care and represent the medical system whether they like it or not. That said, as you read *doctor*, consider how the entire medical system might also be implicated.

In Parsons's 1975 revision, the sociologist explained that there are three primary criteria for "accepting the social role of being sick":

one, the illness is not the sufferer's fault but is instead imposed upon them; two, the sufferer can claim exemption from their usual day-to-day activities, such not going to work or school; and three, if the illness is severe, the patient must seek help within the institutionalized healthcare system. That last one, Parsons said, is further admission from the patient that they don't genuinely want to be sick and that they agree that medical intervention is required to help cure them, or at least properly manage their illness.[48] All told, the sick role gets assigned when the patient seeks medical care and continues to follow them around until they get well—if they ever do.

Beyond the sick role itself are the forces of the doctor-patient relationship which, according to Parsons, is defined by an asymmetry of power. On one end of the seesaw is the mighty heft of the doctor role. They are granted a socially superior status because they've been certified to be the keepers of other people's health, a role "grounded in responsibility, competence and occupational concern." On the other side of the seesaw is the patient. They are almost weightless, their legs flailing in the air because they are "unburdened" by the weight of power and decision-making. Instead, they are expected to defer to the doctor and follow their advice with a certain degree of motivation in order to achieve health (or, at least, the best possible functioning given the circumstances). In this metaphor, the only way for the patient to put their feet back on the ground is if the doctor gets off the seesaw; no amount of power puts them on equal footing with their doctor. For incurable conditions such as endometriosis, getting grounded is most apt to happen when one of the two parties gives up on the relationship.

Although many alternate theories to Parsons's sick role have come and gone over the decades, asymmetrical power remains a defining feature of medicine. The degree of asymmetry worsens if the patient is part of one or more disadvantaged groups because they're likely to have less agency and control of their medical interactions. However much our society wants to believe that individuals have power over their own health, that notion is swiftly undone once they enter the system and become patients—and almost all of us enter the system eventually. Within institutionalized medicine, power is a necessary component of care delivery. The hierarchy dictates that doctors are the experts, and patients are the recipients of the doctors' expertise. This dynamic exploits fear, driving home the idea that patients will only comply with healthcare directives when they are sufficiently afraid of the consequences of not complying. The messaging patients get is clear: *if you don't do as the doctor says, something bad will happen to you.*

We have all purchased stock in this view of medicine. Even collaborative care and trauma-informed healthcare models hinge on asymmetrical power dynamics in the doctor-patient relationship, though the asymmetry may be less pronounced if the doctor chooses to acknowledge and respect patient experience and knowledge. Regardless of medical model, physician power is fed by the widespread acceptance that doctors are inherently trustworthy[49] and that they are altruistic[50] (see: every single Facebook post, news article or inspirational meme that has called healthcare workers "heroes"). But if doctors are merely selfless caretakers, why do countless endometriosis patients feel like they've been abandoned?

My knee-jerk reaction when first reading Parsons's definition of the sick role was that endometriosis patients simply do not fit the mold. Like square pegs in medicine's round holes, we defy the criteria he laid out because many of us remain high functioning despite our pain. We go to work, school, the gym and social outings even while feeling like death warmed over. As for the seesaw of power, endometriosis patients diverge from normal patient behavior because many of us have learned not to trust doctors who've repeatedly failed us. We're the ones who get off the seesaw. By not giving them our unfailing devotion, we reclaim some of our power.

But a few weeks later, I came back around to this interpretation and challenged my own thinking. I'm not sure endo patients start out intentionally rebellious; rather, we become that way out of self-preservation. In reality, I think, we *wish* we could be exempt from the travails of modern life. But we're not, because our pain is seen as a consequence of weakness rather than of extraordinary suffering. Because our world has been fed the script that female existence is defined by pain—periods, childbirth, sexual violence, plain old misogyny—we are expected to tolerate greater amounts of suffering. Women of color are expected to be able to bear even more pain than white women. We have little to no appreciation for how fat, disabled or gender non-conforming people might experience pain. When witnesses see someone struggling, they don't typically think, "Wow, that person must be in incredible pain"; instead, they assume we are lacking in the tenacity, endurance and even intelligence required to live our frivolous little lives with grace, and that our forfeiture is failure. And so I've changed my mind: we fit into the sick role. It's just not as neat and tidy as medicine would like.

Endometriosis is not our fault, although there is a not uncommon belief out there that we are at least a *little* responsible for it. From failures to procreate early and often to us being too promiscuous, there is a wide range and a long legacy of blaming people for their own endometriosis. (More on that later.) Meanwhile, our illness is typically not considered a legitimate reason to take leave from our responsibilities. After all, we hear, our pain is not special; every vagina bleeds. And when we do seek out institutionalized healthcare, we spend years visiting doctors before we are diagnosed—not because diagnosis is particularly hard, but because we spend a significant amount of time not being believed. Belief, too, is meted out unevenly, with white patients believed more easily than Black or Indigenous ones. In emergency departments and doctors' offices, trans people face double-barreled disbelief: their health problems and their gender identity.[51] In one Ontario-based study pulling from data collected in 2009–2010, 21 percent of trans people said they avoided emergency departments because they didn't think they would get good care.[52] Denial and mistrust only reinforce our positions in the sick role: the more we are misunderstood, the more we seek understanding, the more we are accused of performing sickness to get attention—all while our disease progresses, making us sicker.

If this isn't an obvious power trip, I don't know what is—and yet it happens all the time. Denise returned to her doctor at the age of thirty-four after she started having pain during the week leading up to her period. Instead of investigating further he just prescribed her another five naproxen: one a day for five days of PMS and five days of menstruation. Meanwhile, I've personally received sixty-tablet refills of the same drug at the same dosage without anyone batting an eye.

Was Denise's doctor being stingy because he didn't believe her when she said she could barely walk some days? Or could it be sexism combined with internalized racism leading him to assume she could grin and bear it? Denise was sensitive to the fact that if she lost her cool, her doctor—who was also Black—would write her off as an Angry Black Woman. And it was also true that he had been taught to practice medicine within a system forged by white supremacy and misogyny. The power dynamics here were multilayered and complicated, and Denise did her best to muddle through. "At the time I was like, 'Whatever, I'll take what I can get.' But now I realize that he didn't want to give it to me. I still have no idea what the connotation is. All I know is that the non-racialized people got bottles," she says.

The next time she saw him, she couldn't just grab a script and run. Since the ten-naproxen visit, her periods had become weeks of sheer agony. Not only that, but now her belly button was also bleeding. She'd first assumed it was scar tissue leftover from her teenage appendectomy. But when her doctor's nurse practitioner looked more closely, she could see a nodule protruding from Denise's belly button.

Worse, it seemed the nodule was attached to a much larger mass in her belly. This could be cancer, the nurse warned. With the C-word hanging thick in the air, Denise watched her doctor transform into an unrecognizable figure before her very eyes. "He was a totally different man when he thought it was cancer," she tells me. He rattled off a laundry list of specialists she could see, tests she could do. He called her cellphone in his off-hours to ask how she was doing. He was a medical shapeshifter. Why was he snapping into action now, Denise wondered, but not when she had presented with excruciating pain?

Denise dutifully played the role of patient, undergoing a gamut of tests. X-rays of her belly and chest showed fluid in her lungs and what looked like a tumor. They stuck a long needle in her back to extract the fluid and biopsied the mass in her lung.

When she finally made it back to her doctor's office to get her results, he'd reverted back to his natural state.

"It's not cancer," he told her flatly. "It's endometriosis."

He wouldn't get the glory of saving her from certain death. Instead, he would have to deal with a patient who kept whining about period cramps and bugging him about painkillers. In what felt like an act of retribution, he refused to sign the paperwork she needed to get time off work and wouldn't prescribe more than ten naproxen.

What else could Denise do? She fired him. By doing so, Denise was able to claw back just a little bit of power from the system that had failed her. But did she win? Though she'd never heard of endometriosis before, she left the office that day knowing two things. One, she was extremely sick. Two, if past experience was any indication, getting proper care was going to be extremely hard.

◆

When it comes to healthcare, the sick role isn't the only place in which inequality thrives. Asymmetry of power is woven into all relationships within medicine where one person is deemed the superior. A shockingly high number of medical students report being bullied and harassed by their superiors.

Although the use and abuse of power against patients is not well studied, it has been looked at among medical professionals. Surveys show as many as 85 percent of med students reported being mistreated by more senior healthcare workers—mistreatment that includes sexism and racism.[53, 54] One research paper on the abuse of power in medical training spells it out like this: "The chief barrier [. . .] is unprofessional conduct by medical educators, which is protected by an established hierarchy of academic authority."[55] This reality suggests that medicine is defined by a culture of abuse. While that's terrible for healthcare workers, patients bear the brunt of this chain of abuse because they are the weakest, most disempowered links.

In any other situation, we'd be considered naive fools to think cycles of abuse don't replicate and trickle down into other relationships, especially those defined by asymmetrical power. When it comes to medicine, though, our society has a massive blind spot. We don't want to believe patients are mistreated—*doctors take oaths to protect them, for chrissakes!* Many of our fellow citizens are willing to make excuses for some doctors' egregiously awful behavior toward patients because we want to believe in their altruism. In fact, they hold the *most* trusted profession in the world.[56] Case in point: people still defend Norman Barwin, a fertility doctor in Canada who for decades secretly used his own sperm to impregnate patients without telling them he'd switched their samples.[57] Even after this abuse was made public—after years of people whispering about it—one patient wrote on RateMDs.com: "Dr. Barwin was my doctor for more years than I can count. He was compassionate, accessible and lovely. His motivation was to help. Those who discredit him forget that they wanted babies and they got them."[58]

When you're up against such a powerful machine and its numerous apologists, even male patients struggle to call out a doctor for bad behavior and have their complaint heard. In this misogynistic world, it often feels like women and gender-diverse people don't stand a chance. That seems especially true for those of us with female-coded chronic illnesses, and extra-extra true for those afflicted by the mystery that is endometriosis. That's because endometriosis is a black box. No one knows what's going on inside that box, and it feels like no one ever will.

This lack of knowing and the corresponding lack of effective treatments short-circuit our relationships with medicine by challenging doctors' sick role scripts. As patients, we expect our primary care physicians to either know how to test for endometriosis or at least promptly refer us to someone who does, and yet many don't.[59, 60] In the spirit of deference, we keep going back, hoping for better, but are continually disappointed. It's like having a bad boyfriend: he treats you like trash, yet you keep making him dinner. Eventually you decide you'd rather eat alone than put up with his shit.

The same breaking point happens for endometriosis patients, and some people do abandon attempts to get institutional care. However, those who hope to get some kind of treatment need to keep engaging with the medical system in some capacity, even when we lose our trust and faith in it. In those situations, what often happens is that we begin trusting ourselves and other chronically ill people more than we trust our doctors. We read medical journals, join support groups and become activists, these little rays of empowerment chipping away at our doctors' socially superior positions.

When our doctors finally catch on to that, they usually react in one of two ways: they give up some of their power in order to work more collaboratively with the patient, or they reassert the rules of engagement that give them the balance of power.

Here's an example of such digging in. I spent the summer and fall of 2021 requesting my medical records from as many doctors' offices and hospitals as I could remember visiting. I filled out, faxed and emailed what felt like a couple dozen forms. But when I got to the office of my GP at the time, I was told I would have to either mail or hand-deliver my request form.

Could I fax or email it? I asked.

No, they don't give out their fax number or email, they replied.

I wasn't just annoyed by the inconvenience of going to the mailbox. I also couldn't comprehend such an old-school way of operating, especially during a pandemic. And so I did what any other pain-in-the-ass journalist would do: I found their fax number online and used a free online fax service to send in my form.

Now I admit that maybe this was a jerk move. I was clearly thumbing my nose at their stupid rules. What doctor's office on this planet won't accept a fax? Medicine is almost single-handedly keeping the fax machine alive! But my act of rebellion could not stand. The doctor personally called me twice shortly after receiving the fax; both times, I missed the call. She didn't leave a message. If only she had gotten back to me this quickly when I called about a health-related matter! A few days later she called again. Why was I refusing to comply with their protocol? she demanded. Did my unwillingness to drive a one-hour round-trip to deliver the document in person mean I wouldn't show up for doctor's appointments?

In the end, I gritted my teeth and mailed the form. Sometime later they called to say they'd received my letter and would send me an invoice to pay the fifty-dollar requisition fee—online. And when I received my file, it didn't consist of a bunch of papers tucked into a manila envelope. It was stored digitally on a USB flash drive.

I think they probably failed to see the irony.

It seemed obvious to me that this wasn't about the method of delivery at all. It was about who makes the rules and who has to follow the rules, and how my defiance broke the rules. But it was also much more than that. It was part of the larger "problem" of noncompliance among patients, particularly those with endometriosis.

Endometriosis itself challenges the medical system in ways it does not like to be challenged. Because there's no known cause or cure, doctors who are not well versed in the benefits of endometriosis excision—which is to say, most of them—are often left to their own devices to "solve" a patient's misery. The clinical standards for endometriosis care continue to revolve around hormonal therapies, but those interventions do not eliminate the disease. Rather, they often cause a host of side effects, ranging from loss of sex drive to depression. And so patients often end up doing a lot of legwork and research to figure out how to help themselves, which can include trying out various interventions outside of traditional medicine, from doing acupuncture to smoking weed to getting their chakras unblocked with reiki.[61] The wellness industrial complex exists *because* people feel ignored and unaided by medicine—and that makes endometriosis patients a target market for a range of products and services, some more legit than others. People buy jade eggs and yoni steamers because their doctors have shown them that they can't—or won't—do any better.

To a desperate person, seeking nontraditional interventions feels like active participation in one's own healthcare. To doctors, though, it often looks like ignoring proper medical advice, as Kate Seear suggests in a research-based analysis ingeniously titled "'Nobody Really Knows What It Is or How to Treat It,'" about noncompliance among endometriosis patients.[62] Seear argues that a patient failing to comply with healthcare directives is often seen by doctors as a frantically waving red flag that says, "We've got a social deviant here!" It is seen as risky behavior that demands immediate re-education.

Doctors' attempts to control that behavior are an extension of power asymmetry. But wherever there is power, there is also resistance. Seear articulates that women exercise their agency and resistance in different ways than men do, namely through acceptance of their bodies, nonaction, sabotage, rebellion and by lamenting things they can't change. A different study on trans people accessing mental healthcare in Sweden shows similar power dynamics: "Seeing rela-tionships with healthcare providers in almost adversarial terms, participants took back their power by directing what they would speak about and what they would not."[63]

With endometriosis specifically, doctors often give patients laundry lists of burdensome and expensive self-care and risk-avoidance measures: do yoga, eat organic food, see a physiotherapist and maybe a psychologist, take antidepressants, avoid parabens, use unbleached tampons, take vitamins, eat more fiber, don't eat dairy, get eight hours of sleep, and most importantly *do not* let this disease control your life.

Who on Earth has the time and the money for all this?

To avoid endometriosis becoming a second full-time job, patients have to make choices to maintain any semblance of sanity and balance. And so, Seear explains, we just kind of wing it. We might try some, or maybe all, of a doctor's suggestions but only adopt the habits and coping mechanisms that suit us best. Most patients look at this trial-and-error process—which includes their experiences with medications and procedures—as part of a rich trove of personal medical knowledge. And that's where we run into problems: unless it is validated by a doctor, it's not considered knowledge at all.

"The failure to give serious consideration to the possibility that patient noncompliance is a form of expertise," writes Seear, "may reinforce the idea that when patients do not comply, it is a problem of communication from experts *to* patients, rather than a problem inherent to the message that experts themselves are trying to transmit." In short, when doctors see willful noncompliance, they think the patient hasn't understood their directives when, in fact, the patient understands and disagrees. Other research notes that medical noncompliance among trans patients is often an outcropping of lived or current violence in their lives—and that discriminatory medical care can be a source of violence.[64,65]

Seear's research goes even further by arguing that endometriosis patients' noncompliance is not only an outcome of self-knowledge but equivalent to some level of scientific and medical expertise. When patients use noncompliance as a form of "rational action motivated by a desire to avoid additional risks to which they will be exposed through compliance"—say, declining a medication proposed by a doctor that could cause terrible side effects—it's because we have some kind of evidence to support our reasoning. To the patient, it's a way of exercising agency in a situation in which we feel powerless. It's also a way for us to rightfully question the effectiveness of what a doctor is proposing, when they have repeatedly demonstrated a lack of knowledge about our illness. In the end, we come to know the reality of our disease better than any outsider could: there is no cure and no effective pharmacological treatment, and even surgical treatments aren't guaranteed to save us.

And yet, in these kinds of situations, practitioners *still* see our risk avoidance as risky in itself. I can understand why they see it that way, to some degree: they work within a medical model—and really a world—that likes to blame sick people for their poor health. Mainstream society feels completely comfortable moralizing sickness by judging, say, a smoker who gets lung cancer, an alcoholic who gets cirrhosis of the liver, or a sex worker who gets HIV/AIDS.[66] Parallel to that are rebellious patients who refuse certain treatments, with empowerment considered their vice. "Individual people are expected to control their bodies and to contain them within their physical boundaries; sickness is a failure of self-control and rationality," write researchers from the School of Public Health and Preventative Medicine at Australia's Monash University, in a paper on medicine's social construction of endometriosis.[67]

Women and people assigned female at birth are expected to exert even more self-control. Amid all this is the fact that doctors don't know why endometriosis occurs in some people and not others, the

Monash researchers continue. A lack of answers drives many patients to do their own research (some of it good, some of it not), driving an even bigger wedge between doctor and patient. After all, the power our society gives to doctors is founded on the notion that they know more about health than the rest of us—hence why any research a patient brings to an appointment is so commonly dismissed out of hand. As the Monash researchers put it, "Women with endometriosis present a threat to medicine's claim of knowledge of the body, and [. . .] instead of acknowledging the inherent limitations of androcentric medical knowledge, fault is established within women."

There it is. Instead of admitting the system is not calibrated to give endometriosis patients the care they need, actors within the system shift blame and responsibility onto patients themselves, and then hate it when we take the reins.

◆

For better or worse, the people overseeing endometriosis are gynecologists. This disease, despite affecting organs and tissue far outside of the reproductive system, has been the domain of gynecology since it was first detected.

The thing about gynecology is that, generally speaking, it's never been great. In fact, its history is probably worse than you can imagine. From the time of the ancient Greeks and Egyptians to the Middle Ages to the Enlightenment to the industrial revolutions and the modern era, gynecology has been various shades of fucked up.

Gynecology is a field of medicine founded on the historical premise that it should be men who tell women how their bodies work. In North America in the mid-1800s, doctors and medical associations used the law and Catholicism to make women fear midwives and stop using them for birthing and abortion, simply because they wanted the two most lucrative aspects of midwifery for themselves.[68] Before this turning point, most gynecological care was performed by midwives, witches and healers, many of whom were immigrants or women of color.[69] After this transition, gynecology became dominated by white men and their chauvinistic beliefs.

Since then, that approach has been systematized and handed down to medical students of all genders and ethnicities. As we saw in Denise's case, we can't assume that non-male, non-white medical and nursing staff will be different from or "better" than the typical white, male healthcare worker. They are, after all, trained and conditioned to work in a medical system—and a larger society—that presume that white and male is a default setting; worse, that presumption is so deeply ingrained in the practice of medicine that it's almost impossible to see unless you know how to look for it.[70, 71] As Helen King expertly details in her 1998 book *Hippocrates' Woman*, "From the 19th century until the present day, gynecology has been the branch of medicine which most strikingly manifests the inequality intrinsic to traditional patient/doctor relationships in Western culture."

"The sick role is feminized," King continues, "while the doctor embodies what are considered to be the masculine virtues: in gynecology, all the patients are women, and the majority of those deciding what counts as disease and how to treat it are men."[72]

Today we see a greater diversity of gynecologists—but that has not bred a better system.

At 58.9 percent, there are currently more women gynecologists than any other gender in the United States, a reversal that when first reported yielded dozens of alarmist news articles about men being pushed out.[73, 74] Of course, many of those articles presented the news as some kind of reverse sexism in action, as if men are disappearing because women are taking over. But data suggests another force is at play. Instead of being pushed out of gynecology, it seems like the real cause is that men are abandoning ship. Consider this scenario: in the U.S., OBGYNs earn less than almost all other surgical specialties, and women OBGYNs are paid at least $36,000 less per year than men.[75, 76] As more men opt to pursue higher-paying specialties, the wage floor for women OBGYNs is not rising to compensate; it remains frozen in the wage gap, devaluing the specialty overall.[77] In addition to that, those who specialize in minimally invasive gynecologic surgery—i.e., the people most qualified to perform endo excision—appear to earn even less as a whole, with female specialists earning an average of $52,087 less than their male counterparts.[78]

This devaluation of non-obstetric gynecological expertise is having real-world consequences on patients. Consider that a biopsy of a penis gets a surgeon 45 percent more money than a biopsy of a vagina.[79] If you were trying to earn a good living, which procedure would you do? These payment discrepancies are a significant reason why right now half of U.S. counties don't have one single OBGYN in them, and why the OBGYN shortage is expected to grow to 22,000 missing doctors by 2050.[80] When performing gynecology is systemically punished, the people who do pursue it do so out of a sense of duty (or vanity, or both).

In and outside of gynecology, female physicians and medical academics face sexism around every corner. Across medicine in general, women are published (and cited) less frequently in journals than men.[81] In the U.S., they are at least 60 percent less likely to receive National Institutes of Health funding[82] (and receive less funding when they do), and they don't conduct clinical trials as frequently as men do.[83] In a number of areas including female pelvic medicine, they also receive fewer payments from Medicare, and when they do receive Medicare money, they receive less of it.[84] Oh, and female physicians earn about $2 million less than male physicians do over the course of a forty-year career.[85]

In medical academia, women are less likely to receive professorships and leadership positions.[86, 87] According to one recent analysis of U.S. public medical schools, 16.7 percent of med school department chairs were women; the adjusted average annual salary difference between female chairs and male chairs was more than $67,000.[88] Another analysis done specifically on department chairs in obstetrics and gynecology showed that 38 percent of chairs were women and that they earned $183,200 less than male chairs.[89]

Beyond numbers, that last analysis also reports that most of those obstetrics and gynecology chairs don't operate much anymore and tend to be male, which makes it doubly difficult to relate to current students and residents. "Men with a primarily nonsurgical clinical practice may be ill equipped to mitigate the institutional gender bias experienced by women gynecologic surgeons," say the researchers.[90] Meanwhile, 2018 figures indicate 82 percent of residents in obstetrics and gynecology were women,[91] but only 46.4 percent of female students said they received mentorship for leadership roles, while 57.1 percent of male students said the same.[92] With these figures, it should be no mystery why there is a dearth of female leadership in gynecology. Even the American College of Obstetricians and Gynecologists has failed to model female leadership—and it's a college wholly dedicated to vaginas and uteruses. The college has had just six female presidents since its founding in 1951; Luella Klein, the first woman to hold the top position, claimed it in 1984.[93] Neither her, nor the five women after her, could be called a specialist in endometriosis.

And so, even if there are more female gynecologists, they're disadvantaged in every way possible by the same systemic misogyny that punishes endo patients. With this abysmal showing, you'd at least think that female doctors would be more attuned to the struggles of their patients.

There is some evidence that suggests female doctors spend more time with patients and are more willing to collaborate with patients to some extent.[94] A study out of Canada showed that female patients are more likely to die when operated on by a male surgeon than by a female one.[95] However, internalized sexism is also extremely real, and healthcare is no exception. There, it cuts both ways: from patient to doctor, and doctor to patient—although in a relationship defined by asymmetrical power, both directions do not hold the same weight. "A key feature of sexism, as with oppression against any group, is that there is an institutionalized power differential between the oppressor group (men in the case of sexism) and the oppressed group (in sexism, women). Oppression is popularly described by the formula: oppression = prejudice + power," write the authors of a paper called "The Fabric of Internalized Sexism."[96] "Internalized sexism is not merely sexism perpetrated by women upon women. Sexism involves two distinct groups, one of which is systematically denied power by the other"—for example, a patient denied power by a doctor (either as an individual or as a proxy for the medical system). And because sexism is so widely and routinely practiced throughout medicine, it filters down into the stream of everyday language and operations, where it becomes insidious and invisible.

All this means that having a female doctor when you have a female-coded disease is still no guarantee that you will be treated any better than if you were treated by a male.

Given the current rarity of trans doctors, it's hard to draw a parallel on the topic of trans doctors' internalized transphobia interfering with their treatment of trans and non-binary patients. What we do know is that among trans patients, encountering transphobia in a doctor's office is almost a given; two in three trans patients in the U.S. worry their health evaluations are influenced by their gender or sexual orientation. The same research says refusal and abuse of trans patients of color is even more routine.[97]

The truth is, however progressive modern gynecologists of any gender may personally be, it takes guts and intention to subvert the oppressive edges of institutionalized medicine and its internalized discrimination.

As far as the written record is concerned, gynecology has existed since at least 1825 B.C.E., when the world's oldest known gynecological text, the Kahun Gynaecological Papyrus, was published in Egypt.[98] The document associates nearly every possible female health complaint to the womb. Blinding eye pain? "It is discharges of the womb in her eyes." Pain in the legs or butt? "It is discharges of the womb." Tooth pain? "It is toothache of the womb."[99] The papyrus describes how those with "wandering wombs"—the uterus was believed to roam around the body—should fumigate their vaginas with that evening's dinner, like some kind of Bronze Age yoni steam.

Beginning in fifth century B.C.E., Greek physician Hippocrates—the namesake of medicine's vaunted Hippocratic Oath—and at least eighteen unnamed Hippocratic writers wrote a number of medical texts widely circulated throughout the world of antiquity.[100] Greeks in this period did not perform autopsies or human dissection,[101] so their understanding of the female reproductive system was primarily based on animal biology and on the imaginations of men. The seminal Hippocratic text *Diseases of Women I* borrowed that Egyptian concept of the wandering womb and said that an empty uterus could wander around the body, to the extent that it could choke a person and even kill them.[102] It also put forward the notion that people who have never given birth suffer more intensely from menstruation than those who have had babies. Giving birth, therefore, is seen as a way of making periods less awful. Sound familiar?

This early reasoning for pregnancy being a solution to pain was based on the assumption that pregnancy leaves the uterus distended. Bigger uteruses meant more room for menstrual blood, as if the blood was just sloshing around inside people's bellies like jugs of red Kool-Aid. The smaller uteruses of never-pregnant people, meanwhile, were too tight of a squeeze for all that liquid.[103] According to Hippocrates, the ancient Greeks theorized that those individuals had more pain because the pressure of the liquid turned them into sentient water balloons, with wombs stretched thin and ready to burst with blood.[104]

Back then, they also believed the reason women menstruated and men didn't was because women carried more moisture in their bodies due to their more sponge-like skin, which was itself caused by their less sweaty, more sedentary lifestyles.[105] They reasoned that men had thicker skin because they toiled away all their moisture by building acropolises and crushing grapes with their feet, while women who got to stay home and chill expelled their excess moisture through menstruation.

The Greeks hadn't yet figured out the whole endometrial lining thing.

Ancient practitioners of prescientific medicine in the Greco-Roman world were fascinated and mystified by menstruation.[106] Hippocrates's theories about the womb were elaborated upon by his contemporary, Plato, and by Galen and Aretaeus of Cappadocia a few centuries later. Aretaeus is known for calling the womb "the seat of womanhood itself"—an idea that endures in medicine and in larger society.[107] Along with other philosophers of the time, these men concocted wild theories of the womb and its mysteries. The uterus, desperate to bear fruit, wandered around inside a woman's body hunting for semen.[108] If it could not find any, it would become angry and close up women's breathing passages and compress her intestines, causing disease. The uterus, however, was attracted to fragrant smells, and fumes wafted into the vagina could lure the uterus back into its rightful place. If that didn't work, repulsive medicines taken by mouth could force down a womb that had traveled too high inside the body.[109]

Over the next fifteen centuries,[110] a variety of men (and a few women, such as Metrodora) made a wide variety of revisions, assertions and accusations related to the uterus. Greco-Romans, Egyptians, Western Europeans and Arabs entertained an almost comical repertoire of ideas. The uterus caused convulsions. It was demonically possessed. It was animalistic in nature and had its own free will. Menstrual blood and other "moisture" had to be regularly expelled to ward off "the vapors" (otherwise known as anxiety and depression).[111]

Women with any kind of physical or mental complaint—so, almost all women—were said to be hysterical. The notorious pelvic massage was one treatment, in which doctors supposedly masturbated their patients either with their hands or by aiming a high-powered hose at their vulvas. Bloodletting was another, in which doctors put leeches inside of vaginas to cure pelvic pain.[112] "In one unsettling account," notes one horrifying tale of endometriosis care, "a practitioner advised others to be sure to count their leeches, as they had been known to occasionally wind up lost inside the uterus."[113]

Of course, women and their husbands were told by physicians that sexual intercourse could solve most of these womb-related woes. No wonder men fetched the doctor whenever their wives "took ill."

The biggest break between ancient concepts of gynecology and more modern ones came during the 1800s. It was the post–Scientific Revolution era, but more importantly, it was the era of slavery in North America.

As medical historian Deirdre Cooper Owens notes in *Medical Bondage: Race, Gender and the Origins of American Gynecology*, the 1808 ban on importing enslaved people made Southern plantation owners especially interested in ensuring that the Black women they had enslaved remained fertile and free of venereal disease.[114] As bearers of future laborers, they could fetch higher prices on the slave market. "Slave owners used these men's medical assessments to ascertain whether a woman would be an economically sound investment," Cooper Owens writes.[115] Even so, enslaved women— even pregnant ones—were still worked to the bone, tortured with physical and sexual violence, and starved of nutrition. That made them more prone to gynecological problems such as fistulas, which often manifest as holes between the uterus, bladder, colon or rectum causing incontinence.[116] They usually result from sexual violence or the birthing process.

Fistulas are how James Marion Sims got famous.

Sims, the one-time "father of American gynecology," was a white man born in South Carolina in 1813 who wrote in his unfinished, posthumously published autobiography, "If there was anything I hated, it was investigating the organs of the female pelvis."[117] Sims wrote that he started his medical career as a general practitioner but found it deeply unfulfilling and readily admitted in his book to being a mediocre doctor. Still, he craved recognition from his peers, which he went on to receive; Sims invented the modern speculum, and the 1852 publication of his pioneering paper, *On the Treatment of Vesico-Vaginal Fistula*, got him invitations to perform surgery on European royalty.[118]

Before all that, though, he was most famous for experimenting on enslaved women. Sims, a supporter of the Confederacy, detailed throughout his memoir that he traded his medical services with plantation owners to receive enslaved women with fistulas, whom he kept in a backyard hospital in Alabama. There he made dozens of attempts to surgically close the fistulas of a handful of Black women. He operated on them without first giving them anesthetic, despite the 1840s emergence of ether and chloroform.

Sims met his first fistula patient when she was seventy-two hours into her first labor.[119] It was 1845 in Alabama, and seventeen-year-old Anarcha Westcott's baby was stuck in her pelvis, Sims wrote in his autobiography. He used forceps to extract the baby, and Anarcha survived—only to be promptly stricken ill by two "incurable" fistulas. He sent her back to the plantation, telling the owner that Anarcha wouldn't die, but she'd also never get better. Shortly thereafter, Sims learned of Betsey and Lucy, two other enslaved women in similarly desperate circumstances, but also declined to treat them. It was only when a "respectable" white woman, Mrs. Merrill, was thrown from her pony and complained of intense back and pelvic pain that Sims reluctantly decided to investigate by way of a vaginal exam. He ordered his patient to get on her knees and elbows, then tugged at her uterus with his fingers until something strange happened: "I could not feel the womb, or the walls of the vagina. I could touch nothing at all, and wondered what it all meant. It was as if I had put my two fingers into a hat, and worked them around, without touching the substance of it," reads his autobiography. And then suddenly Mrs. Merrill queefed, a gust of air rushing out of her vagina causing "an explosion." It dawned on Sims that filling the uterus with air would let him clearly see into it. Excited by this prospect, he asked the plantation owners who enslaved Anarcha, Betsey and Lucy if he could have them with the promise he wouldn't accidentally kill them.[120]

Lucy was his first surgical case. Of her, he wrote: "The whole base of the bladder was gone and destroyed, and a piece had fallen out, leaving an opening between the vagina and the bladder, at least two inches in diameter or more. That was before [Sims adopted anesthetics], and the poor girl, on her knees, bore the operation with great heroism and bravery. I had about a dozen doctors there to witness the series of experiments that I expected to perform."[121]

Over time, he found another half-dozen enslaved women from around the country with similar symptoms, and he brought them to his backyard hospital where he operated on each of them and also made them work as his surgical assistants.[122]

In 1853, he moved to New York City to establish a women's hospital.[123] The first hospital, with thirty beds, was located inside a rented four-story house on Madison Avenue between East 28th and 29th streets.[124] Though he found himself without enslaved women on whom to operate in the Yankee North, he quickly found a new supply of surgical subjects: Irish immigrants seeking refuge during the potato famine. They arrived at ports up and down the East Coast aboard coffin ships infested with typhus and rapists, with many of the Irish in New York City settling in tenements in the Lower East Side neighborhood of Five Points, not far from Sims's hospital.[125] Americans were not fond of this new immigrant community, and this anti-Irish sentiment spawned the idea that these new immigrant women were probably as strong and fertile as Black women, which meant they could withstand the same amounts of physical pain. To Sims, these perceived qualities made them excellent candidates for experimental gynecological surgery.

Mary Smith was the first patient to seek help at the charity ward of Sims's new hospital, in 1855.[126] She had a massive fistula caused by a difficult labor back in Ireland. She had sailed from Europe with a large pessary—a wooden ball the size of a fist—inside her vagina, put there to keep her bladder from falling through the vaginal wall. It had been there long enough to become encrusted with phosphatic deposits, likely caused by years of leaking urine.[127] "This miserable object was operated on over 30 times, almost always [positioned] on the knees and chest, each operation lasting from two to three hours, without ever taking an anesthetic, and she suffered during a period of nearly five years before even partial retention was gained. For a long time, she was the 'show-case' for demonstrating the mode of operating," wrote Sims's protégé Dr. Thomas Addis Emmet in 1884 of their work on Smith.[128] Like Anarcha, Lucy and Betsey before her, she lived and worked at the hospital.[129]

Amid mounting political tensions that would ultimately lead to the Civil War, Sims went off to Europe in 1859 to teach doctors there his version of modern gynecology, while Emmet stayed behind and continued to operate on Smith. It was during Sims's absence that Emmet was able to mostly repair Smith's fistula, five years after efforts began.[130] Upon Sims's return to New York, however, the doctor picked up where he'd left off with his experiments on Smith. He promptly undid Emmet's work by unintentionally lacerating her bladder while attempting to remove stones from it.[131] Ultimately, Sims abandoned Smith and she died two years later, destitute and incontinent.[132]

Sims and his colleagues justified their experiments, saying their subjects were of low intelligence, and that they were dishonest and prone to exaggeration.[133] The doctors were righteous in doing their experimentations, they reasoned; after all, discoveries made in that work could be repurposed to treat white women—under anesthetic, of course.

Sims reveled in his newfound celebrity, and he thoroughly enjoyed showing off his expertise. Sometimes dozens of people would stand around him in his operating room to watch as he operated on his Black and Irish subjects. These brutal procedures brought onlookers from around the country. In Europe, he'd been influenced to use anesthetic; sometime after his return to New York in 1871, he began using chloroform, though he used it sparingly, preferring to reserve the drug for obstetrics cases.

Four years later, the board of the New York Woman's Hospital, which Sims had helped establish, told him he could no longer have more than fifteen spectators as a way of respecting women's desire for modesty. He resigned on the spot in an egotistical fit. The appendix of his book, written by Emmet after Sims's 1883 death, argues that if the women consented to fifteen spectators, their consent for any number of spectators was implied and should be automatically assumed. Besides, the argument continued, they'd be unconscious anyway; they wouldn't know how many people had watched.[134]

After Sims died, his likeness was cast in bronze[135] and eventually wound up in Central Park, facing the New York Academy of Medicine. It was removed in 2018 amid protests, with plans to relocate it to his grave.[136] Memorials to Sims still stand in his home state of South Carolina, as does a statue of him at the Alabama capitol in Montgomery.[137] In late 2021, after years of lobbying from local activists, a new monument went up in Montgomery. Called *The Mothers of Gynecology*, statues of Anarcha, Betsey and Lucy welded by local artist Michelle Browder stand not too far from where they suffered at the hands of Sims.[138] The statue, writes Browder on her website, "will act as a first step toward teaching and reimagining the true story of the nation, facing the injustice of the past and honoring the courage of overlooked heroes."[139]

As Sims worked as a gynecologist, so too did a number of other physicians. The earliest editions of medical journals such as *The Lancet*, the *Journal of the American Medical Association* and the *British Medical Journal* mention various vaginal, uterine and cervical phenomena. The 1800s brought the professionalization of medicine, a movement that simultaneously sought to uncover scientific truths and generate income.[140] This wasn't exclusive to gynecology, but it was a particularly easy discipline to exploit, seeing as physicians' competition were mostly female midwives who were easy to discredit by virtue of their gender and ethnicity.[141]

Midwives—virtually all of whom were women, most commonly Black, Indigenous and immigrant women[142]—weren't only birthing guides; they also handled a number of gynecological problems, including abortions, which at the time were legal and routine.[143] Physicians—virtually all of whom were white men—were looking to get out from under enduring accusations of quackery. Until the later part of the 1800s, they were better known for purveying elixirs and snake oils than for curing disease.[144] The push for the professionalization of medicine saw an involuntary transfer of the domain of female health from midwives to doctors.[145] This transfer was hastened by the development of tools such as speculums and forceps, and of anesthetics such as chloroform, ether and opium—innovations that enabled physicians to lure pregnant women away from midwives with the promise of an easier birth. These incentives turned out to be extremely powerful. By the turn of the twentieth century, physicians delivered about half of the babies born in the United States.[146]

But American physicians didn't only win business by offering expectant mothers a more compelling option. They also did it by vilifying midwives and lobbying for the criminalization of abortion—except when medically necessary, in which case the procedure would be performed exclusively by doctors. As expertly detailed by Leslie J. Reagan in *When Abortion Was a Crime*, they did this for two main reasons: one, to claim an elevated position in society by quashing non-physician practitioners, and two, to make more money. Considering abortions and birthing were two of the most sought-after (and lucrative) health services of the time, physicians thought *they* should be the ones making that money. To secure their dominance, physicians' associations began attacking midwives as unlicensed know-nothings who posed a serious threat to the life and safety of mother and child.[147]

In 1857, the American Medical Association (AMA), led by Dr. Horatio Storer, began lobbying for the criminalization of abortion at every stage of pregnancy.[148] Up until then, it was only illegal after "the quickening," or the first time a pregnant person felt the fetus move.[149] Storer, a fervent antiabortionist who considered the practice infanticide, introduced ideas of morality, patriotism and preservation of the white race as guiding principles on the debate.[150] He stoked fears by pointing to declining birth rates among white middle-class women and the growth of immigration, facts he juxtaposed against the backdrop of abortion rates rising 300 percent within the nineteenth century.[151] If these trends were permitted to continue, it would surely lead to the decline of civilization, he argued. The subtext was, of course, that controlling the means of reproduction had the added advantage of controlling women (which is why I advocate for endometriosis being included in conversations about reproductive freedom).

"In giving abortion new meaning," writes Reagan, "[medical doctors] provided a weapon that white, native-born, male legislators could use against the women of their own class who had been agitating for personal and political reform. Regular physicians won passage of new criminal abortion laws because their campaign appealed to a set of fears of white, native-born, male elites about losing political power to Catholic immigrants and to women."[152]

In the throes of all this, the Catholic Church decided in 1869 it would condemn abortion.[153] State after state began passing anti-abortion legislation, and in Canada abortions became punishable by life in prison. The criminalization of abortion was the final nail in the coffin: medicine had finally taken over women's health, the field swiftly becoming populated by male physicians. But that was not exclusionary enough.

At the turn of the twentieth century, the AMA commissioned a report on the state of medical teaching in the U.S. and Canada as part of professionalization efforts. In 1910, the Flexner Report condemned medical schools for improperly training future doctors and specifically called out obstetrics, describing it as having "the very worst showing."[154] The report denigrated the practice of sourcing medical trainees from the lower rungs of the socioeconomic ladder and criticized how affordable medical school was at the time—a factor, the Flexner Report noted, that made it too easy for people of undesirable classes or racial backgrounds to attend, which caused an infiltration of incompetence.[155] Most Black medical colleges closed shortly after the publication of that report.[156, 157] From there, medical school tuition steadily climbed, creating an additional applicant filter.

The repercussions of this are still felt today. In 2018–19, just 6.2 percent of American medical school graduates were Black,[158] though Black Americans represent 13.4 percent of the U.S. population.[159] A lack of ethnic and racial representation in medicine is harmful to chronically ill people of color, because it absolves the system of responsibility for delivering culturally appropriate care, and that in turn promotes racial biases and health inequities. In the Canadian government's own words, "In recent years, racism has been increasingly recognized as an important driver of inequitable health outcomes for racialized Canadians."[160]

In historical revisits of the social and institutional upheaval of the 1800s and early 1900s, one crucial change has been conveniently buried: the over-medicalization and pathologization of women's bodies. Just as Helen King wrote, the sick role became feminized: men were strong and heroic; women were weak and frail. Even the birthing process—something people had been doing since the dawn of humanity in caves, jungles, shacks and teepees—became a sterile, hospital-centered event.

And then came along John A. Sampson.

Sampson was a member of the 1899 graduating class at Johns Hopkins University in Baltimore. By the time Sampson's residency under gynecologist Dr. Howard Kelly came to a close in 1904, he'd written eighteen articles on surgery and gynecology.[161, 162] He became fascinated by the condition he later named endometriosis, which had until then been predominantly viewed as a physical manifestation of hysteria.[163]

Sampson theorized that endometriosis was caused by retrograde menstruation, in which endometrial tissue and cells he referred to as Müllerian mucosa exited the uterus through the fallopian tubes, which caused seeds of disease to spread through the pelvic cavity. He also suggested that epithelial tissue and menstrual blood could escape from hemorrhagic/chocolate cysts (so named for their dark red-brown color) and cause adhesions.[164] "If bits of Müllerian mucosa carried by menstrual blood escaping into the peritoneal cavity are always dead, the implantation theory, as presented by me, also is dead and should be buried and forgotten. If some of these bits are even occasionally alive, the implantation theory is also alive," he wrote in a 1940 article in the *American Journal of Obstetrics and Gynecology*.[165] In the same article, Sampson also noted that retrograde menstruation couldn't explain every instance of endometriosis and suggested alternate theories could be at play. It's since been shown that most menstruators experience retrograde menstruation.[166]

Sampson's theory of implantation was derived from work on just two hundred or so patients,[167] and yet it would go on to become the most influential idea in the treatment of the disease, instructing the care of millions of people over time. Almost instantly canonized, Sampson's theory has gone mostly unchallenged in nearly one hundred years of clinical practice,[168] seemingly because no one has mounted a compelling enough alternative theory to knock it off its pedestal. It became the backbone of treating endometriosis, and to this day is still difficult to subvert—but lord, has Dr. David Redwine tried.

Redwine, a pioneering endometriosis specialist who retired in 2012, abhors that Sampson's theory is still the most widely accepted explanation of endometriosis. Talking to me from his home in Arizona, he calls Sampson's retrograde theory "the most dangerous theory in the history of medicine" because it is a "fantasy" that could, and should, have been dispelled decades ago. That it wasn't has harmed "tens of millions of patients" whose treatment was based on the theory of reflux menstruation as the origin of the disease, says Redwine.[169]

Spurred to action by his first wife's experience with both the disease and with ineffective medical treatment, Redwine opened the Oregon Institute of Endometriosis in the small city of Bend in 1987.[170] There, he noticed that the disease he read about in textbooks barely resembled the actual experiences of patients. "The old classic textbooks talked about the classic black powder-burn lesion, but I was turning up lesions of all kinds of colors, no color at all, etcetera, and these lesions became more obvious with time," he tells me. "I thought, 'My gosh, you know, that's kind of crazy.' You might think that something is seeding à la Sampson's theory of reflux menstruation, when actually something that was there already is changing in appearance and becoming more obvious."

He says his textbooks also talked about something he dubbed dandelion spread, an idea based on Sampson's theory that compares endometriosis cells to the white spores from a spent dandelion: they easily blow away and project seeds into other fields, creating more dandelions. "If every month, new cells come out of the fallopian tubes, the pelvis should fill up like a pasture filling up with dandelions," Redwine explains. But when he did a pelvic mapping study to test this idea, he found it wasn't true. Across 130 or so patients with endometriosis, he found older patients didn't have more disease, even though they'd had more menstrual cycles than younger people.

"I was taught all through medical school and internship and residency that endometriosis spreads by dandelion spread with reflux menstruation. I didn't know what to believe, except I didn't believe in Sampson's theory, because it just didn't make sense," says Redwine. Sampson's theory also doesn't explain how or why the disease has been found in fetuses and premenstrual girls, or how the rare male develops endometriosis.[171] It also does not account for the occasional instance of a person developing the disease after they've gone into menopause.

For so many doctors, though, Sampson's theory seemed like a logical explanation for what had been such a cryptic, impossible-to-understand disease. His definition of endometriosis helped remove it from its black box and ultimately gave doctors a straightforward course of action: if the disease is caused by menstruation, controlling or eliminating menstruation could control the disease. This is why hormonal birth control became such a dominant force in the treatment of endometriosis; in fact, the pill's first federal approvals were not for reproductive control but for "menstrual disorders,"[172] and the first physicians who prescribed it did so to treat endometriosis.[173] Today, hormonal contraceptives are the first-line treatment for endometriosis.[174]

And yet, while hormonal contraceptives may lessen some pain and bleeding, it hasn't been proven that these drugs slow or stop disease progression.[175, 176] This is part of the reason why it takes so long for doctors to diagnose the disease; many patients try birth control and other drugs and interventions for at least a few years, during which time diagnosis usually isn't pursued.[177] For many doctors, especially non-specialists, using prescription drugs to reduce menstrual symptoms is seen as a victory, even if they produce a litany of other side effects. Nearly every single one of the dozens of people with endometriosis (and/or polycystic ovary syndrome) that I interviewed for *BLEED* tried at least one form of hormonal birth control before stopping because of side effects or ineffectiveness.

Meanwhile, hormonal birth control is a US$20-billion industry.[178] Much like how doctors took over gynecology, the pharmaceutical industry has taken over endometriosis care.

◆

Although Sampson's theory is still the prevailing justification for modern clinical care of endometriosis,[179] it's becoming increasingly clear in the research arena that endometriosis is incredibly complex and could have multiple causes. Many researchers are embracing the idea of endometriosis as a multifactorial disease with possible abnormal immune, hormonal and genetic functioning.[180] At least one group of researchers has argued there is some connection between childhood sexual or physical abuse and an increased likelihood of endometriosis.[181] Others have suggested there could be an environmental component to the disease, with pollutants such as dioxins to blame.[182] Dioxins are almost everywhere, including in pads and tampons, and even microscopic amounts can accumulate inside of us, with the World Health Organization noting that their half-life in the body is between seven and eleven years.[183]

These are all interesting ideas, but the links to immunity are particularly fascinating.

Autoimmune disease is generally caused by your immune system attacking healthy tissues because it can't distinguish them from foreign cells.[184] There are dozens of autoimmune diseases including psoriasis, lupus, rheumatoid arthritis, multiple sclerosis, Graves' disease and Hashimoto's disease.[185] Often, people don't have just one autoimmune problem; it's actually quite common to have at least two.[186, 187] These diseases cause inflammation and persistent fatigue and can be quite painful[188]—symptoms deeply familiar to those with endometriosis.

Researchers have been digging for information on the relationship between endometriosis, the immune system and autoimmunity for the better part of three decades. There is some evidence that people with endometriosis—considered a chronic inflammatory process[189]—are at a higher risk of having autoimmune problems, and that having an autoimmune disease can make a person's endometriosis more aggressive.[190] A literature review from 2001 concluded that current endo treatment options aren't great, and that treating it with therapies for autoimmune diseases holds promise—and yet, twenty years later, this approach has still not been adopted.[191]

I ask Dr. Jörg Keckstein, an Austrian gynecologist and professor with more than forty years of experience treating and researching endometriosis, what he thinks of the link to autoimmunity.[192] When looking at endometriosis tissue under the microscope, he tells me, you can see considerable amounts of fibrosis—that is, the result of the still-unexplained phenomenon in endometriosis that causes repeated tissue injury and repair.[193] "The fibrosis gives you a picture of how the immune system reacts," Keckstein says. But it's a bit of a chicken or the egg situation. There's clearly some interaction between endometriosis and the immune system, he continues, "But what was first? We cannot say." He suggests the immune system influences the severity, symptoms and localization of endometriosis, and that there may be a correlation between endometriosis and Hashimoto's disease (which affects the thyroid).[194] However, stone-cold, irrefutable proof of correlation and causation between endo and autoimmunity continues to elude researchers.

What researchers do know is that there is *some* kind of link. While endometriosis may never be officially categorized as an autoimmune disease, the immune system appears to be deeply involved in this illness.[195] Multiple studies indicate that people with endometriosis often have some kind of immune dysfunction.[196, 197]

Macrophages—defined by the National Cancer Institute as complex white blood cells that surround and kill foreign micro-organisms, remove dead cells and stimulate other immune system cells[198]—are a dominant force in endometriosis and are found in abundance inside of lesions.[199] In 2020, researchers explained that macrophages are "at the center of this enigmatic condition" because they enable endo lesions to grow blood vessels and nerves, as well as generate pain symptoms.[200]

Amid all the divergent ideas and uncertainty, we know one thing for sure: endometriosis is much, much more than a bad period. Let's have a moment of silence so we can tell all our gym teachers of yore to suck it.

Still, in clinical practice, Sampson's theory and the drugs and interventions built on it still prevail. Redwine suggests potentially millions of people have been improperly treated for endometriosis in consequence.[201] Some never even get a proper diagnosis. Minimally invasive laparoscopic surgery, which is performed in an operating room under general anesthetic, is still considered by endo specialists (but not currently by medical colleges) to be the gold standard for endo diagnosis. Even the finest imaging available right now often can't show the entire scope of a person's disease, and a lot of ultrasound techs and non-specialist doctors haven't been adequately trained to detect endo in basic ultrasounds.[202] Typically, some level of excision is done at the same time as diagnosis, but surgeons don't know exactly what they'll find until they're peering around your insides. That means they can't predict whether your surgery will be thirty minutes or five hours, a factor that makes it tough to book adequate OR time and streamline patients. It also introduces an economic problem: in many places, including the U.S., gynecological surgeons are paid the same flat rate no matter how long or complex the procedure is.

Some specialists are beginning to push for higher-resolution imaging to be used to at least partially map out disease location and severity before surgery, but the practice has not yet been widely embraced. And it certainly doesn't help matters that the endometriosis guidelines from the influential European Society of Human Reproduction and Embryology were revised in 2022 to say drugs, and not surgery, are the new gold standard.[203] All these contradictions muddy the waters around endo, and that enables and excuses failures in care.

This confusion—buoyed by the fact that the medical system does not fairly compensate gynecologists with endo specialization and skills in minimally invasive surgery—means a lot of people who become generalist OBGYNs don't bother doing much to treat endo at all. In 2021, just 2 percent of all obstetrics and gynecology graduates globally chose to specialize in pelvic medicine during residency. Even fewer went on to specialize in minimally invasive gynecologic surgery.[204, 205, 206] It seems many OBGYNs prefer to go the route that earns them the most money for the least amount of effort: delivering babies.[207]

This dramatic shortage of doctors specializing in endometriosis pushes patients back onto GPs who, in addition to not understanding endo, often see chronic pain patients as "malingerers" who eat up their time with exaggeration and psychosomatic pain. In fact, these patients are people who, by unwittingly taking on the sick role, have been subjected to a deeply flawed system predicated on unequal power dynamics.

How is all this possible? Why is it that, for some reason, we're beholden to an unproven theory, taking medications that don't help us in the long run, arguing with doctors who don't believe us while waiting years—and often decades—for diagnosis and surgery? It defies logic—unless, of course, you consider that it's not meant to be logical at all. It's simply that a lot of people in the system aren't interested in addressing non-male pain.

3. OPEN UP AND BLEED

the mental dimensions of pain

At thirty-five, I was diagnosed with complex post-traumatic stress disorder.

I'd long struggled under the shapelessness of depression and anxiety, two shadowy figures that came in and out of my life with seemingly no rhyme or reason.

On a gray December morning in 2019, I arrived at the mental health hospital where a doctor would finally tell me what was wrong with me. I trudged out of the slush and into a brightly lit beige linoleum hallway; I took a seat outside of a closed door, all the while thinking about what I was doing here. Was I really mentally ill, or was I just upset from years of trauma and gaslighting? Had the pain and suffering of endometriosis shaped my psychology, or was it more about my inability to get proper care?

I won't pretend that my fraught healthcare journey was my first experience with trauma. My life so far is split into two eras: the Before Times from birth until seventeen, and the After Times, from eighteen to present day. The turning point was when I left my mother, choosing my own survival over hers. It proved to be the right choice; she died a decade later.

Watching the Before Times play out in my memory is like leafing through a photo album full of portraits of trauma. I'm two. I get hit for having an accident in my bed. I'm three. Police lights swirl around the dark living room after my mother tried to kill herself. I'm four. She makes me a peanut butter and brown sugar sandwich. The bread is covered in mold. I'm five. Yelling, breaking the dresser mirror, attempting to throw the 1980s television out the second-floor apartment window. At dawn, my older brother and I escape by walking to our grandparents' house together. Divorce ensues. I'm seven or eight. The adults have been up all night drinking Ouzo and probably taking drugs. When daylight breaks, he decides to drive me home. He squeezes the boxy, baby-blue sedan through a narrow passageway between the rental bungalow and a chain-link fence. I get in. She demands I get out. She punches a glass door, shattering it. I ask the neighbors to call the police. I'm ten. I tell the school nurse my mother drinks too much. She sends a social worker to my incensed mother, who punishes me for my transgression by giving me the silent treatment. I never tell anyone again. I'm eleven. The most vibrant red pours out of me and continues to do so for seven or eight days. My belly hurts inside and out, the skin swollen to the touch. "You're a woman now," they tell me. I am in agony.

And so it begins. Walk-in clinics, birth control, naproxen, shrugged shoulders, missing school, missing life, a generation of busywork. I didn't know it then, but I would spend the next twenty-four years of my life looking for relief.

These little blips play in my mind like split-second videos, as if I'm watching a home-video montage in my mind. I know viscerally that these things happened to me, but a part of me wonders if some of them happened at all. Can my memory be trusted?

I've made the choice to keep most of this movie's cast anonymous, and in a sense who did what doesn't really matter to me. What I'm really reckoning with these days is how an obviously vulnerable kid like myself, with so much early exposure to the medical system, was thrown away.

The worst part is that I was not alone: many endometriosis patients start seeing doctors as children. On average, kids start their periods around the age of twelve, although it's becoming increasingly common for children to get it as young as eight or nine.[208] Not everyone with endo immediately feels symptoms, but many do; my first period was wickedly awful. The icing on this demonic cake is that you're *bleeding out of your vagina*—truly, the most embarrassing thing for a kid to articulate to anyone, let alone a doctor. Because of that, we may not tell the truth about just how terrible our periods really are. This is how we fulfill the sick role early on: learning to defer to doctors in ways that emulate our relationships with our parents, trying not to be too dramatic, trying to appease the adults.

Once that pattern is established, it is very, very difficult to break. For children who are victims of neglect and abuse, the consequences are even more dire because we have already been exposed to poisonous power dynamics. In the U.S., one in seven children experience abuse or neglect every year, most often at the hand of a parent—and that's just the reported cases.[209] Girls represent 51.6 percent of these reported maltreatment cases, according to a 2020 report.[210] When a child experiences frequent maltreatment, their nervous system often trains them to avoid future maltreatment by any means necessary. Unfortunately, this makes them more vulnerable to future abuse,[211] as they learn to defer or ingratiate themselves to more powerful people. They may also develop a form of post-traumatic stress that causes anxiety to overtake interpersonal relationships. Although the 2020 report on child maltreatment does not correlate type of abuse by victim sex or gender, similar government data from Canada shows that girls are more likely than boys to experience family violence (representing 57 percent of victims).[212] Meanwhile, research on maltreatment among

LGBTQ+ youth shows that "while all individuals who experience childhood maltreatment may face challenges with healthy development and functioning as young adults, these risks are likely to be exacerbated for young [LGBTQ+] people."[213] These realities can have devastating long-term consequences on how a person learns to navigate power differentials.

A 2018 research paper published in the journal *Human Reproduction* suggests a correlation between endometriosis and early life abuse. After surveying 3,394 cases of confirmed endometriosis, those researchers concluded that people who experienced severe and repeated forms of abuse had a 79 percent higher chance of developing endometriosis.[214]

Child abuse isn't the only area of trauma that's relevant here. Experiencing or witnessing other types of trauma can radically transform a person's ability to cope with certain situations, particularly ones that feel dangerous. Unequal power is integral to intimate partner violence and sexual assault as well, and those affect cis women, trans and non-binary people much more frequently than they do cis men.[215] Trauma also proliferates through exposure to the healthcare system, as it did for me—I came into it pre-traumatized, but some medical encounters added new layers of trauma.

And yet there is no accounting or appreciation for trauma when it comes to delivering healthcare to marginalized people. Rather, as patients we are expected to override our fears and feelings of powerlessness, and then get blamed when we can't. Sometimes it feels like medical professionals—wrapped up in the belief that they give everyone equal treatment—lose sight of the fact that health is not merely a molecular phenomenon but is wrapped up in our life experiences. In the sick role, chronically ill people are treated as children but are held to adult-sized standards of accountability. We are expected to give up our autonomy on health decisions, but we are held responsible for our poor outcomes. If you become anxious or depressed about medical stuff and around medical people, that is a reflection of your failure to control your emotions. Never mind the pile of scientific research that shows physiological and neurological links between chronic pelvic pain and depression (which we'll get to in a bit). Also never mind that repeated adversity in medical settings affects how people cope with their chronic illnesses and how they behave in the doctor-patient relationship.[216] If we become adversarial or refuse to follow a doctor's orders, the chances are good that we'll be viewed as mentally ill.

And then what becomes of people with genuine mental illness?

In the summer of 2021, I spoke with Tara, a thirty-six-year-old white woman with undiagnosed PCOS.[217] We'd connected through social media, after she saw my tweet that I was looking to speak to people with endo, PCOS and other pelvic disorders about their medical experiences. When we speak on the phone, she tells me how her suspected PCOS triggered rapid weight gain during her teens, and how that and a bundle of mysterious symptoms saw her start taking antidepressants at age thirteen. On top of all this, she thinks she developed an eating disorder, putting further pressure on her self-image and self-esteem. Being told to lose weight by doctors when she went in with PCOS symptoms certainly didn't help.

It was through these experiences that she learned early on that doctors are not to be trusted. When I ask if she's ever told a doctor why she struggled with anxiety in medical settings, she pauses, then says, "I should preface everything by saying I am suspicious of the medical system.

"I'll tell my doctor, 'This is a system, and in the system, you have more power than me. So, at the end of the day, your job is to help me, right? That's your job. So we have to have these boundaries, that has to be understood, because I have to fight the system. And if fighting the system means that I have to fight you, then that's what you have to accept as being part of the system. It's not personal. I have to get the help that I need.'"

When I ask her how doctors have responded to that, she answers that most of them just kind of nod along. One time not so long ago, though, she went to a hospital in a state of mental crisis. When she tried to establish her boundaries, she says they put her in a room with a social worker who tried to keep Tara from leaving until she could meet with a psychiatrist. She says the social worker was hostile and that the conversation quickly became confrontational. Tara panicked; all this was a major trigger for her anxiety about healthcare. The hospital staff refused to admit her because of her behavior and security escorted her off the premises. "They put it on me by saying, 'You're refusing to see the social worker,'" she says. She left the hospital and walked down the street and around the corner to the fire station, where they called an ambulance. When the paramedics arrived, she asked them to take a statement about what had transpired. At that point, she was operating mostly out of spite: she wanted a written record of their refusal to treat her.

There is a reason why it seems every doctor's office has a sign saying they have zero tolerance for yelling or abuse. Objectively, I agree no one should fear for their safety. But a healthcare facility is not a café or a bookstore or a grocery store. It is a place where people are more likely to feel vulnerable and stressed, and where emotions often run high. Do they only deserve care when they speak and behave properly? Who decides what "proper" looks like?

When Tara and I speak, some time has passed since her hospital run-in. With this mental distance, I ask her how she interprets that experience now. "I don't trust healthcare providers sometimes," she replies. "You know, it's a system, it's a business, it's a job for a lot of people, and I respect that. It just means that you have to go in with boundaries and expectations."

Trauma can be cumulative, and those events at the hospital justified and reinforced her existing fear of doctors. The next time she tries to get care for any reason—PCOS, a mental breakdown, stepping on a rusty nail—she faces the very real possibility of being triggered again. In her case, personal traumas have created a self-fulfilling prophecy in which she fears becoming anxious, so she becomes anxious—a crime that might get her forever labeled "hysterical." And once you've got that sign tied 'round your neck, it's very, very hard to convince someone to take it off. In Tara's case, we can easily see what a world of difference trauma-informed care could make. This nascent movement in healthcare is one that considers how a patient's past and present circumstances might affect their sickness and healing.[218]

We could all use at least a little more understanding and compassion.

Unfortunately, right now it's still a real trip being a person with a chronic illness and health-related trauma. Unless you are independently wealthy and can hire the best doctors around, being chronically ill puts you at the mercy of the system—and nothing breeds anxiety and uncertainty more for a person with complex trauma than being thrust into a stressful situation over which they have little to no control.[219]

In the process of writing BLEED, I spent a lot of time thinking about trauma—about how it's generated, how it affects how the world sees us, how being misunderstood can halt healing or even retraumatize us. It's all so cyclical. Abuse and abandonment breed fear and uncertainty, which breed anxiety. A lifetime of anxiety becomes a personality, becomes a traumatized person, becomes a lightning rod for future abuse.

Typical post-traumatic stress disorder (PTSD) is caused by one traumatic event or situation. The loss of a loved one. A difficult childbirth. A sexual assault. A car crash.

Complex PTSD is repeated or prolonged trauma. Childhood neglect. Domestic abuse. Human trafficking. Living in a war zone.

And, I think, medical gaslighting.

In circumstances outside of medicine, such as in intimate relationships, gaslighting is rightfully recognized as emotional abuse. In a 2019

American Sociological Review article, sociologist Paige L. Sweet theorizes, "Gaslighting is effective when it is rooted in social inequalities, especially gender and sexuality, and executed in power-laden intimate relationships. When perpetrators mobilize gender-based stereotypes, structural inequalities and institutional vulnerabilities against victims with whom they are in an intimate relationship, gaslighting becomes not only effective, but devastating."[220] Not only is a gaslightee emotionally abused and manipulated within the relationship, but the gaslighter also often succeeds in telling people around the woman—and it almost always is a woman—that she's just a "crazy bitch," writes Sweet.

It makes me think of my own circumstances.

I was extremely independent from a very young age because being alone was my key coping mechanism in a life of chaos. I learned to be my own companion early on, but I hadn't been given the tools to be my own advocate. That meant that a lot of my traumas got locked up inside me, only seeping out at inopportune times in inappropriate ways—and that, of course, made me look strange and maybe even crazy. At the same time as these connections were being forged, I also began suffering symptoms of endometriosis, which made me a fixture in walk-in clinic waiting rooms. I'd been trained that people go to the doctor when they are unwell. But when I would get into the doctor's office, my words either froze in my mouth, or they came tumbling out in nonsensical jumbles.

What is clear to me now, but was not obvious to me then, is that my family trauma and medical trauma merged early on. Going to doctors who didn't seem to care about my suffering reinforced the neglect and abandonment I felt at home. I was desperate to connect and to be understood, but I had been trained to be stoic and to hide personal problems from the outside world. This especially played out in healthcare settings, where I was asked to disclose personal information about my most shameful bodily functions at times when I felt most vulnerable.

I had a right to feel vulnerable. I was always a chubby kid, and no one has ever let me forget it. Kids at school, family, friends, coworkers and complete strangers have all felt it was their duty to let me know I was fat, just in case I hadn't noticed it myself. Doctors were no exception, and they started telling me to lose weight from the very beginning. The message was clear: if my life did not revolve around losing weight, I would never be worthy of kind, compassionate care. At the same time, my menstrual pain just would not stop—and so I kept going back and re-exposing myself to the abuse. I *needed* a doctor to do something about my excessive pain and bleeding. The more I went back to the walk-in clinic, though, the less they seemed to care. I felt ignored and helpless. I was just a teenager, and there was nothing I could do about a medical system that kept telling me I was fine when I very clearly wasn't.

As I grew up to become a chronically ill adult, it became very hard to shake that asymmetrical parent-child relationship in medicine. As a kid, I had so desperately wanted doctors' approval and validation, but rarely got even the most basic concern. The older I got, the angrier I felt about that. I developed a new defense mechanism to prevent me from exploding with rage: dissociation. Being able to mentally escape a room I could not physically leave became a way to lessen the force of impact. From then on, every doctor's appointment followed the same script: first, mounting anxiety and fat salty tears; then, when my anxiety spilled over the top of my emotional cup, I shut down. I actively avoided eye contact, instead fixating on a benign object in the room. My eyelids grew heavy with hopelessness and my head filled with white noise. This involuntary sequence helped prevent me from freaking out, but it also made it nearly impossible to be taken seriously.

My therapist has since informed me that dissociating is a normal trauma response.

I wonder why more doctors don't know that.

Getting medical help can be traumatizing. Unfortunately, chronic illness doesn't care if you're traumatized. It has a way of taking over your life and becoming a full-time job. There are always forms to fill out, calls to make, research to do, waiting lists to join, alternative therapies to explore—and that's on top of experiencing the actual illness.

Nobody likes doing this busywork. I'd rather do my taxes than go to a doctor's appointment. Still, we're pushed into doing it because the bar to qualify for "good care" is constantly raised.

With endometriosis, that can look like trying different types of hormonal contraceptives, each experiment taking three to six months of our lives. Maybe we try Motrin or Advil, then Tylenol, then naproxen, then naproxen plus Tylenol, then more naproxen. We get invasive pelvic exams, transvaginal ultrasounds and colonoscopies, and referrals to specialist after specialist—except, somehow, an endometriosis specialist. These non-endo-specialized doctors decide to try other hormonal drugs, ones that throw us into a state of fake menopause, ones that if taken for too long do irreparable damage to our bones. When that doesn't work, we might get sent for surgery—except it's not the excision surgery you need but a uterine ablation, where they burn the lining of your uterus but typically do nothing about the lesions *outside* the uterus. Worse, the scar tissue caused by the ablation can be a breeding ground for new endo lesions. Still, they might try that surgery a couple times, and if the disease comes back (which it almost always does), then they might try the other, more effective surgery in which the disease is cut (excised) from surrounding tissue. But excision is now harder to do because of all the scar tissue the first surgeries left behind. That means a longer surgery and a longer recovery. And if it comes back after all that? God help you, because only prayer is going to save you now.

All of this is expensive, time-consuming and exhausting. Still, we do it, because the alternative is doing nothing, and that would be admitting what the doctors have said all along: that our pain, in the grand scheme of things, doesn't really matter.

So we become even more engaged in getting to the bottom of our pain by doing research and joining online groups where thousands of people share their own horror stories. That makes you aware of the unfairness, and that makes you mad. But if you challenge your doctor, they think you're uncooperative and maybe even mentally ill. Maybe you've been exaggerating this whole time. The more you press, the less it seems they want to help. And so you start looking for other doctors who might give you answers. The ultimate cruelty is that the more you get passed around, the more diffuse your paper trail becomes, until there is no institutional memory about you at all—except your own memory. But, of course, you cannot be relied upon to tell your story faithfully and accurately. Each new doctor wants to send you for the same tests so they can see the results for themselves.

If you are tired just reading this, imagine what it's like to live it.

Perhaps the very worst part of all this is that you're expected to navigate healthcare's maze of bureaucracy and endure rampant gaslighting while remaining good-natured and polite—all while feeling like hot garbage. It's like getting stabbed in the abdomen as an onlooker yells out, "Don't exaggerate! I don't think that stabbing hurts as much as you say it does."

I got my full-time job in endometriosis at the age of twenty-six, when I decided I wanted a hysterectomy. It felt like a pretty rational conclusion: I didn't want kids and I didn't want a period. I brought my ingenious solution to my GP, but she immediately shut it down.

Instead, she sent me for my first ultrasound.

For the uninitiated, a transvaginal ultrasound goes a little something like this: a stranger—the tech—brings you into a room and tells you to take off your pants and underwear, to cover your lower half with a thin paper sheet, then to lie on an examination bed with your heels in stirrups. Then the stranger comes back in, sometimes with a second stranger, and covers a transducer wand—basically, something that looks like a twelve-inch vibrator—with a medical condom of sorts. In my most recent ultrasound, the tech put a glove over the tip of the wand, using one of the fingers to create a barrier while the other empty fingers flopped around. They tear open a little single-serve pouch of medical lube, apply it to the wand, and say, "This may be a little cold." Then they insert the wand into your vagina and press on your uterus and pelvic region to help the wand "see" inside you.

As you may expect, these exams are painful and embarrassing for a lot of people. They can feel extremely invasive and traumatic even for people without a history of sexual trauma, especially if you're not forewarned about how the ultrasound works. I wasn't the first or last person to go into an appointment expecting the kind of ultrasound pregnant ladies on TV get, only to instead get the take-off-your-pants kind. It is one of the most intimate exams a person can have, yet it's treated as if it is as routine as a blood test. Even more frustrating in my case was that the ultrasound didn't show anything. Sure, I had a chocolate cyst full of old blood on an ovary, but it was nothing to write home about.

Surely doing six more of these ultrasounds over the next six years would help, right? Predictably, every time I went for another ultrasound, nobody found anything diagnosable. Each time, I was sent home with the same naproxen I'd been taking since I was fourteen. I was never referred to a gynecologist.

When I received those first ultrasound results, I felt as though I'd been condemned to a life of pain. I grew used to the shadow of doom, though: I got my period and I hated it, and I got it again and I hated it more. Still, I kept living as best I could. Sometimes a whole year and maybe even two would pass before I brought it up again to a doctor, until a blockbuster period sent me knocking on a doctor's door. That would set off a whole new cycle of testing and disappointment and naproxen. But instead of becoming boring and rote, each new transvaginal ultrasound caused a sense of mounting moral injury. This process was the furthest thing from trauma-informed healthcare. It was *traumatizing*. Worse, all the tests seemed to do was discredit my suffering.

Why did I keep submitting myself to this medical busywork?

In March 2016, I drew a line.

I hadn't gone to the hospital intending to draw this line, but the circumstances demanded it. After this transvaginal ultrasound, I would begin demanding to know what my doctors thought they would accomplish with the test that the previous ones had not.

It had started as a fairly routine appointment: I took off my pants and underwear, put on a hospital gown, then laid down on the exam table. A technician burst into the room without so much as an introduction and got right down to the task at hand, starting with an external ultrasound. Cold and uncaring, she guided the trans-ducer across my jelly-covered stomach and abdomen and stared at her monitor. Next, the transvaginal ultrasound began. By then I'd become grudgingly familiar with them, so I just laid there and hoped it would soon be over.

But then she noticed something on the monitor. She announced she would show some images to a doctor then left the room, leaving the transducer wand inside of me, with its bottom half and the cord hanging out of my vagina. She'd left the door open in her haste—the door that faced a busy hallway in a busy hospital in the middle of a weekday afternoon. I squeezed my thighs together as hard as I could to regain a little dignity, but nothing could shield me from the fact that my unfortunate situation was completely visible to all those who walked past.

The technician reappeared a few minutes later with a male doctor in tow, bringing an unannounced guest to my pelvic ultrasound party. Instead of saying hello or introducing himself, the doctor beelined for the monitor, then pointed to something on the screen. "Hmm, I didn't see that before," the tech told him.

"What is it?" I asked. They wouldn't tell me. They wouldn't even look at me. The technician grabbed the external transducer and again pressed on my stomach, pushing so hard that I was left with a huge purple bruise. Then it was over.

"The results will be sent to your doctor," she told me and placed a tiny box of tissues on my stomach. "You can clean up, put your clothes on and leave."

I often joke that I have amnesia because of the medical trauma I've endured. In my memory, all I can really remember is the door being left open. It's perhaps a blessing and a curse that I have a lot of written records. The details of this retelling come from an official complaint I made to the hospital's ombudsperson, a message still sitting in my email's sent messages. I wrote: "I felt the entire experience was extremely dehumanizing. It would not have taken twenty seconds longer to be kinder and gentler with me, and to treat me with a little more respect and to extend privacy to me." The ombudsperson said they contacted the head of the medical imaging department before formally replying to my complaint. They answered by telling me my complaint prompted a new policy: "From now on, the endovaginal probe should not be left inside the vagina when the technologist leaves the room to discuss the case with the radiologist unless the patient consents to it. Nevertheless, the patient will have to be warned that the probe might have to be reinserted following the discussion between the technologist and the radiologist. That being said, if the probe must be reinserted, it will be done when the radiologist is in the room."

It didn't change anything about my experience, but I guess I'd won one for the team. The thought of a transvaginal ultrasound still fills my throat with dread.

◆

That feeling crept back into my throat on September 6, 2019, at New Jersey's Newark Liberty International Airport. I'd just landed at my transfer point on a flight to New Orleans, where I would be meeting an old roommate for a little vacation in the city's eclectic Bywater neighborhood before attending a journalism conference in the French Quarter. I was waiting for my second flight that Friday afternoon when my phone rang.

I'd moved to a new city in mid-2017, and with it came new doctors. Since the move, I'd been trying to track down some answers and had just gone for yet another ultrasound. I swiped to answer the call: it was the hospital calling to book me in for a transvaginal ultrasound.

But I'd just had one, I told the receptionist. You want me to come back for *another one*? Did they see something? Why do I have to come back?

The receptionist couldn't tell me who ordered it or why. I wearily accepted the appointment for another ultrasound in two weeks' time. I resented being asked to do more busywork without a justification. Didn't I deserve to know?

That early October day, I wake up a nervous wreck ahead of the 7:15 a.m. appointment. I am so grateful a friend offered to drive me to the hospital and accompany me to the waiting room. It's mercifully quiet, not yet jumping with the day's parade of patients. I am told this ultrasound will be done by a doctor—a *male* doctor. My anxiety spikes. *Great*, I think. We watch the clock as we wait. The hands hit 7:30, then 7:45, then 8 a.m. *Why are doctors always late?* I think, now vibrating with anxious nervousness, my eyes brimming with tears that threaten to escape and my lungs refusing to accept anything other than short, shallow breaths.

The radiology technician pops her head out of the exam room to tell me the doctor will be here soon. I take a seat on the edge of an uncomfortable office chair a good twelve feet diagonally across from her, ready to sprint away. With my back rounded, my shoulders curled in and my autumn jacket tightly tucked under my arm, I cast my heavy eyes downward, unwilling to meet the technician's gaze. *I will burn a goddamned hole into this floor if I have to.*

She demands to know why I am so upset, then tells me my anger is irrational. She is defensive about my defensiveness. My attempts at explanation come out in a jumble of anxiety. *I'm not making sense.* Unable to speak, frustrated tears plunge down my face. Why don't we do this on a day when you are less upset, the technician threatens. *I will always be this upset.* I tell her I'm confused about why I'm here, that I'm traumatized by doctors. She refuses to soften.

Our standoff breaks when the doctor finally arrives. "Please take off everything from the waist down," he tells me. I'd intentionally worn a dress that day so I could stay as fully clothed as possible, as if keeping my modesty was possible in such a situation. I wrap the paper sheet around my legs.

As the doctor and the technician return, suddenly a flood of words comes rushing out: "I just had one of these. Why am I having a second one? The receptionist wouldn't tell me. I spent the last month in emotional limbo. I'm already traumatized. *These exams are harmful to my mental health.* I keep doing them, for no reason! I've been on naproxen since I was fourteen, and I'm thirty-five now! It hasn't helped in at least a decade. I still don't know what's wrong with me. Are you going to be the one who gives me answers?"

This barrage of information softens the technician's face, and the doctor doesn't admonish me like other nurses, technicians and doctors have. Instead, he talks to me while performing the exam, telling me that the level one transvaginal ultrasound—the kind I had undergone all those times before—is not a great diagnostic tool for endometriosis. It's not granular enough to give any kind of useful information of what's happening outside of the uterus, and endometriosis is a disease where tissue grows outside of the uterus.

I read between the lines. *All those awful ultrasounds were just things doctors ordered to make it seem like they were doing something. It was all an elaborate ruse to make me think the system cared.*

What we're doing here, he continues, is a *level two* ultrasound. "This is endometriosis on the bowel," he explains, pointing to the monitor. "That's automatically stage four." And there it is: a diagnosis twenty-four years in the making. I am both unsurprised and vindicated.

I'd spent two-thirds of my life hearing doctors say that losing weight would solve all my problems, as if a hundred brisk walks a week and an all-salad diet would make this disease any less awful. They'd suggested getting pregnant as a way to solve the pain, as if I could just toss the baby in the trash after it served its purpose! All the messed-up things I'd been told had been delivered with a kind of coldness that made them seem rational, and yet they cut into me in some of the most personal, intimate ways. Their words had for so long conspired with my existing traumas to drive home the overwhelming feeling that I had to make myself smaller to fit into the box of people who deserved care.

At that moment, I mentally accused every doctor I'd ever met for letting this disease fester inside of me when they could have chosen to help instead. I imagined the angry letters I would write to them. I wanted to tell them they had failed me, and that I now had proof of it. But a million questions spun inside me at the same time. I wanted to know, had their ignorance let my endometriosis grow this entire time? What if they had caught it earlier? Had I finally jumped through enough hoops to have someone actually help me?

4. TYPICAL GIRLS

intersections

Over the summer of 1996, I got my first period, turned twelve and started Grade 7. It was a perilous time for learning how to "be a woman." As I sat in a bathroom stall at school delicately unwrapping a new pad from its obnoxiously loud pink wrapper, it never crossed my mind that perhaps other girls *didn't* have to wear overnight pads during the daytime or have a bottle of Motrin rattling around in their backpacks. I was so fearful of blood leaking through my clothes that I also cut pantyliners in half and stuck them to my underwear above and below the limits of the pad, as extra assurance I would not be embarrassed.

I assumed it was normal. I'd been told by family, doctors, nurses and sex-ed teachers (who were also my religion teachers) that periods are supposed to hurt and be messy. My high school best friend also had awful periods and had to have a massive ovarian cyst removed around the age of thirteen or fourteen. At least, I thought, I wasn't *that* bad. As it turns out, none of this was how it's supposed to be.

If endometriosis is abnormal bleeding and pain, what does "normal" look like exactly? I wouldn't know a normal period if it slapped me in the face, so I asked Dr. Olga Bougie to explain it to me.

"Oh gosh, it's funny, I was training medical students, and a male medical student was like, 'How painful are these supposed to be?

What are we supposed to ask patients?' That's a great question," says Bougie, a minimally invasive endo surgeon in Ontario as well as a prolific researcher.[221]

Because pain is subjective, there's no single normal but rather a normality scale, she continues. "It's influenced by many other things besides potentially having a pathology like endometriosis. We often look at if it's affecting your quality of life. So, you know, having a painful period, [but] taking an Advil and being able to go to school or work and not having that disrupt your well-being and quality of life is one thing," Bougie says. "But, you know, many of the patients that I see—and from what we know—many are scheduling their life around their periods."

Not being able to go to work, school or even run the most basic errands is a red flag, she continues. "That's really not normal."

As a teen, Donna diagnosed herself with dysmenorrhea, an umbrella term for painful menstruation.[222] Now forty-three, she's still operating under that assumption. That's because most of the doctors she's seen haven't ventured beyond that initial diagnosis, even though endometriosis is the number-one cause of secondary dysmenorrhea in teens,[223] followed in no particular order by adenomyosis, fibroids and PCOS. (The difference between primary and secondary dysmenorrhea comes down to pathology, moving to the second level when doctors diagnose the pain.) Guidelines in Canada—where Donna lives and works as an antiracism consultant—say that endometriosis is found up to 73 percent of the time in teens whose pain is not controlled by anti-inflammatories and hormonal contraceptives.[224] Guidelines set in the U.S., meanwhile, note that if teens with dysmenorrhea don't see improvements after three to six months of hormonal birth control and anti-inflammatories, their gynecologist—assuming they have one—is supposed to investigate further to find the source of their pain.[225]

As you may expect, almost no one experiences this streamlined path to diagnosis and treatment. Donna certainly didn't.

"I think because of my age, a lot of my concerns about my period were dismissed as me just being a teenager not wanting to be sidelined with a period. But it was more than that," says Donna. Like many other teens, she routinely missed school because of her periods, choosing to stay curled up in bed with a hot water bottle instead of scribbling down algebra equations in a classroom. No one seemed alarmed by her regular absences. Around the world, menstruation is the leading reason for why kids miss school, whether that's because of pain, lack of toilets, lack of sanitary supplies or period shaming from peers.[226, 227]

In Donna's adolescent years, her pain got to a point where she had to gobble double doses of naproxen every two hours to get any reprieve at all. Despite this intense pain, the frontline treatment for painful periods—hormonal contraceptives—weren't even suggested to her until she got to university. Even then, multiple doctors told her an intrauterine device (IUD) was "too dangerous" for her without explaining why, leaving her to question whether that warning had anything to do with her being Black or being in a bigger body. Without answers, routine treatment or even a proper diagnosis, Donna was left to fend for herself for years when it came to her periods.

It felt unfair in so many ways, most of all because she'd always known she didn't want kids, yet she could never convince a doctor to consider a hysterectomy. She remembers one physician telling her that no one would ever perform a hysterectomy on such a young person (she was seventeen at the time), and that her pain was just her lot in life as a woman. Worse, when she sought a second opinion, that doctor "literally laughed," she says. "He said, 'No doctor will do it. You don't know what you want. What if you want to have kids one day?'"

And although she replied that she would never change her mind, she still has a uterus today—and, as promised, no kids. One thing she does finally have, though, is an IUD. Like many other Black women who've faced medical discrimination, she opted for the longest-acting birth control available to her when she was eventually given the choice.[228]

By then, she was already in her forties. "Basically it's eliminated my period, and for me that's the best possible outcome," she says.

The amount of time patients with pelvic pain problems spend fighting for care cannot be overstated. While her peers enjoyed their carefree youths, she fought through her teens—then twenties, thirties and into her forties—to have access to basic healthcare.

Realizations like these make me wonder how my life could have been different if I had known as a teen what periods were supposed to feel like, and if more of the doctors and nurses I saw understood and communicated better about the boundaries of normal menstrual pain. Maybe it wouldn't have taken me twenty-four years to get a diagnosis. A vast majority of endo literature, from the annals of academia to *Cosmo* articles, focus on the adult experience of pain— but by the time we're adults, we've already been ground up by the normalization machine. How life-changing would it be to take teenagers' menstrual pain seriously?

In the case of Trinity Lillian Graves, it may have saved her life. Instead, her obituary reads: "Died unexpectedly. She suffered years of daily chronic pain from endometriosis." Graves took her own life in August 2021, at the age of eighteen.[229] As her mother Sarah Austin explains in a first-person account on EndoFound.org, Graves's short life was overwhelmed by endometriosis and adenomyosis pain for which her doctors had no answers. (Adenomyosis is a profusely painful condition where endometrial tissue that is only supposed to line the inside of the uterus starts growing into the muscle wall.[230])

"We had the distinct pleasure of working with 12 unqualified, ill-equipped medical professionals: gynecologists, adolescent health physicians, GI physicians, mental and behavioral health clinicians who collectively were insensitive, minimizing and dismissive. As a group, they were not particularly well trained, they didn't understand the symptom profile, they were not used to complex cases, they did not present options, and they inspired no hope," writes Austin.[231]

Adolescence is a tumultuous, challenging and exciting time in people's lives, says Bougie—and teens are only just beginning to find their identities and voices. That makes it all the more difficult to communicate to a variety of doctors just how miserable they are, especially if—as girls often are—they're taught that it's inappropriate and even shameful to talk about their private parts. "They're kind of in this transition zone, and sometimes they'll see a pediatrician, sometimes they'll see a family doctor, or sometimes a gynecologist who primarily sees adult patients," she explains, adding that a lot is left unsaid by everyone involved when a teen doesn't have the same language and confidence as an adult to explain their symptoms. "All those kinds of subtle things have an impact."

Contrary to common myths predicated on Sampson's theory of retrograde menstruation, adolescents can and do have advanced endometriosis. But because of their age and relative inexperience with menstruation, their pain can easily get dismissed. "Their periods get normalized, they get put on the birth control pill and they don't have [endometriosis] investigated as a potential diagnosis," says Bougie. That's why she thinks studying endo in teens is critical to evolving our entire understanding of the disease: "We can't address and move forward in the journey of endometriosis without looking at the teens."

That includes looking at the mental health consequences of chronic pelvic pain. The *Journal of Health Psychology* notes that research and the clinical approach to endometriosis in teens tends to focus on the emotional elements of the condition: helplessness, disappointment, frustration, anxiety, depression, diminished self-confidence.[232]

Western medicine is not well suited to this task. It can see an illness as physical or mental, but it does a really, really bad job of understanding the connections between the two. The way the human body is perceived today in science-based medicine has been heavily influenced by Western philosophy and the concept of dualism—particularly the mind-body problem.[233]

Since ancient times, philosophers in Western and Eastern traditions have tried to reconcile how our anatomy and our minds (i.e., thoughts, emotions, intelligence) influence each other. And since then, no one has agreed on anything. That said, the most popular modern Western interpretations of the mind-body problem were shaped by René Descartes, a seventeenth-century philosopher and mathematician who saw the body as a machine and the mind as the seat of consciousness.[234]

Descartes lived during the Scientific Revolution, when chemistry, biology, astronomy and physics first took on a more scientific and less mystical bent. Investigations into the human body and mind eventually led to the establishment of pathology, gynecology, psychiatry, neurology and other specialized disciplines. As medicine became more scientific, society became more medicalized, two simultaneous phenomena that reinforced the imperative to treat the body and the mind as two separate entities.

Today, this division makes less and less sense. We are slowly realizing that we are not well served by keeping the mind and the body separate in medicine. I particularly love this summary of it, written by Mathew Gendle at North Carolina's Elon University: "The fact that modern Western medicine has one set of practitioners for 'mental' disorders and an entirely separate set of professionals for all other types of health complaints is nonsensical, and the failure to recognize the reality that 'mental' illnesses are, in fact, biological diseases fosters an environment that 'others' patients and stigmatizes substance dependency, as well as behavioral, thought and perceptual disorders."[235]

In Trinity Lillian Graves's case, doctors taking her pain *and* mental anguish seriously may have made an enormous difference. Sadly, though, our healthcare systems still tend to manage one problem at a time—which means it is fundamentally set up to fail people with chronic illness. Most doctors are unable to fully grasp just how interconnected pain is when it comes to the body and the mind. They also fail to see how an illness like endometriosis can have ripple effects all around us; for instance, how the disease can profoundly affect our partners and damage our relationships.

"The experience of cyclic and chronic pain, combined with a lack of proper recognition by health professionals, may generate varying degrees of psychological and interpersonal impairments, which are as much a source of distress for the patient and her partner as the pain itself," write the authors of a paper on the psychosocial impact of endometriosis.[236] "Furthermore, pain problems of the reproductive tract may carry an even heavier psychosocial burden in comparison to other chronic pain problems common in women because of their deleterious effect on fertility, sexuality and romantic relationships."

Sometimes this is because of a breakdown in intimacy, because pelvic pain can make sex excruciating. Sometimes it's about moral harm, when a partner can't hold on anymore to someone so physically and spiritually injured.

Perhaps the worst injustice of them all is how any manifestation of mental and physical fallout—getting depressed, getting fat, getting mad—becomes pathologized into its own form of illness that medicine *is* willing to treat.

◆

When you think of a typical endometriosis sufferer, who do you envision?

If you imagine a white cis woman, you're not alone. Endometriosis has been called the career woman's disease, the scourge of the private patient and has been closely associated with white, middle- and upper-class women since it was first named in the 1920s. For the longest time, it was believed that only white women got the disease.[237] In 1948, Joe Vincent Meigs, one of the most influential— and notorious—figures in endometriosis, told the American College of Surgeons that endometriosis would lead to the decline of the white race. The *New York Times* ran an article the night of his eugenics-tinged October 20 speech, its headline blaring "SOCIAL ILL IS LAID TO ENDOMETRIOSIS: Women's ailment restricting the propagation of intelligent class."[238] The article explained Meigs's view that because the disease was so prevalent among educated white women who delayed marriage and childbearing until they became totally infertile, it was only a matter of time before civilization declined.

Meigs, wrote the article's author, "said that, unless checked, the ailment pointed to the eventual displacement in social dominance of healthy and intelligent people by the weak and unintelligent but fecund class which had produced history's leading dictators." To counter this phenomenon, Meigs proposed restrictions on birth control and subsidies to encourage white women to marry and reproduce as young as possible.[239]

Endometriosis is so deeply aligned with whiteness that Black women with pelvic pain have for decades been consistently misdiagnosed as having pelvic inflammatory disease (PID), which is caused by sexually transmitted infections.[240] The emergence of PID as a catchall for Black gynecological problems confirmed a bias that society had held since the antebellum era: that Black women were sex-crazed "jezebels" (a bias has also been used to justify sexual violence against Black women).[241] We haven't escaped the racism sown into Black women's gynecological care. In fact, PID misdiagnosis in Black women is still prevalent today, more than forty-five years after Chicago OBGYN Dr. Donald Chatman's discovery that at least one-fifth of those diagnosed with PID actually had endometriosis.[242]

There's little wonder why, as a Black gynecologist, Dr. Melvin Thornton often finds Black patients in his office after years of systemic denial elsewhere.[243]

"It's hard to get it resolved," Thornton tells me over Zoom on a break between patients. He explains that the modern experience of medicine, particularly for working-class and low-income people, looks a lot like ten minutes at a walk-in clinic office, endless waits in urgent care and no follow-ups. In these scenarios of transient healthcare, people's files follow them wherever they go—and if their chart says they have PID, getting another doctor to challenge that diagnosis is very difficult. Thornton saw it himself while working in a Los Angeles county hospital.

"They keep getting labeled and labeled and labeled. And you look at your records and they've never had a positive culture for gonorrhea, chlamydia. Never, y'know?" he tells me. The first doctor makes an initial assessment, diagnoses PID, prescribes antibiotics to take care of it and sends the patient away. When the STI tests come back negative, the patient often isn't informed of the results— that whole "no news is good news" thing. Meanwhile, Thornton says, the diagnosis code in their file stays the same: PID. Of course, with a chronic condition like endometriosis, it's only a matter of time before a patient seeks medical attention again. When the next doctor sees the PID code in their chart, a whole new cycle begins: wrong diagnosis, ineffective treatments, no follow-ups. Thornton sees this playing out almost exclusively in lower-income communities of color. There, a doctor might look at your race and class and fill in the blanks—a judgment call based on bias, not medicine.

To untangle all the various layers of discrimination in medicine requires looking at its systems with an intersectional lens.

In 1989, lawyer Kimberlé Crenshaw coined the term *intersectionality*,[244] arguing that Black women face racism and sexism, and that the sum of these two isms is not simply 1+1=2, but that it creates a whole new form of discrimination specific to Black women. As such, Crenshaw explained, Black women experience violence and discrimination in ways that Black men and white women do not—like how Denise's problems weren't well understood or treated by her doctor, even though they were both Black. If maleness and whiteness are the defaults, Crenshaw wrote, "Black women are protected only to the extent that their experiences coincide with those of either of the two groups." They may find solidarity with other Black people or among women, but neither group really speaks to the full experience of being a Black woman.

Of course, discrimination isn't only about race and sex, especially not in a medical system defined by power imbalances. Discrimination is rampant throughout the entire ocean of the medical experience, and we are all swimming in it to some degree.

Ethnicity, gender, sexual orientation, age, socioeconomic status, dis/ability and body size are some of the things that push us away from the coast. Some people are further out than others. A slender, well-adjusted, straight, middle-class white woman might be ankles-deep in the water. A fat Black queer woman or a white teen mom on welfare might be a few miles from shore. Meanwhile, an Indigenous trans person with treatment-resistant depression and a hereditary heart condition may find themselves struggling to tread water in the deepest depths of the sea. Yes, we are all at risk of drowning—but some people are more likely to go under than others. So many people within medicine fail to see that some people need more help coming to shore, that a life preserver tied to the end of a twenty-foot rope only helps people up to twenty feet away. A lot of privilege and a bit of luck help you get hold of this floatation device. As for the people who drown, well, they just couldn't be saved.

Endometriosis patients are already disadvantaged by the fact that we have a feminized chronic illness in a misogynistic world. All the other things that compromise our ability to get fair treatment are an undertow, dragging us further into the ocean. "What's that saying? We're all in the same storm, but we're not in the same ship?" Heather Guidone asks me.[245] She's been a patient advocate for thirty years and works as the program director of Center for Endometriosis Care, the Atlanta, Georgia, home base of renowned surgeons Dr. Ken Sinervo and Dr. Jeff Arrington.

Endo sufferers come from around the continent, and even the world, to seek care inside of this squat rectangular medical building north of downtown Atlanta. More often than not, they arrive at their wits' end and a lot sicker than they need to be. Guidone tells me these patients regularly need four or five hours of surgical excision work because of how extensive their disease has become after years of neglect. Many have been forced out of jobs or school. They've usually tried hormonal birth control and other hormone-suppressing medications, only to find they delivered more harm than good. "The average person [coming] through our doors has had at least two hormonal therapies and two surgeries," she says. Now they're at the point of despondency, almost afraid to ask for help one more time because they've been burned so many times previously. Guidone tells me it's gut-wrenching.

"I don't want to say it's a travesty of women's health because I want to be inclusive in that messaging, but there's definitely a gender component," she tells me. She routinely meets patients whose primary care providers have spent years ignoring or trivializing their feelings and concerns about their disease and how it's affecting their lives. Guidone and I joke sarcastically about what those doctors must tell patients: "So what if you can't have pleasurable sex? I don't care," she mocks. "That's not your lot in life. You're not supposed to be feeling good about it; you're supposed to have a baby and shut your mouth."

Discrimination can be this painfully obvious. Often, though, it's small acts of laziness or slips of coded language that pile up over time, Donna tells me. "I think sometimes when we think about discrimination, we think about these big overt acts where you were made to feel small. And I don't think that that is often what discrimination [in healthcare] looks like. It *can* be those big things, but I think you can still get a base level of care that's not great, but it's not terrible," she explains.

"And so it's not necessarily that, you know, someone called me a name or said, 'You're too fat or you're too Black' or whatever. It's that when you have a system where doctors inherently feel that they are doing right just by being doctors, [they tend to say], 'Okay, I'm going to treat you for what I see,' as opposed to listening to what you say," continues Donna.

I ask her why she thinks she got such subpar care for so long. Was it obvious to her that she was being discriminated against? And if it wasn't overt, how could she tell?

"I didn't realize that the level of care I was getting was basic and just ho-hum until I [got my current doctor] and I realized what good care looks like," she answers. "It's not to say that all the other doctors before were mean or harsh—but they were just doing the minimum. And I think the only reason I was able to get resolution in a place where I'm happy now is because my doctor had empathy; she asked the right questions, and it turns out that she had the exact same experience with the exact same condition." Because the doctor understood what Donna was experiencing, she was able to refer her to the same professionals she had personally seen to help address her own pain.

Most people with endometriosis (or PCOS, or other poorly understood chronic diseases) would consider that a lucky break. We know, perhaps better than anyone, that caring for women remains a radical concept in medicine. Even more radical is caring for people even if they're trans, non-binary, Black, Indigenous, disabled, fat, mentally ill, poor, queer. Even if they don't ever want kids. All of us deserve good, compassionate, individualized medical care regardless of how we move through this world and regardless of what or how we contribute to society. Presently, though, it feels like the only thing intersectional about endometriosis care is the discrimination with which it is delivered.

Aside from discrimination, people with more complex cases of endometriosis have to jump over additional hurdles to win care. I interviewed Denise (whom you met in the Oh Bondage, Up Yours! chapter) when she was forty-two. By then, she'd had multiple surgeries and had the scars to prove it. The lesion around her belly button turned out to be the size of an orange. After receiving a diagnosis of thoracic, diaphragmatic and umbilical endometriosis, she also discovered she had thymoma, a type of chest tumor that often affects people with autoimmune diseases, as well as supraventricular tachycardia, a cardiac condition that causes an abnormally fast heart rate.

With these new conditions, she joined a not-insignificant number of patients who have both thoracic endometriosis and heart and pulmonary problems. "You know when your lungs collapse during your menstrual cycle? I also have that," Denise tells me. This type of endometriosis—the kind found outside of the uterus, ovaries and fallopian tubes—is called extrapelvic, and it can cause endo lesions to grow on the cervix, vagina, vulva, skin, intestines, urinary tract, brain, eyes, lymph nodes, lungs and other locations. When the lungs routinely collapse in lockstep with menstruation, that is called catamenial pneumothorax.[246]

Wendy Bingham, founder of the American nonprofit organization Extrapelvic Not Rare, says that because disease outside of the reproductive system can masquerade as other problems, it can go undiagnosed for a very, very long time.[247] For instance, a significant number of people with endometriosis are first diagnosed as having irritable bowel syndrome (IBS), with many enduring needless colonoscopies in consequence.

Despite being cis, white and fit, Bingham personally waited thirty years to find out she had endometriosis. She is fifty-three when we speak; she was diagnosed in her mid-forties. She tells me a big part of the diagnostic delay was because she didn't always have terrible period pain or excessively heavy periods. She hadn't even heard of endometriosis until her late twenties, when she began studying anatomy at physical therapy school. It was then when Bingham had her first documented pneumothorax, or lung collapse. A colleague who himself had a history of collapsed lungs told her to keep an eye on it and see whether the pneumothorax might align with her menstrual cycle. When she thought about it, her collection of health issues *did* seem to have suspicious timing with her period, but she'd never really kept notes.

Getting more information about this possible link was next to impossible. It was the late 1990s. Even the most basic information about endometriosis couldn't be found in most libraries, and the only internet access available sounded like an exploding fax machine.

A couple years later, at thirty-two, Bingham gave birth to a son. Conventional wisdom told her she wouldn't have a period while she was nursing, but it came back just three months later. "The day before I had my cycle start, I had a big lung collapse," she tells me. "After that, I went through a couple years where every month was like that. I could be at a grocery store and know my period was gonna start because I felt it in my chest. The room would get really dark; I'd get really shaky and almost kind of lose touch with reality. And then I felt that dribbling in my chest. And when I would tell doctors that, they just were like, 'You're completely crazy.'"

In her forties, things really started to change. Moving across the country, changing jobs, changing doctors, a son with ADHD— Bingham's stressors were adding up. She was hit by extreme fatigue, and an electrocardiogram (EKG) found she had a very low resting heart rate. She'd been a runner all her life, averaging fifty miles a week, but suddenly felt she couldn't run at all anymore. She brought her symptoms to a cardiologist, who demanded to know if she thought she could run an eight-minute mile. He asked the question eight times; she said no the first seven times but changed her answer by the eighth. "I guess I can," she told the doctor. He smirked with the satisfaction of having proven her a liar.

Really, though, even the mere thought of running an eight-minute mile made Bingham exhausted. So, she got a calendar and started tracking her symptoms, pain scale and the effects on her functional abilities. After a few months, she noticed a direct correlation between her pain, her respiratory problems and her period. She was diagnosed with thoracic endometriosis three decades after the onset of her symptoms, and at forty-six was finally operated on, giving her considerable relief.

In another country and on another timeline, Denise was only just finding out about her own extrapelvic endometriosis. This wasn't purely a gynecological disease, she learned. It is a systemic, invasive disease that can travel throughout the entire body, leaving painful lesions on critical organs, nerves and other body parts far, far away from the uterus.

Even after getting a diagnosis and multiple surgeries, though, Denise is still fighting to get the severity of her endometriosis recognized. When we speak, Denise tells me her new family doctor—a white woman—started off their relationship by making Denise jump through hoops to get time off from work and by denying that her chronic hip and leg pain has anything to do with endometriosis. Instead, she insisted Denise see a chiropractor out-of-pocket. If Denise didn't go to the chiropractor, the doctor would withhold the medical notes she needed to get paid time off from work. A year after our initial interview, though, Denise says the doctor has come around and has even worked with a specialist on the paperwork she needed to get disability benefits. But she's also only provided Denise with a tightly controlled amount of naproxen, leaving her to maintain her role as a drugstore painkiller mixologist.

It's frustrating to Denise that she had to fight so hard for so long just to get a baseline amount of a drug that barely dulls her pain, when the people in her overwhelmingly white endometriosis support groups easily get narcotics like morphine and oxycodone. She can't help but wonder if her race has anything to do with it.

Medical workers are less likely to take the pain of Black people seriously and prescribe them painkillers—even if they show up to the ER with bone fractures.[248] This medical discrimination exists across all ages among Black people; even Black children with appendicitis are left unmedicated in far bigger numbers than white kids.[249] Black women, and particularly low-income Black women, are less likely to have their pain believed and treated than white women of any socio-economic status.[250] If they do receive painkillers, they often receive lower doses, fewer pills and no refills.[251] It's so obviously discriminatory that a number of comedians have joked that Black people were saved from the opioid crisis because doctors wouldn't prescribe them OxyContin or other narcotics.[252] Though many Black Americans still report difficulty getting pain management in recent years, more have been dying from opioid overdoses since the 2010 passage of the Affordable Care Act (Obamacare).[253] Research from Yale University highlights that previous low rates of opioid use in Black communities were at least partly because of the exclusion of Black people from health insurance and healthcare.[254] Still, despite better access to medical services, Black Americans remain less likely than white people to be insured. Hispanic Americans are even less likely.[255]

Meanwhile, an endo-related distinction among Black patients (as well as Indigenous patients) is that they are more likely to get an abdominal hysterectomy, even when they qualify for a minimally invasive one. The abdominal surgery leaves large scars, is more painful and has longer recovery times.[256, 257, 258, 259]

As for Denise, she doesn't even *want* opioids. She just wants to be believed when she says she's in abject agony. She's learned to circumvent her GP as much as possible to limit the amount of gaslighting in her life. "My gynecologist is my go-to person, but my GP should be more understanding," she says.

When I ask Denise how she feels about the ways she's been treated, she takes a deep breath and sighs. She considers herself a positive, upbeat person, and she shows up to most of her doctors' appointments put together in professional work attire and a full face of makeup. She wonders if the way she looks and talks conveys to them that she isn't suffering—that if she isn't crying and wearing stained jogging pants, that she is somehow in less pain than she says she is. And so she feels she needs to communicate more assertively to her doctors, but she's still figuring out how to do it without stepping out of sick-role bounds. When we first speak, she tells me she's thinking of writing her doctor a letter to ask why she won't prescribe more naproxen. What she really wants to do, though, is ask her point-blank: "How do you see me? What is it about me that portrays a person who is not ill?"

When we touch base a year later, she still hasn't sent the letter. She's just been so distracted by and overwhelmed with managing her day-to-day health problems, that it's been tough thinking about the bigger picture.

She still plans to write it.

◆

In medicine, what we look like matters a lot, especially when it comes to chronic pain conditions.

Unlike other health problems that can be detected in blood, urine and through radiology, pain is invisible. That means doctors have to rely on the patient's interpretation of their symptoms—something that study after study shows many healthcare practitioners are not willing to do. This has been described by academics as epistemic injustice; in medicine, it happens when a patient's knowledge and understanding of their condition is not considered credible because of their practitioners' prejudices.[260] "If the stereotype is to think women are more expressive than men, perhaps 'overly' expressive, then the tendency will be to discount women's pain behaviors," noted researcher Elizabeth Losin in a media release about her paper on gender bias and pain.[261, 262] "The flip side of this stereotype is that men are perceived to be stoic, so when a man makes an intense pain facial expression, you think, 'Oh my, he must be dying!'"

Trans people have long been vulnerable to epistemic injustice. Throughout the 1960s, '70s and '80s, people who wanted hormones or surgery to help them transition had to follow a very specific script to qualify for care. For example, a trans woman would have to dress up as a woman to her doctor's appointment and tell the physician she was attracted to men. Patients also needed to say they hated their bodies. If they didn't comply to these rules, they'd usually be denied gender-affirming care.[263] "This kind of testimonial injustice was supported by the interaction of anti-trans prejudice with mental health stigma: the positioning of trans people as by definition experiencing a psychiatric disorder—'gender identity disorder'—made them vulnerable to having their reports of their own experience dismissed on the spurious grounds that mental health problems made them unreliable or even deceptive," write Miranda Fricker and Katharine Jenkins in 2017's *The Routledge Companion to Feminist Philosophy*.[264] For trans people, this type of epistemic injustice remains firmly rooted in healthcare, in and outside of the search for gender-affirming care.

Essentially, in a society that overwhelmingly regards cis men's versions of events as definitive truths, conventional wisdom dictates that anything less compelling than their knowledge must be taken with a grain of salt.

Take a small study published in 2016 in the authoritative journal *Pain* that showed disheartening results about the relationship between sex, pain and doctors' judgments.[265] One group of thirty-four pain clinicians and another group of twenty-nine medical students were given twelve fake letters from GPs asking for their opinions on treatment for their chronic pain "patients." The letters were accompanied by twelve videos of the fake patients, six of whom were male and six of whom were female. Each video was five to ten seconds long—just long enough to make a first visual impression.

After seeing each video, the clinicians and med students were asked to rate whether the person in the video was exaggerating or minimizing their pain, and whether they would prescribe each patient opioids, analgesics or antidepressants. As you may have guessed, participants assumed males had more pain than females, that females had lower pain tolerances and that females were both more likely to exaggerate their pain and less likely to hide it. Regardless of their pain estimates, even females who described enormous pain were less likely to be prescribed any painkillers, opioid or otherwise.

In addition to all this, the clinicians and students had to categorize who they thought was trustworthy and who wasn't, and how trustworthiness would affect their course of treatment. Low-trust females, but not low-trust males, were disadvantaged on every question put to the participants. Meanwhile, all categories of females were deemed less trustworthy than low-trust males. The authors of the paper noted that the way patients dressed and looked had a lot to do with whether they were perceived as trustworthy. This tracks with individuals' stories, and reams of empirical evidence, that the way you look affects the care you receive, especially when you present as female or as having "female problems."[266, 267, 268, 269] If you have pink hair, a nose ring or shabby clothes, you are just looking for drugs. On the other hand, a reasonably attractive and put-together person may also have their pain disbelieved, because you can't be dying if you remembered to put on mascara. Becoming a trustworthy patient therefore becomes an exercise in finding a middle ground that most appeals to doctors: not too grungy, but not too fancy. Ideally white and thin.

Complementary research has observed similar conundrums. A 2016 experiment published in *Pain Medicine* showed stigmas regarding patients' ethnicity, chronic pain and history of drug use made doctors less likely to believe and trust their testimonies.[270] A 2017 *Journal of Bioethical Inquiry* paper charged that when doctors ignore the lived experiences of chronic pain sufferers, the overarching message becomes that whatever the patient has to contribute to their diagnosis and care is not nearly as valuable as the doctor's perspective—a dynamic that completely erodes trust in healthcare.[271, 272]

These studies are part of an overwhelming body of research, from various researchers in various journals around the world, that establishes that women are systematically disadvantaged and criticized[273] when it comes to having their chronic pain understood, respected and treated. Researcher after researcher after researcher has found what women know to be true: that our pain is not taken seriously, sometimes to the extent that we're accused of exaggerating or even outright lying. There is so much evidence of this, and yet the issue is still treated as a conspiracy theory within medicine. The fact of the matter is that women are too often sent to the psychologist's office, while men get sent home with painkillers.[274, 275] And if we do get medications to help manage our pain, we often receive less-effective treatments or smaller doses than men would. This phenomenon has been described as a paradox and an "expression for hegemonic masculinity and andronormativity in healthcare"[276]—or, in simpler terms, as a system that believes cis male experiences and values are the norm, and which treats all female experiences as less awful than those of males.

And, recent research out of the University of Alabama at Birmingham indicates that cis and trans women experience similar levels of chronic pain, that their pain is greater than that of cis men, and that trans women may be even more sensitive to certain types of pain than cis women.[277]

Our pain starts being downgraded when we are young and naive, and intensifies the more marginalized we are and the further we stray from the cis-masculine norm. This has become so pervasive within healthcare that it is an invisible pillar of the system. Most practitioners would deny they were guilty of such discrimination. Beyond medicine, our society as a collective likes to believe we are born without bias and that discrimination is an intentional act some people choose to perform. Instead, bias lives inside of us all. While it's true that not all biases are harmful, pretending they don't exist at all only compounds discrimination. Unfortunately, the medical system has world-class expertise in denial and gaslighting—meaning it has a special proficiency in being discriminatory while saying it's not.

Almost nobody outside the boundaries of the "normal" patient gets a pass when it comes to medical discrimination. Take, for instance, fat people.

Weight stigma has deadly consequences, and so many stories exist of people dying from a range of illnesses that went undiagnosed and untreated because of their weight.[278] "There is not a single patient with significant obesity who has not experienced weight bias, whether it's comments from doctors or nurses, the way waiting rooms are set up, or privacy issues," said Dr. Yoni Freedhoff, a Canadian obesity specialist, in a 2019 article in the *Journal of the American Medical Association*.[279] "Weight bias is ubiquitous in society as a whole. Doctors are part of society."

When I ask Beth Allan, a thirty-nine-year-old white cis woman with undiagnosed PCOS, how she's experienced medical discrimination, she identifies weight stigma immediately: "My experience has been that doctors are very firmly focused on my body size, and are often not willing to have any conversations about anything until my body is not the size that it is."[280] Between her parents and the medical system, Allan has always been under pressure to lose weight—never mind that PCOS makes it extremely difficult for people to lose weight in the first place.

When Allan did begin exercising, she did it nine times a week for two to four hours at a time. She also developed an extremely restrictive diet that she calls "big time disordered eating and exercise anorexia stuff." She did ultimately lose fifty pounds, but even then, her doctor would only treat exercise-related injuries, offering things like cortisol shots to keep Allan at the gym "because I wasn't in a small enough body."

As for her suspected PCOS, her doctor's solutions have been "lose weight, stop eating carbs, try the birth control pill, take an SSRI [antidepressant]. That's it," she tells me. After Allan regained the weight she'd lost, her doctor told her she would only consider pursuing a PCOS diagnosis if Allan joined a weight management clinic.

Fatness is a wedge that divides patients and practitioners because it is seen as a personal failure to control oneself, and self-control is used as a metric by which to measure worthiness of care.

In Ted Combs's case, though, fatness was the key to affirming his gender and sexuality.[281] For many years, Combs was grateful that his PCOS meant that his periods came few and far between. He grew up in a religious rural Midwest community that he says was 100 percent white until his early teens. Although Combs, who is also white, didn't know he was trans or pansexual (attracted to people regardless of gender) until going off to college, he always knew he was different in a town that didn't like difference. His home state also has long-standing conscientious objector laws, which allow medical professionals to decline services to which they are morally opposed, including gender-affirming care for trans people. (In some areas, doctors even refuse to perform basic healthcare if it involves trans patients.)

When we speak, Combs is thirty-nine. Twenty years ago, he was diagnosed with PCOS. Shortly after that, he learned that being overweight helped him reduce his risk of pregnancy—assuming he was fertile, of course; 70 to 80 percent of people with PCOS are not.[282] Unfortunately, doctors really liked to tell Combs to lose weight, a thought that terrified him. "Every time I'd start losing weight, I would get maybe ten pounds down and panic. Then I'd stop and maybe gain like five pounds of it back," he tells me. Many doctors—and, let's face it, many people in broader society—believe that if our lives don't singularly revolve around losing weight, we simply don't care about our health at all. Imagine what they'd think of *intentionally* regaining weight?

Combs's experience with discrimination primarily finds itself at the intersection of fatphobia, misogyny and transphobia, although he wasn't out as trans for most of his PCOS journey. When he finally realized he was trans later in life, it was at a time when health insurance regimes in the United States excluded gender-affirming care.

Combs desperately wanted a hysterectomy to end his PCOS suffering, but was sensitive to the optics, and didn't want to give the state any reason to say no. He didn't want to give the state any reason to say no. "If things were coded as a medically necessary hysterectomy but they knew you were female-to-male trans, a lot of the insurance companies were known to say, 'Oh, no, this is actually a transition-related thing and you're just coding as medical,' and then deny it," Combs tells me. (A nondiscrimination provision was enacted in 2016 prohibiting trans discrimination in the Affordable Care Act, then got rolled back under Trump, then got reinstated under Biden.[283, 284])

Around the age of thirty-five—after having a *two-year* long period—Combs finally asked for the hysterectomy. The gynecologist laughed in his face. "He said, 'We don't do that on healthy women your age,'" Combs recalls. He couldn't believe the doctor's reaction. Instead of a hysterectomy, he got sent for a dilation and curettage (D&C) to scrape out the impossibly thick endometrium that had caused him to bleed for most of the past two years. He was frustrated by his lack of options. "We actively stated we do not want children. And you're doing a D&C to end a two-year period! How the fuck is that normal?"

By then Combs was severely anemic from constant blood loss, for which the doctor prescribed a double dose of iron and birth control, which made Combs feel sicker. "[After] I had the D&C, within a week or something I was already having a period again. It was so bad I didn't really want to leave the apartment because I was afraid I'd flood over," says Combs. That period also stretched on for two years. On top of that, the birth control pill he was taking made him completely miserable. "I was curled on the sofa and crying, like, 'I don't know how much longer I can do this.' And my spouse was like, 'You're done [with] that med.' We felt like I was taking poison. It was drastically having major negative effects on my mental health."

Combs moved to another state to do his PhD, and everything changed. His student insurance from the university had trans-inclusive coverage. Although Combs needed the surgery because of pain and blood loss, having trans-inclusive insurance meant fewer chances of having the procedure denied. The school year began in September; he saw a doctor in October and had the hysterectomy in December.

I ask Combs how he feels looking back at everything he's been through. "In some ways, it's kind of vindication—'See? I told you it was medically necessary to have a hysterectomy!' I didn't tell that to the doctor, but it was more of a 'I knew I was right. I knew I needed this,'" he replies, referring to the doctors who'd denied his hysterectomy requests. It's a bittersweet victory, in some respects. In the year since we first spoke, Combs discovered the extreme anemia he experienced may have contributed to current cardiac issues.

What does he want people in the medical system to learn from his experience?

"Listen to people when they tell you something's going on with their body and what they need, because people know their bodies."

For people who are systemically denied bodily autonomy in one way or another—abortion, gender-affirming care, voluntarily sterilization and so on—it's tragically common to be treated as a know-nothing, even about your own body. For Combs, being trans meant he was subjected to transphobia (on top of misogyny and fatphobia) when seeking care for his PCOS—a reality that made seeing some doctors a dysphoric experience. "The presence of external female characteristics [like breasts], that was fine with me. But the internal functioning—having a period and having a feminine disease—was an issue when it came to dysphoria," he says.

It's not unusual: having a female-coded disease can be a major source of stress in trans and non-binary people, not only because of the biological organs and processes involved, but because of the one-track mind so many doctors have when it comes to treating feminized health problems. As one person told CBC News in 2021, "Sometimes it's exhausting having to explain to everyone and having to educate everyone, not only on gender but also on endometriosis, especially since it's a super-gendered disease. It's like a double battle."[285]

◆

History feels so long, but the study of gynecology reminds us that just two hundred years ago, doctors used bloodletting and opium douches to ease painful menstruation. Less time has passed between today and Abraham Lincoln's 1863 Emancipation Proclamation than the entire duration of American slavery.

Some aspects of the science and technology used in gynecology have improved with time. We have vaccines for the most common strains of human papillomavirus (HPV), which is a major cause of cervical cancer. We can be screened with regular Pap smears, also to prevent cervical cancer. We have ultrasounds, minimally invasive robotic surgery and even lasers that can rejuvenate tired vaginas.

Yet medicine also relies on old inventions like forceps and speculums to perform some of the most routine gynecological care. In an *Atlantic* article about the speculum's lack of reinvention,[286] journalist Rose Eveleth notes that the speculum used today is almost identical to the one developed in the mid-1800s, by James Marion Sims. "As you can imagine, the female anatomy hasn't changed that much," a product manager for a medical device company told Eveleth.

That may be true—but consider why the device was invented: to help Sims more easily perform exams and experimental surgeries on enslaved Black women, whom he did not anesthetize. Did he *really* care about their medical experience or their pain? That medicine still uses the speculum—a device so many vagina owners have come to loathe[287]—when a number of studies and pilot programs[288] have shown Pap smears can be done without them and could even potentially be DIY'd at home,[289] is evidence that established medicine still doesn't care enough about the patient experience to do better. If we unroll that idea further, we can more easily see that perhaps we haven't really changed our ideas about who deserves kind, compassionate, accessible care and who doesn't. A U.S.-based study published in the peer-reviewed *Journal of Community Health*[290] showed that cost, anxiety, fear of finding cancer and anticipation of pain were major barriers to booking Paps—factors that were prevalent among Hispanic and Black study participants, two groups with the highest likelihood of developing and dying from cervical cancer.[291, 292] An American LGBTQ+ healthcare organization also found that only 27 percent of trans men got Paps, compared to 43 percent of cis women—an issue frequently caused by being un- or under-insured and by the potentially dysphoric element of gynecological exams.[293]

Like the speculum, the moral and social dimensions of gynecology have not progressed nearly as quickly as many patients—and some practitioners—would like.

◆

Today's society is a little better versed about discrimination than we were even ten years ago. The Black Lives Matter movement has crossed the threshold between counterculture and the mainstream, shedding light on the harms that Black people have endured throughout history. #MeToo opened our eyes to the sexual violence that permeates female, trans and non-binary experiences. The LGBTQ+ rights movement has gained incremental ground on equality and human rights. It feels like people are more aware of systemic injustice than ever before, especially when it involves the judicial system.

Discrimination inside medicine is less well known. Despite a bestselling book and biopic about her, not everyone knows about Henrietta Lacks, a poor Black woman from Baltimore who in 1951 unknowingly had cells taken from her as she lay dying from cervical cancer at Johns Hopkins Hospital.[294] Those cells, known as HeLa, have since been commercialized well into the billions of dollars and have been on the frontiers of medicine, used in the development of the polio and HPV vaccines,[295] as well as in AIDS,[296] cancer and COVID-19 research, among other scientific pursuits. Her cells were even shot into space.[297] There are more than 100,000 papers in the National Library of Medicine featuring work involving HeLa cells, and those cells have generated billions in pharmaceutical profits with no compensation as of yet given to the Lacks family. Only since 2013 do researchers have to acknowledge the family in their publications.[298]

And not everyone knows about the Tuskegee syphilis study,[299] a forty-year-long experiment in the American South that deceptively recruited Black men by bribing them with meals, free medical exams and burial insurance in order to study the effects of untreated syphilis. Even after it was discovered that penicillin cured the STI, the drug was withheld from the 399 syphilitic men in the study.

It should be well known that somewhere in the range of 70,000 and 200,000[300]—and possibly more—Black, Hispanic, Indigenous, poor and disabled people have been forcibly sterilized throughout history in the U.S. alone and that as recently as 2020, women held in U.S. migrant detention centers reported forced sterilization.[301] More people should know that some countries demand that trans people get sterilized in order to have their gender identities legally recognized.[302]

A documentary called *Belly of the Beast*[303] reports that between 1997 and 2013, more than 1,400 female prisoners in California were sterilized.[304] (In 2014, a ban on using sterilization as prisoner birth control was passed by the state, although rumors abound that the practice persists.[305]) Most people probably don't know that right now, menstruation is being used to gain control over the bodies of youth and adults with intellectual and physical disabilities. Stopping disabled individuals from having their periods and/or being able to reproduce by coercively sterilizing them or giving them contraception is currently legal by caregiver request in a number of places, including most U.S. states.[306, 307]

All of these programs are instances of state-sanctioned medical violence against people of color and people with disabilities, with women and gender-diverse people bearing the oversized burden of the violence. Worse, they're just the tip of the iceberg. Around the world, untold numbers of people have been violated by state- and institution-run programs designed to compromise people's health and reproductive freedoms. And these aren't purely historical harms. It continues to this day.

When it comes to endometriosis, the experiences of people of color are vastly understudied in medicine and science. One rare paper on the subject, co-written by Dr. Olga Bougie whom we met earlier, points out that because the main symptom of the disease is pelvic pain, and because endometriosis and its treatment are so heavily influenced by psychosocial factors, people from non-white ethnic and cultural backgrounds likely have different clinical presentations than white people.[308] "Race affects provision of healthcare at all levels and, in the case of endometriosis, likely influences access to care, specialist referral, diagnosis and treatment offered," writes Bougie and her fellow researchers. The most likely consequence of this is that endometriosis is vastly underdiagnosed and undertreated in Black women, and probably other women of color too.

◆

The physician's assistant asked Kellyn Pollard five or six times whether she wanted an STI test. Pollard was already on the exam table, and the PA's fingers were already inside her when she asked, then asked, then asked again. Pollard declined each time, saying there was no need, and besides she already had so much pelvic pain that she really didn't feel like having her cervix jabbed with a bunch of extra-long Q-tips. But the PA kept insisting: "Are you sure you don't want that? Are you sure? Because, I mean, it kind of seems like you need it."[309]

Pollard refused again.

"Okay, well, we're going to do it anyway."

Pollard is twenty-seven when we speak. I found her through an article she wrote about her endometriosis journey for the *Black Wall Street Times*, an independent news publication named after the affluent Black Oklahoman neighborhood of Greenwood—dubbed Black Wall Street—which was destroyed by white rioters in the 1921 Tulsa Race Massacre.[310] Pollard is from Oklahoma but several years ago moved to Texas, where she works in clinical research administration. The article she wrote is entitled "Am I Crazy?: A Black Woman's Journey with Endometriosis."[311]

Pollard has asked herself that very question many, many times in the seventeen years she's had endometriosis symptoms.

The day that she found herself on the exam table, the PA had a medical student with her. Poking at Pollard's IUD strings, she explained to the student that "they can be hard to find in people like her." *People like her?* What did that mean, Pollard wondered, squinting into the light above the exam table. "I just felt like a specimen, not a patient. The way she was talking about things while she was down there, making it sound like what I had was different than any other woman," she tells me. "That was one of those moments, like, 'Am I crazy? Am I tripping? Or is this really happening to me?'"

Pollard's endometriosis symptoms began as soon as her period did, at the age of ten. Migraines came on so intensely she would vomit, and she bled so heavily she routinely left in the middle of class to change her pad and tampon. At twelve, her pediatrician put her on birth control—first the regular three-weeks-on, one-week-off kind, then a pill marketed as giving its users "seasonal" periods once every three months. It did lighten her periods, but she still got them every month. Still, she figured it was better than suffering the full force of her period.

She spent the next eight years trying out different birth control pills, looking for that elusive, magical one that would make her pain-free. By twenty, though, massive clots in her period blood told her something bigger was happening to her. A few months later, she went under the knife. When her eyes snapped open in the recovery room, the first thing she could think was "My uterus is on fire." The anesthetic had worn off after her first laparoscopy, leaving her with a belly full of flames. She'd had an ablation, the nurse told her; the surgeon had burned off some lesions but had mostly left her extensive scar tissue intact. Oh, and she also had stage two endometriosis, they informed her. She was sent home with a script for a narcotic to manage the postoperative pain.

She bled for four months straight. Not long after, she moved to Texas.

By the time she got a gynecologist in her new town, she'd developed burns on her stomach, thighs and back from overusing heating pads, their warmth sometimes the only relief of the day. In Texas, a second surgery excised some lesions but not all. Pollard was disappointed when her pain persisted. She then sought out an endo specialist recommended by a friend, but he didn't help either. "That is the doctor who, despite my two laparoscopies and all of my doctor's notes, was like, 'You don't have endo; it's in your head. I'll prescribe you Lyrica, and then we need to put you on another antidepressant and probably change your birth control.' And that was it. No examination from him, nothing. [The experience] was sitting in his office while he basically told me I was crazy," Pollard recounts.

She left his office dejected, with no plans to take the drugs he prescribed, let alone ever see him again. Why waste her time and money on another dead end? Plus, she *knew* she wasn't crazy. "No. I'm not sick in my head. I'm sick in my uterus," she remembers saying to herself.

Still, gaslighting has a very tricky way of seeping into the mind. As her pain persisted, she began wondering if maybe focusing on it *was* making her suffering worse. Maybe it really was phantom pain? Maybe she *did* need to have her brain chemistry altered.

"It kind of reversed all the progress I had made in those three-ish years; acceptance, getting a diagnosis, trying to make headway and making a management plan—all of that to just be thrown out the window," says Pollard.

Unlike Denise, Pollard *was* prescribed opioids. Every time she turned up at the ER in agony, doctors assumed she wanted oxycodone, hydrocodone, morphine or codeine, and they obliged without doing anything more to investigate her pain. But Pollard already used an opioid medication, Tramadol, as her everyday pain management drug. What she really wanted was answers: why was she in so much pain, and who was going to help her?

She's still waiting. Although a third laparoscopic procedure in 2018 "cleaned her out," she still often finds herself in agony. When we speak in 2021, she's on a break from a newer drug called Orilissa meant to reduce endometriosis pain. (More on Orilissa later.) The downside is the relief it can provide is fleeting; Orilissa is only supposed to be taken for twenty-four months over the course of a person's entire life because it can cause irreversible bone loss. Pollard later clarifies in an email that she and her doctor decided to continue using the lower dose of Orilissa for another year after the initial twenty-four months, because it was the only thing that really helped her pain. (She did blood work first and will have a bone density scan done after the year is up to make sure they haven't turned to dust.)

Before going back on the bonus round of Orilissa, Pollard was taking gabapentin for nerve pain, plus oral birth control at the same time that she had a Mirena IUD. After restarting the Orilissa, she cut out the oral birth control. These combinations of drugs are, by her doctor's own admission, a bit of a crapshoot. Her doctor recently told her, "I don't think you'll get worse, but you're not going to get better."

When she tells me that, I am both surprised at the doctor's frankness and devastated for Pollard. At twenty-seven, she was told her condition may never improve. I ask her how it felt to be told such a thing.

"That was really hard to hear," she answers.

Pollard doesn't know exactly what the future of her endometriosis looks like, but she knows the enormous price she's already paid. Between massive medical costs, damaged relationships and the time she's spent begging the medical system to care about her, Pollard's losses are already overwhelming.

5. NERVOUS BREAKDOWN
the great birth control swindle

On an early summer day in 2019, the eve of a vacation to Canada's Maritimes, with the warm air and golden sunshine brushing against my cheeks as I biked, I thought about veering into traffic.

It wasn't the first time I'd ever thought about it. It wasn't even the first time I'd thought about it that June. A week earlier, I'd accompanied my boyfriend to a lake in a nearby conservation park so he could go standup paddleboarding. I intended to lay out a blanket and rest on the sandy beach, but the shallow water and nearby picnic tables were filled with families and shrieking children. I was overcome by anxiety. This beach had too many people, too many children, too many witnesses to a potential panic attack. I took off for the woods.

I quickly found a secluded path I could have all to myself. A perfect aloneness. The further I walked, the more the screams of children splashing in the water became muffled by thick vegetation. Tall green sugar maples, American beeches and eastern hemlocks enveloped me in a vivid green canopy, creating a blanket of silence broken only by the creaking of the forest and the occasional twig snapping underfoot. Alone on the trail, I began humming an upbeat Ramones-y rhythm to keep my swirling thoughts company.

A lyric materialized in my imagination, so I opened my phone's recording app—the same one I sometimes used to record interviews. I warbled into the mic:

I don't care if the bears attack
I don't care if I'm hit by a truck
I don't care if I fall off a bridge
I don't, I don't, I don't
I don't care

This morbid tune was pretty catchy and I was impressed by my creation. I decided to sing it to my boyfriend when he returned from paddleboarding.

He was not amused.

I was struggling hard through an intensely busy month, balancing a trip to New York City with one of my closest friends to see Bikini Kill, getting laser tattoo removal in Montreal, attending a friend's birthday dinner, interviewing a variety of people and writing freelance articles, attending spin class a couple of times a week and hitting the gym in between.

To an outside observer, life looked pretty normal—privileged, even. Instead of curling up in bed and staying there all summer, I carried on with my busy, productive life out of fear of acknowledging how sick I really was. Overworking has been my go-to coping mechanism since I was a teen, first as a way of escaping my household, then as a way of escaping my body.

But really, I'd been dead inside for weeks. However quiet I seemed on the surface, my mind was a storm of anxiety and my mood weighed down everyone around me. I felt broken beyond repair, maybe more broken than I'd ever felt. This bout had come on suddenly, like a switch had been flipped: one day I felt okay, and the next I wanted to jump off a bridge. Nothing in my life had really changed . . . except that IUD I'd had inserted less than two months earlier.

In 1970, Illinois physician Dr. Herbert Ratner testified at U.S. Senate hearings to evaluate the reported harms of hormonal contraceptives. The doctor told the story of a woman who had started having suicidal ideas after going on the pill—the first time she'd ever entertained such thoughts.[312] She told her husband, a pharmacist, how she felt. "He assured her that this could not be so because such complaints were not included in the list of side effects on the package insert which accompanied the medication," Ratner recounted. That woman eventually went off the medication, and her suicidal ideation vanished shortly thereafter. At the same hearings, psychiatrist Dr. Francis Kane told the panel about his study in which 139 private patients without any history of psychiatric care were asked how the pill made them feel. Ten percent said they felt great. Meanwhile, a whopping 64 percent said they felt different from their pre-pill selves, and 34 percent of them said they were depressed.[313]

These were some of the earliest public mentions of a seemingly causal relationship between the pill and depression. Fifty-three years later, the psychiatric side effects are still being debated. Just a few years ago, a study done at Northwestern University's department of medicine in Chicago unequivocally stated that hormonal contraceptives do *not* cause depression.[314] "When you review the entirety of the literature and ask, 'Do hormonal contraceptives cause depression?,' the answer is definitely no," Dr. Katherine Wisner, one of the paper's authors, told the university blog.[315] In 2021, a study based on Swedish health registry data said more or less the same thing.[316] (Interestingly, that Northwestern study also notes that 60 percent of medical residents reported having no training in prescribing contraceptives for people with "severe and persistent mental illness.")

Plenty of studies and first-person accounts say the opposite. For instance, a one-million-person population study done in Denmark and published in 2016 in *JAMA Psychiatry* concluded that people using hormonal contraception have a 70 percent higher risk of depression than those who've never used it.[317]

And then there was what I knew from my own experience.

Around 2016, I started seeing my first gynecologist. She worked one day a week at a hospital pain clinic, and I'd enrolled there just to see her. From our very first meeting, she seemed convinced an IUD would solve my pain and bleeding.

The idea of an IUD put me on edge; I'd gone off the pill eight years earlier because of the mental health effects it had on me. That last pill I tried gave me the wildest of mood swings without any rhyme or reason. One minute I'd be smiling and joking, and the next I'd be in tears. Sure, it helped lighten the bleeding and took the edge off the pain—but it also made me anxious as hell. I didn't think that it was fair that I should have to pay for that relief with my mental health.

I also couldn't shake the feeling that the pill had somehow erased part of my personality, or that it had compromised my ability to enjoy my life. I'd been on it since I was fourteen. I'd graduated from high school and university while on the pill. My first jobs, first romantic relationships, first tattoos, first solo international trips—all these monumental life moments had been colored by birth control and its effects on my body and mind. I began questioning whether I was meant to be a depressed, anxious mess, or if it was the pill making me that way.

My mind settled when I stopped using hormonal birth control at twenty-six. My emotional peaks didn't feel so precipitous, and the valleys didn't feel so bottomless. In that first year after going off the pill, I started feeling better about myself and better about being alive.

Then my period returned with a vengeance. It was seven to nine days of bleeding and cramps, sometimes so intense I felt like I was either being stabbed in the guts, or having my uterus and intestines twisted into balloon animals. Going to the bathroom, getting on a bicycle or even sitting in a wooden chair sometimes nearly made me faint from shooting pains.

The first time the gynecologist mentioned the IUD, I shrugged it off. The second time, I told her about my mental health concerns and said I'd think about it. The third time she brought it up, I mentioned the Danish study[318] and how people were more likely to be depressed with an IUD than with other forms of birth control. Couldn't I just get a hysterectomy instead?

No, she answered. She wouldn't even consider surgery until I'd tried the IUD. I had nothing to worry about, she told me; the IUD only secreted hormones locally, meaning they'd only hang out in my uterus and nowhere else. She wrote out a prescription for one and slid it across the desk. "It's up to you," she said.

Was it, though?

I felt trapped: getting a hormonal device implanted inside me threatened all my mental progress—but so did the excruciating pain.

Medical literature dating back to the ancient Greeks has suggested some people experience menstrual cramps as painful, or sometimes even more painful, than labor. By that logic, I was having at least twelve babies a year. Worse, all of this was preceded by a week of intense PMS that often left me completely exhausted, soaked in a puddle of inexplicable sadness and struggling to locate my thoughts in a haze of mental fog. I felt awful for at least two weeks of every single month, and I spent the other two weeks of the month rushing to catch up on everything I'd let lapse. Then the cycle started all over again.

Heather Guidone of Atlanta's Center for Endometriosis Care sees the push toward pharmaceuticals and away from surgery every day.[319] "There's this marked shift away from specialty surgery and multidisciplinary care and more of this heavy pharma-dominated push [in our branch of medicine]," she says. That's not to say no one is helped by medication; for some people, birth control and other hormone modifiers can be lifesaving. It's more about the portrayal that these drugs are benign, or at least that their side effects are a sacrifice people have to make in order to receive care. "What it's being presented as is sort of like the emperor's new clothes," says Guidone, cribbing a line from her colleague Dr. Jeff Arrington. "'Well, you don't need surgery for diagnosis or treatment; you can just take this pill or this injection that's gonna ruin your bone mineral density, probably destroy your liver, gonna make you suicidal, probably screw up your hormones for good long time and kind of make you feel like shit.'

"That's very scary to me, because now you're taking options away. That's not informed consent. You cannot keep some treatments from a patient because of your preference or your priority."

It felt like an IUD was being forced on me. In the most black-and-white view of the situation, yes, I had a choice: I could say no and walk away. But if I did that, I'd lose my gynecologist and any chance I had of eventually getting the hysterectomy. Was that really consent? By then, I saw the hysterectomy as a pain elimination strategy *and* a way to divorce the medical system. If my periods kept me coming back to the doctor, then having no period at all would let me stay away.

I brought her IUD ultimatum home and tossed it on top of a pile of papers on my desk. I had to think about it. I certainly couldn't forget about it, though. That damned piece of paper tugged at my resolve every time I got my period. I even buried it under sticky notes, bills and other scraps of paper, but even with it out of sight I could feel it weighing on me. I thought about it whenever I burned my abdomen with my hot water bottle, downed more than my daily allotment of naproxen or filled my menstrual cup in less than an hour.

I was angry when I caved. I was furious at the doctor, at the IUD, at my body, at the fact that I couldn't just make myself better. Something had to give, and it felt like the easiest course of action was to acquiesce. If the IUD experience was awful, then at least we'd have an answer and could move on. And if it wasn't awful, maybe that was enough.

Either way, I'd grown physically and emotionally exhausted from the monthly gut stabbings and crimson monsoons. I needed to know if there was something for me on the other side.

◆

For most of history, women have been "hysterical."

The way we think of hysteria now—as mental suffering, specifically women's mental suffering—is often attributed to the Greeks because of the word's etymology: *hystera* meaning uterus[320] and *hysterikai* describing suffering from the womb.[321] However, health historian Sabine Arnaud set the record straight in a 2015 book wholly focused on the coining, concept and diagnosis of hysteria.[322] In fact, Arnaud writes, it was a handful of Frenchmen and a Scot in the late eighteenth and early nineteenth centuries who were mainly responsible for consolidating—and conflating—a variety of different conditions under the single pathology of hysteria. As the field of neurology developed, the men determined that hysteria had much less to do with physical ailments than with psychological ones.[323] Hysteria ultimately came to serve as a catchall for undesirable feminized traits. From the Middle Ages to the Renaissance to the Enlightenment, hysteria has been molded to incorporate many different diseases and reflected the culture of the era, though each usage shared something in common: they used hysteria to pathologize women's bodies and minds and downgrade their power—especially the power of willful, rebellious women. These shapeshifting definitions of hysteria solidified views that women were weak and frail of mind and body, and therefore deserved lower social stature and diminished agency.[324]

Hysteria has almost exclusively been used to describe women. For instance, French physician Augustin Fabre wrote in 1883, "All women are hysterical, and every woman carries with her the seeds of hysteria, because hysteria, before becoming an illness, is a temperament, and what constitutes the temperament of a woman is rudimentary hysteria."[325] Some believed men could be vulnerable to hysteria, too, though they were less likely to experience it, and those who did were commonly perceived as effeminate or homosexual. Rather, instead of hysteria, men more likely suffered from melancholy and hypochondriasis and later neurasthenia, a condition described in the book *Hysteria beyond Freud* as "the neurosis of the male elite."[326]

That Sigmund Freud, an Austrian neurologist and the creator of psychoanalysis, is the person most commonly associated with hysteria in popular culture belies the misogynistic shoulders on which he stood. Still, while he certainly didn't invent the idea, he did reorient how hysteria was perceived by the dominant culture, and that development went on to fuel a pharmacological revolution after his 1939 death.[327] Freud viewed hysteria not as a disease of the body or brain, but rather as a physical manifestation of early sexual trauma, then as the outcome of repressed sexual fantasies and the denial of self-fulfillment.[328] Though he believed people of any gender could be hysterical—a controversial idea at the turn of the twentieth century—he still thought women were the ones predominantly prone to it because they tended to be more passive in nature.[329]

Freud's thinking on hysteria as a neurophysiological disease that could be induced by trauma, and not merely womb troubles, was substantially influenced by his contemporary, French neurologist Jean-Martin Charcot. Charcot worked at Salpêtrière Hospital in Paris, originally opened in 1656 as an internment center and asylum for sex workers, feminists, the poor and other social deviants.[330] It was there where Charcot received frequent delegations of visiting doctors, researchers and other observers, including Freud in 1885—men who came to see the way patients could be hypnotized into reproducing fits of hysteria.[331] (Note that at this point, painful periods were still associated with hysteria.) Salpêtrière had a photographer on staff for this very reason. In episodes recorded on film for posterity, patients would scream and collapse into a heap on the ground or into someone's arms, their heads bobbing as they lost consciousness.[332, 333]

Freud sourced much of his early thinking on hysteria from Charcot and kept a lithograph of *A Clinical Lesson at the Salpêtrière*—the most famous painting of Charcot—in his office for decades.[334] Freud wrote prolifically on female sexuality, both on its own and in comparison to male sexuality, yet his personal views on women were disappointingly reflective of the time. For that, he has been rightfully excoriated. Second-wave feminists from Simone de Beauvoir to Germaine Greer viewed Freud's ideas on women with substantial hostility. One critique of Freud's influence on society, Eva Figes's 1970 feminist polemic *Patriarchal Attitudes*, notes, "Of all the factors that have served to perpetuate a male-orientated society, that have hindered the free development of women as human beings in the Western world today, the emergence of Freudian psychoanalysis has been the most serious."[335]

Freud remains partly responsible for the ways medicine treats women—and basically anyone who isn't a straight cis man—today. Eventually, the idea that hysteria was a psychological response that could be controlled or even cured caught on. It began with rest cures and talk cures, but those were later overruled by pharmacology—an easier, faster solution to heal the mind. As Andrea Tone writes in *The Age of Anxiety*, "Psychoanalysis had normalized neurosis as a medical disorder and set the stage for the psychopharmacological revolution that followed."[336] In a world coming to understand science as truth, the development of psychoanalysis gave new legitimacy to the pathologization of women, which in turn abetted the view of women as, essentially, defective men. The pathologization of queerness followed in similar footsteps, with people like Hungarian psychoanalyst Sandor Rado arguing that the only norm was heterosexuality and that all other orientations were phobias shaped by bad parenting (a concept also used to pathologize gender non-conformity).[337] As the founder of the U.S.'s first psychoanalysis school at Columbia University, Rado was influential in the development of psychoanalysis's anti-queer bent and its pathologization of LGBTQ+ people.[338]

In the years following Freud's death, hysteria was redefined as nervousness and psychic tension, then as anxiety and then as depression. The beginning of this evolution coincided with the return of World War II soldiers, including many with shell shock, as well as the rise of postwar capitalism and the meteoric growth of the pharmaceutical industry.[339]

Especially in North America, this confluence of factors seemed to flood mainstream culture with great malaise. In the book *Prozac on the Couch: Prescribing Gender in the Era of Wonder Drugs*, author and psychiatrist Jonathan Metzl explains how mainstream American culture struggled to find its footing amid women's growing economic and social capital—and how psychoanalysis, then psychiatric drugs, helped stall their advancement. "The conflation in psychoanalysis of individual and cultural anxiety provided a ready means for validating middle-class masculine inquietude," he writes.[340]

This helped spread the pathologization of femininity, and "by the mid-1940s, Freudian ideas were used to justify an entirely domestic femininity and to mark a woman's ambition as a symptom of mental illness."[341] That influence extended into the following decade, giving Freudian-derived psychoanalysis "near-hegemonic" power in defining anxiety, depression and other mental illnesses to Americans.[342]

Psychoanalysis alone could not cure these problems, and lobotomies and electroshock treatment were too barbaric—or so said the burgeoning pharmaceutical industry. Although barbiturates were the first class of drugs created to ease people's minds, the postwar era saw them swiftly replaced by tranquilizers and benzodiazepines, which were seen as less dangerous (but which are now recognized as highly addictive). Antipsychotic Thorazine, classified as a major tranquilizer and dubbed the "chemical lobotomy," debuted in the early 1950s as a brute-force cure for emotional problems (including homosexuality, which was then considered a crime).[343] However, it was too strong for some of the more prevalent nervous conditions, and so pharmaceutical companies developed minor tranquilizers that patients could take more liberally.[344] Miltown, the trade name of anti-anxiety drug meprobamate, became an overnight success. It was a cure for the realities of modern life, and Americans ate them up, filling one prescription per second by 1957.[345] As Tone writes, Miltown helped normalize the everyday use of psychiatric drugs, particularly by women.[346] It also, in Tone's words, "shifted the practice of frontline psychiatric diagnosis from the psychiatrist to the family doctor"[347]—a change that bestowed upon non-specialists the power to medicate anyone who behaved "abnormally."

Miltown's success led to the rapid-fire proliferation of other minor tranquilizers. Librium, manufactured by Roche, was the first benzodiazepine to enter the market.[348] It was soon followed by a slew of others. And then Valium hit in 1963,[349] blowing most competitors out of the water and entrenching psychiatric medication in the lives of everyday people living everyday lives.[350] These drugs were marketed aggressively to doctors, with ads in medical journals and sales rep visits to medical offices encouraging doctors to prescribe them more widely—including to people who displayed no obvious psychiatric symptoms at all.[351] How women came to fill twice as many tranquilizer prescriptions as men has been mythologized through pop culture, with the Rolling Stones suggesting housewives needed a "mother's little helper" to help calm them down. However, fascinating literature on this subject—including the below-quoted article by Metzl—suggests that the popularity of tranquilizers among women was a way for them to manage the rampant sexism they endured at all turns, from being returned to their domestic duties after their wartime jobs ended, to their diminished position in the nuclear family, to an overarching culture that reinforced that good females are the ones who submit to the patriarchy.

As Metzl writes, "Popular culture extolled a 'new femininity'—really an old maternity—not by a picture of a woman in rolled-up, working sleeves, but rather by a mother at home with her children. One might say [. . .] that a sudden onslaught of cultural pressure sought to return the repressed, married and out-of-work female back to the home as a mother. Magazines glorified the domestic sphere above all other pursuits. Articles told women to 'Have Babies While You're Young.' They asked women, 'Are You Training Your Daughter to Be a Wife?' And informed their readers that 'Really a Man's World Is Politics' and that life was fulfilled by 'The Business of Running a Home.'"

Metzl further argues that American mothers became the scapegoat of seemingly all social problems in the postwar era and were denigrated for adopting "non-feminine" traits like aggression, independence and power. In his estimation, they turned to prescription drugs to cope with misogyny.[352]

The real story is that in the earliest days of tranquilizers, drug companies had no reason to advocate for medicating women specifically and exclusively; their primary objective was making money by having as many people as possible use the drugs. However, they massively profited from existing biases against women. Doctors saw drug ads primarily featuring women which contained coded language about how female anxiety was abnormal and did the drug companies' dirty work for them by overprescribing to women.

A person couldn't be blamed for assuming they did this to keep women docile and compliant; we could draw some convincing links between the steep incline of Valium prescriptions during the sexual revolution and the women's liberation movement. However, this overprescribing to women wasn't necessarily a concerted effort to quash female resistance. In reality, it was more insidious than that: doctors of the era had unquestioningly inherited a medical system designed to benefit white men. That resulted in an overwhelming tendency to serve chauvinistic interests by pathologizing and psychologizing female traits and women's lived experiences. And so, even without a big evil plan to medicate women, rampant sexism made it so that was exactly what happened. As Patrick Radden Keefe details in his incredible book *Empire of Pain*,

> A typical ad for Valium read, "35, single and psycho-neurotic." An early ad for Librium showed a young woman with an armful of books and suggested that even the routine stress of heading off to college might be best addressed with Librium. But the truth was, Librium and Valium were marketed using such a variety of gendered mid-century tropes—the neurotic singleton, the frazzled housewife, the joyless career woman, the menopausal shrew—that as the historian Andrea Tone noted in her book *The Age of Anxiety*, what Roche's tranquilizers really seemed to offer was a quick fix for the problem of "being female."[353]

All this history is pertinent to endometriosis because of its eons-long association with hysteria. Even today, many physicians' views of endometriosis patients are colored by assumptions and accusations of mental illness, which often leads them to suggest and prescribe antidepressants and other psychiatric drugs, rather than pursue care for the underlying disease. The psychic ligaments stretching between pain and depression in chronic pain sufferers cannot be ignored, and yet they so often are.

Researcher after researcher has found what so many women know in their gut to be true: that we have more pain than men do and that our pain is not taken seriously, sometimes to the extent that we're told we're making it up.[354] We get sent off to the psychologist's office while men get painkillers.[355] If we do get medication to help manage our pain, we often receive less-effective treatments or smaller doses than men would.[356] In this, we can see how "hysterical women" are belittled in the healthcare system. The problem is, many female patients are still treated as hysterical to some degree—and if females are prone to hysterical exaggeration, how can we trust them to be truthful about the extent of their suffering?[357]

◆

Nancy Petersen is the founder of the massive Nancy's Nook Endometriosis Education group on Facebook, which counts more than 150,000 members worldwide. She's also a retired nurse with endometriosis who spent a number of years working with surgeon Dr. David Redwine.

Petersen, who is eighty-one when we speak, tells me endometriosis patients have almost always been considered to have some kind of mental problem.[358] "Kate Weinstein wrote a book about thirty years ago about endometriosis,[359] and her data at that time showed that 75 percent of patients had been dismissed as neurotic. She didn't sort it out by ethnic groups or origins, but it was kind of across the board," Petersen explains.

When Petersen joined Redwine in the mid-1980s to create the endometriosis treatment program in Oregon—right around the time Weinstein's book came out—she discovered a similar finding in her patient surveys. "My survey tracked Kate Weinstein's work exactly: 75 percent of our patients had been dismissed as neurotic, and, in fact, every one of them had biopsy-proven disease," Petersen notes. Even Redwine's then-wife had been written off.

"It was kind of an alarming piece of information for me: that these people who are living difficult lives struggling with peritoneal-quality pain are being told that it was a mental health issue."

It seems hysteria has been repackaged for the new age.

On a sunny April day in 2019, I plucked that piece of paper off my desk, went to the pharmacy and accepted my fate. The pharmacist handed me a box so comically large it felt like a public admonishment, as if my jacket was emblazoned with "IUD" in scarlet lettering. I hid it inside a black tote bag and headed to the sexual health clinic, where I joined the other sluts and perverts in the waiting room. Everything about the experience felt shameful. Desperate to avoid eye contact, I did what everyone else was doing: I stared at my phone until my number was called. That they didn't yell out my name was one small gift of anonymity in a clinic where everyone ends up getting their genitals touched.

Upon my summoning, I was ushered into a small windowless room. The walls were brown. The door, brown. The counter, the exam table—it was all just a rainbow of various shades of brown. And there was just so much furniture, much more than necessary. I felt confined as I dutifully sat in the corner in an old office chair squeezed between the counter and the wall. I fished my little medical notebook out of my purse and clutched it in my clammy hands. I noted how the exam table was placed right in front of the door, just like at my ultrasound a few years ago.

A few minutes later, there was a knock on the closed door. The doctor who entered was an unthreatening blond woman of whom I was completely terrified. My voice trembled as I obediently answered her questions and asked my own. I let her know I was there under duress, that I'd basically been backed into a corner and that I was desperately afraid this tiny plastic device was about to fuck up my whole universe.

In an effort to calm my nerves, she repeated what the gynecologist had told me. "The IUD only works locally in the uterus, so there shouldn't be any systemic effects," she explained, warning that insertion could be painful but mercifully quick, and that there could be some light bleeding and cramping for a few days, but after that I would be on my way to five years of being period-free. I solemnly nodded. She left the room to let me disrobe from the waist down. I took my shoes, leggings and underwear off—I had again worn a dress to remain as clothed as possible—and then sat on the table. She returned carrying a small metal tray with a speculum and some other tools and told me to lie down with my heels in the stirrups.

"Painful" was a massive understatement. As a heavily tattooed person with stage-four endometriosis who once had a stage-diver fall directly onto my face at a Dropkick Murphys concert, I thought I knew pain. But no, getting that tiny T-shaped demonic device past my cervix and into the uterus was by far the most excruciating experience of my life. Worse, the doctor narrated her difficulties. The cervix was flipped. Or maybe I had a tilted uterus. Hmm, well, something is wrong, she muttered as she wrestled to get it properly placed. Every time she moved it, I imagined it ripping holes through the walls of my uterus. It was anything but the quick procedure she promised. After breaking the IUD I brought to the clinic, she left to fetch a new one. Alone in the room, I wondered why I couldn't have just procured the IUD here, since they obviously had some in stock.

She returned with a new gigantic box and continued to poke at my cervix. All told, it was twenty solid minutes of the most nauseating, breathtaking agony. I gasped for air and gripped the edge of the table with my right hand so hard my knuckles turned white: I wondered if I would faint.

And then it was over. She left the room to let me get dressed, as if she hadn't spent the past half-hour staring directly into my vagina. In tear-soaked mourning, I put my underwear, leggings and shoes back on. My sunglasses hid my bloodshot, puffy, terror-filled eyes as I slinked out the clinic's door. At least this part is over, I told myself. Hopefully I won't have to come back to this place.

I was back six weeks later, begging for them to take it out.

The reason why birth control is so commonly prescribed to people with endometriosis is because our pain normally spikes during ovulation and menstruation. That's partly because of how tissue, adhesions and scar tissue outside the uterus cause restriction, inflammation, swelling and pain.[360] The thinking goes that if we can prevent ovulation and menstruation, patients can avoid some of the pain. But the pill doesn't only prevent these two events.

Hormonal birth control works by suppressing some hormones by increasing others. Most forms—the pill, patch, vaginal ring, injection, IUD, etc.—contain synthetic estrogen and progestin (synthetic progesterone). Some contain only progestin, since progestins are more active ovulation blockers.[361] They suppress the pituitary gland's ability to release follicle stimulating hormone (FSH) and luteinizing hormone (LH), which prevents ovulation.[362]

Synthetic estrogens are typically made from actual estrogen, while the progestins found in contraceptives are predominantly sourced from testosterone.[363] A newer progestin called drospirenone is derived from spironolactone, which is the chemical name for water pills, an ingredient in hypertensive drugs[364] and a drug used by some trans people to spur breast growth and feminization.[365]

Synthetic estrogen and progestin are meant to mimic our natural hormones by binding to the body's compatible hormone receptors. Receptors are "docking molecules" inside or on the surface target cells. When the hormone and the receptor meet, it sets off a chain reaction that causes changes to cell activity.[366] And it doesn't only affect our reproductive systems. In her book *This Is Your Brain on Birth Control*, psychologist and researcher Sarah E. Hill notes that a chief difference between natural progesterone and synthetic progestins is that the latter don't only bind to progesterone receptors.

"These testosterone molecules have been tinkered with in a way that makes them look like progesterone to your progesterone receptors [. . .] However, they're not a perfect match," Hill writes. When these testosterone-derived progestins are introduced to our bodies' hormone receptors, they don't fit the way naturally occurring progesterone would. They also bind to testosterone receptors, which can cause masculinizing effects like skin breakouts, weight gain, hair growth and even diminished verbal fluency. This imperfect binding activity, Hill continues, "means that the hormonal message delivered by the pill will be at least somewhat different from the [endogenous] hormonal message."[367] Backing up Hill's work, South African researchers remarked in the journal *Steroids* that progestins bind to multiple receptors, not only the one for progesterone; therefore, they wrote, "it is plausible that synthetic progestins exert therapeutic actions as well as side effects via some of these receptors."[368] For instance, some trans men and non-binary people may enjoy the masculinizing effects and period suppression of testosterone-derived progestin.

Progestins typically work by keeping the reproductive cycle in some version of the luteal phase—the moment in our cycles when progesterone is normally high and estrogen is low.[369] People who take the pill continuously without stopping for a week to get withdrawal bleeding[370] keep their hormones relatively stable throughout their cycles. In some of the earliest studies on the pill, this was called pseudopregnancy.[371]

Unfortunately, stability isn't always a good thing. For instance, the absence of hormone spikes can affect the biological sexual response, which explains why some people accuse the drugs of killing their libido.[372] And that's just one change we might notice when we go off the pill. Throughout her book, Hill argues that going off the pill makes us feel as though we're exiting emotional hibernation.[373] And there are big reasons for that, the biggest one of all being that hormonal contraceptives affect how our brains and biology work.[374, 375] For instance, some recent research has found that the volume of the hypothalamus—a hormone-producing region of the brain that links the endocrine and autonomic nervous system and regulates involuntary physiological functions including heart rate and stress response[376]—was smaller in people using hormonal contraceptives.[377]

One of the most important changes that we know of is that hormonal contraceptives can blunt our ability to respond to stress. That's because hormonal contraceptives appear to interfere with the functioning of the HPA axis, an abbreviation used to explain how the hypothalamic, pituitary and adrenal glands work together to respond to stress and to regulate cortisol, our main stress hormone.[378] The HPA axis is influential in many of our bodily systems, including our metabolic, cardiovascular, immune, reproductive and central nervous systems. However, not everyone has the same base level of HPA axis functionality. Having substance abuse problems[379] can influence how our HPA axes work. So can childhood trauma and abuse, chronic illness and periods of intense psychological stress as adults.[380] These experiences can make it harder for us to manage stress.

Research shows hormonal contraceptives increase cortisol levels at the same time as they blunt cortisol response.[381] To the body, stress isn't only a missed deadline or a dangerous situation; it's also a component of exercise, excitement, life enjoyment and part of how we seek out partners. Blunted cortisol response dampens our response to good stress, too, which can make us anxious and depressed.[382]

It can also make it harder for us to adapt and cope with things in our lives that are genuinely stressful. If our bodies become flooded with cortisol but can't respond to it, it can lead to the HPA axis shutting down, and that can lead to major psychological side effects as well as inflammation problems and autoimmunity.[383] In addition to this, research demonstrates that people with endometriosis tend to have an existing dysfunction of HPA axis that leads to a reduced cortisol response, which itself "was associated with greater menstrual and non-menstrual pain in endometriosis."[384]

The truth is, taking hormonal drugs can cause all kinds of side effects, from depression to sexual dysfunction to sometimes-irreversible loss of bone density. They can alter sleep cycles, metabolism and cognition. They can increase the risk for breast cancer and cardiovascular disease. They can even influence our nervous systems, personalities and identities.[385] And yet barely any of this gets discussed when people with endometriosis are prescribed contraceptives to help manage their pain.

Not every hormonal contraceptive user will experience side effects, and some users willingly accept potential risks. Some may rely on these drugs for actual contraception, while others use them to help alleviate endometriosis pain or to regular erratic periods caused by PCOS. Others may use hormone therapy as part of their gender-affirming toolkit. For whatever reason we use these drugs, we are still owed information about their effects. Medical professionals should not be absolved of their duty to share accurate information on potential adverse reactions with patients before prescribing drugs. Unfortunately, most of the people I interviewed for *BLEED* said they weren't informed about the potential for psychological side effects and were not asked to track their mood changes.

What patients should know is that hormones don't respect the fences built around them. They're going to ring the doorbell of every compatible hormone receptor in your body wherever it may be, whether that's in your brain or your cardiovascular system.[386] "No matter where you administer the hormones," Hill writes, "they all end up in the same place. And that place is everywhere."[387]

And so that thing those doctors kept telling me about the IUD having only local effects? It was complete and utter bullshit.[388] A 2020 case study on the experience of a woman who developed a number of symptoms including suicidal ideation and the heart condition tachycardia after having an old levonorgestrel-releasing IUD removed and a new one inserted the same day suggests we've underestimated the systemic effects of hormonal IUDs and drug-to-drug interactions.[389] Another study, from 2017, suggested that the same device leaked "a sufficient amount" of progestin into the system that it affected HPA axis functioning.[390] Indeed, the package insert for Mirena—one of the world's most popular levonorgestrel-releasing IUDs—notes that depression and/or altered mood accounted for 6.4 percent of adverse reactions.[391] How could depression be a side effect for anyone at all if the drug did not have any systemic dispersal?

Because so little of the bigger health picture is shown to us when we're prescribed birth control, when we begin to notice hormone-led changes in our bodies or minds, we often internalize them. Weight gain, pimples and anxiety are personal failings we have to "fix." We think there's something wrong with us rather than with our birth control, which is probably why a huge number of people on the pill end up on antidepressants. If side effects *are* discussed with a doctor, they're too often viewed as necessary sacrifices to lay at the altar of reproductive autonomy and pain relief.

◆

It's a tough pill to swallow that the birth control many of us rely on can also cause significant health problems. It's made even worse by the fact that health professionals and federal drug agencies tell us these medications are safe.

But what are they basing that on? To get a drug approved, pharmaceutical industry research typically focuses on birth control's relationship with death—and some of them do occasionally cause death—while minimizing non-fatal adverse reactions. In clinical trials for hormonal contraceptives, we can see that some companies don't pay much heed to quality-of-life factors and non-fatal side effects. Many of those trials have such a far-reaching list of exclusion criteria that anyone who doesn't resemble a portrait of perfect health isn't studied at all—meaning that a significant portion of future drug-takers with health problems will have no idea what side effects to expect.[392] So, it may be true that hormonal contraceptives are reasonably safe for most people, in the sense that you probably won't die. But, depending on the type of birth control you're using and its psychological side effects, it might dramatically affect your will to live.

The Danish depression study I brought to my gynecologist to prove that the IUD had systemic side effects is part of a growing body of research on the links between hormonal contraceptives and depression. When I first found it back in 2016, it confirmed that my experience with the pill wasn't just in my head.

Over a Zoom interview, that study's lead investigator, Charlotte Wessel Skovlund, tells me she got the idea for the analysis while working as a researcher for a gynecologist.[393] After a friend of hers who'd recently had an IUD inserted began feeling "stressed," Skovlund asked her employer whether there could be a link. Oh yes, he told her; 7 to 10 percent of women have their IUDs removed because they can't stand the psychological effects the device had on them. "I was like, 'Seven to 10 percent? I think that's really a lot,'" she recalls. Like so many of us, her friend hadn't been warned of the side effects.

It piqued her interest, especially because doctors often talk about the IUD as a miracle solution. "They are telling women that this is the best method because you don't have to bleed, and you don't have to remember to take anything, and it is only working in the uterus; it doesn't get into your bloodstream. And I think that my study proves that that's not true," she says.

Skovlund started from the understanding that mood symptoms are a common reason why many women stop using hormonal birth control. Using Denmark's public health registers, she looked for correlations between prescriptions for hormonal birth control and subsequent prescriptions for antidepressants. The study included one million Danish women between the ages of fifteen to thirty-four, with no prior depression diagnosis, from 1995 to 2013. Healthcare is a universal, government-paid service in Denmark, and each Dane has a personal identification number they use to procure health services and prescription drugs. That unique identifier enabled the team to cross-reference people across multiple databases and compose a longitudinal study that followed them for eighteen years.[394]

Not every depressed person is prescribed antidepressants, and there is a small percentage of people prescribed antidepressants for things other than mental illness. But this study is still a very good examination of the links between contraceptives and depression. As it breaks down the most common forms of birth control, and their dosages and compositions, it makes some stunning conclusions.

Users of the patch were twice as likely to fill a script for antidepressants than non-users, and adolescent patch users were three times more likely. Teens' mental health was particularly vulnerable to the patch, IUD and vaginal ring. Overall, across all prescription contraceptives, users had an average 23 percent higher risk of depression than non-users. However, the study makes an interesting distinction between "non-users" and "never-users": non-users included people who'd previously used hormonal contraception but had since stopped, while never-users had *never* taken the pill at all. So while the difference between users to non-users was 23 percent, the difference in likelihood of depression between users and never-users was 70 percent.

According to Skovlund, that means former birth control users appeared likelier to get a depression diagnosis and start using antidepressants than the never-users, which hinted to her that contraceptives could have much longer-term mental side effects than we've been told.

Skovlund was fascinated by what she found and decided to mine the healthcare system's databases for more insights. In a subsequent study,[395] her team used the same methodology to measure the relationship between contraceptive use and attempted and completed suicides. Compared to never-users, people on birth control with no prior history of depression, antidepressant use or suicidality were almost twice as likely to make a first suicide attempt while on the pill. Like the earlier depression study, teens were more vulnerable, and again the patch and the ring had the highest risks. IUDs and implants also showed high numbers.

This news may be frustrating to people with endometriosis and other conditions like PCOS, since the medical system overwhelmingly relies on hormonal contraceptives to manage our symptoms to such an extent that we often spend years on the pill (and other hormone-modifying medications), waiting for some miracle cure. These contraceptive years are a big reason why many of us wait years and sometimes decades to get diagnosed, never mind that doctors' go-to solution even after diagnosis is still to take birth control.[396]

None of this is to say the pill is ineffective at helping reduce bleeding and pain. For many years, it dialed my symptoms down from eleven on a pain scale to maybe a six or seven. But I also cycled through periods of acute despair and depression that left me feeling numb and worthless. My relationships with friends, family, colleagues and partners suffered. Anger and sadness rotated through me and damaged my empathy filters. I cried all the time and I felt like an asshole. Is having all that twenty-four hours a day, seven days a week, 365 days a year, better than seven to ten days a month of torture? What a choice to have to make.

While it's true that women and trans people are diagnosed with anxiety and depression much more frequently than men are,[397, 398, 399] we saw earlier why that may be the case—namely, being part of a sexist society in which our continued mistreatment and subjugation depends on us being pathologized and psychologized by a paternalistic medical system. *Ahem.*

That association with depression also doesn't control for the fact that women see doctors more frequently than men do,[400] nor for how women tend to describe illnesses using emotional phrases like "I feel" rather than more direct, physical terms. And unlike males who often externalize their depression as aggression or irritability[401] (which aren't viewed as medical problems), women tend to internalize theirs, where it manifests as anxiety and sadness[402] (for which there are dozens of drugs). It also doesn't acknowledge just how much research on contraceptives has been led or funded by the companies manufacturing the drugs and devices being studied. Those companies clearly have a vested interest in coming off as unthreatening as possible, and that may lead them to couch negative outcomes in bullshit jargon that obfuscates research problems.

With so many system failures, a disproportionately huge part of birth control falls on our shoulders. Not having clear, straightforward information about contraception leaves it up to us to figure it out— and that kind of opening creates a lot of room for misinformation and poorly informed decision-making. It's just one more way we become our own doctors and fail to conform to the boundaries of the sick role.

Back on Zoom, I ask Skovlund what she hopes her research will achieve. Evidently many doctors have never even connected the dots between contraception and mental health, let alone integrate those connections into the way they approach care. She tells me that friends of hers who know about her research have started asking their doctors for copper IUDs, which are non-hormonal forms of birth control. These aren't popular with endometriosis or adenomyosis sufferers since they often worsen menstrual bleeding and pain.[403] However, to Skovlund, it shows that when confronted by good information about risks, people choose differently, and their choices are based on a holistic approach, considering what the best option is as a *whole* person, rather than a disparate collection of body parts.

She wishes the responsibility of becoming informed about choices didn't fall so heavily on patients. This approach puts an especially unfair burden on teens, who may not be in the best position to evaluate risks against quality of life. She also wishes doctors didn't treat contraceptives as an inoculation against unwanted babies or as a carefree accessory to a busy life, but rather that they treated them like the serious drugs they are. "That's really unpopular to say [publicly], because then it's like, 'Do you want more abortions or teenage births?'" Skovlund says. "No, I want a better choice for not getting pregnant."

◆

Just six weeks after having the IUD inserted, I had a total meltdown.

I smashed into my mental rock bottom at high velocity just a couple weeks after I made up that song in the woods. By then, I'd been bleeding and having horrible cramps for forty-two days straight. An insurmountable sadness enveloped me and I thought about dying all the time. My resolve to stay alive was tested every time I left the house and had to be *out there*, in the world. My mind was screaming, but I constantly felt at a loss for words. This was *worse* than I imagined. How could the gynecologist have shrugged off the links between the IUD and depression? She worked as a gynecologist in a hospital *pain* clinic. How could she *not* know? Clearly, she believed I was already neurotic to begin with—but even if I was a difficult patient, I couldn't understand her need to circumvent valid concerns and good evidence about the IUD's correlation to depression in order to teach me a lesson in power dynamics. I felt like I'd been set up to fail.

All this was rolling around in my head on the day I decided to get the IUD removed. I remember it was a warm, sunny June day. That morning I woke to a panic attack, one of the worst I'd ever had. I know I biked to the sexual health clinic and back home, but I have absolutely no recollection of my journey. I don't remember what I told the receptionist when I got there, or if I sat in the waiting room or was immediately let into an exam room. It was as if my brain had thrown me into some kind of state of automatism to get me through this. I became wholly focused on one task, and one task only: getting this IUD out of me.

I do, however, remember the dog poster. Taped to the dingy foam ceiling tiles of the exam room was an incredible montage of dogs wearing insane hats. I was completely transfixed. I stared at each dog intently, studying their faces for signs of distress. They were forced to pose for these photos, but they don't seem upset about it, I thought. I assume they got a ton of treats to do it. I scanned the dog poster for at least a dozen minutes while waiting for the doctor to enter the room. In the middle of a panic attack, the dog poster was a strange, soothing balm.

In the middle of my canine meditation, a doctor with a stern and concerned expression entered. Her red hair was pulled back into a ponytail so tight it looked painful. I sat up and blinked, my eyes filmy with tears and puffed up like sad little half-inflated balloons. It felt like I had dozens of sharp little splinters lost under my eyelids, and I desperately and unsuccessfully blinked to focus my gaze and mind. How could I have possibly biked through traffic in this state?

The doctor was a woman I had never met before and have never seen since. I told her I wanted the IUD removed immediately, that it was making me the most depressed and suicidal I'd ever been. She was skeptical. She'd never heard of an IUD causing such intense depression; after all, she said, it only works locally in the uterus without systemic effects. Maybe my IUD had secreted too much hormone at once, she posited.

Or maybe, I could hear her thinking, *you were fucking crazy to begin with.*

She yanked out the IUD and my chest heaved with relief.

Then she jotted down the name and number of a local gynecologist, Dr. Kapper, and handed me the yellow sticky note. A new person to beg for a hysterectomy. "Try her," she told me.

6. WE'RE DESPERATE

to breed or not to breed?

Stephanie Lepage wonders how different her life could have been if only the doctors had bothered to look for endometriosis before her mid-thirties.[404]

There was the family doctor who put fourteen-year-old Lepage on the pill to help control her pain and bleeding. They gave the teen a few months' worth of free samples to help take the sting out of the cost. She paid the rest out of pocket to keep the contraceptive a secret from her mother for as long as she could. No tests or exams, no pain meds, just birth control.

There was that other GP who couldn't find her cervix during a Pap smear. "Dude, I assure you, it's there," she remembers telling him. The exam was so invasive that when her birth control prescription ran out of refills, she let it lapse and quit the pill until she could find another family doctor.

Lepage developed constant pain in her right lower abdomen that was so intense that rolling onto her side would shoot her out of a dead sleep on an almost nightly basis. When Lepage finally got in to see a gynecologist about it, that doctor said it was little more than a red herring. A cyst on the opposite side was merely referring pain—no connection, no pain meds, no problem. She remained in agony for two years without reprieve, living through 730 nights of interrupted sleep and 730 days of constant stabbing until it mysteriously subsided.

There were also times in her life when she avoided doctors completely. She didn't see the point in subjecting herself to their judgment and experimentation, when not one single medical professional over the course of twenty-odd years had been able to answer why her periods brought her such intense suffering.

Lepage, a cis white woman who is thirty-eight when we speak, tells me that knowing what she knows now, it's obvious she had all the classic symptoms of endometriosis. But by her early thirties, she still hadn't been diagnosed. In place of a diagnosis, she had a collection of strange symptoms for which she took hormonal birth control for the better part of eighteen years. On the pill, sporadic pain and bleeding, a flatlining sex drive and painful dryness all chipped away at her enjoyment of life.

Like with me and many other people in our situation, there came a point in Lepage's life where she began to doubt whether the hormonal contraceptives were really helping. They just had so many side effects, and at thirty-two, she wondered whether they were worth it. Maybe her period had become less awful, or at least more bearable than the side effects of hormonal contraceptives she'd been using over the past two decades. The influence of synthetic hormones meant she could no longer recall the difference between Off-the-Pill Stephanie and On-the-Pill Stephanie. After so many years using the pill and the ring, she couldn't remember who she'd been at fourteen—and she couldn't tell how she'd changed since. At the very least, going off the drugs would give her a break and some breathing room away from the healthcare system, of which she had had more than enough. "I'd been on some form of hormonal birth control for almost all of my reproductive life," she recalls. "So I was like, 'You know what, I'm going to see what my body does.'"

In the Before Pill times, Lepage had long, heavy and painful periods. In the After Pill times, her period did change: it became a bit shorter and much more intense. Even now, blood clots come so fast and furious she can sometimes feel them push her tampons out: "I will overflow my menstrual cup multiple times a day. I half-joke that my periods are solid now. They're almost all blood clots because I'm bleeding so quickly." She pauses, then laughs with a tinge of sadness. "Passing a blood clot the size of your palm through your cervix doesn't feel good."

And then another curveball came: she and her partner decided to try to have a baby.

◆

In the Nervous Breakdown chapter, we saw some of the downsides of hormonal contraceptives and how doctors, drug companies and regulatory agencies have successfully passed the buck onto patients who experience side effects—especially if those side effects involve mental health. As we'll see in the pages to come, that attitude has translated to other hormonal drugs.

As far as I can tell, contraceptives were first prescribed to control endometriosis in the mid-1950s, as the first birth control pill was being developed. One of the first to test the drugs on patients was gynecologist Robert W. Kistner.[405]

Kistner, an early proponent of birth control, was a key member of a small group of prominent gynecologists in the 1950s who explored potential uses for the pill beyond preventing pregnancy. Endometriosis, one of Kistner's specialties, was an early use case. He began giving endo patients a combination of estrogen and a progestin in 1956; by 1961, he had given this therapy to 110 people.[406] The drugs were called Enovid and Depo-Provera. In a paper the following year, he explained that he titrated patients up to their full dosages over the course of four to six weeks.[407]

Enovid's original formulation was 0.15 milligrams of estrogen and 9.85 milligrams of progestin per tablet—almost four times as much hormone as later versions of the drug.[408, 409] Though different progestins are at play, consider the scale of these doses: today, popular modern brand Alesse has just 0.02 milligrams of estrogen and 0.10 milligrams of progestin,[410] while Bayer's popular Yasmin contains 0.03 milligrams of estrogen and 3.0 milligrams of progestin.[411] A number of early users of the first Enovid pill died from blood clots and heart failure.[412]

Kistner gave many of his endometriosis patients 40 milligrams of Enovid a day, four times the original dosage, which was itself at least four times higher than it needed to be. A few patients received 60–70 milligrams daily because of persistent breakthrough bleeding, he also wrote. Some received as much as 120 milligrams of it. He concluded his paper by quoting a colleague: "At present it appears that hormone therapy for endometriosis will be the most widely applicable form of management in the future."[413]

How prescient.

For nearly one hundred years, doctors have surmised that becoming pregnant is a way to treat endometriosis. This understanding was originally formed in the first half of the 1900s under Sampson (the reflux menstruation guy), Meigs (the eugenics supporter) and their contemporaries, and it was based on the observation that women with many children had fewer lesions than their less procreative counterparts.

This idea was at the root of Kistner's experiment on endometriosis patients. When the women took Enovid or other estrogen-progestin combinations and stopped menstruating, he called this phase "pseudopregnancy."[414] He found that, in a three-year study following fifty-eight patients who were primarily given those high doses of Enovid, endometriosis went into "remission" for up to thirty months after three to ten months of treatment. In this case, remission meant less painful periods and less painful sex.

Kistner went to bat for contraceptive makers like Enovid's manufacturer, GD Searle & Co., defending the pill against fears and criticisms that it was unsafe for women. In Senate testimony delivered in 1970,[415] he admitted that he had worked as a clinical investigator for "practically all of the companies" that made contraceptives and received funding for that work.[416]

Ultimately, though, the case for using contraceptives to regulate endometriosis was based only on a handful of studies with a few handfuls of women. The pill's continued dominance in endometriosis treatment seventy years later, despite little innovation,[417] shows us the power of drug companies' influence, and how little institutional appetite there is to better understand and treat this disease. Worse, the logic by which these drugs are prescribed has been flawed from the very beginning: hormonal contraceptives don't actually control endometriosis at all. They merely mask the proliferation of the disease while reducing some symptoms.

Reams of scientific evidence show that hormonal contraceptives, as well as hormonal modulators like Lupron and Orilissa (more on them in a bit), don't significantly reduce or eliminate physical disease.[418] They don't even stop the disease from progressing, because endometriosis doesn't solely rely on systemic estrogen: it makes its own supply.[419, 420] Not that that's important to know when treating endo patients.

◆

When Lepage told her doctor she wanted to get pregnant, it was like a light switch got flipped. Her doctor warmly welcomed the news of Lepage's intentions; in her mid-thirties, she *was* getting a bit old.

As she soon found out, however, developing an embryo was far more difficult than she and her partner had anticipated. After six months, Lepage miscarried. She was deeply disappointed by that loss, but as a pragmatic person whose PhD is in embryology and developmental biology, she knew exactly how normal it really was. She pushed it aside as much as she could and kept trucking along.

It was in a Chicago hotel room where she reached a major breaking point.

By then it had been a year since their conception efforts began. A little weekend getaway was more than merited, so she and her partner made the two-hour plane trip from Toronto to attend a friend's wedding.

Unfortunately, her period joined them.

In the months since the miscarriage, she says her period had become "god-awful"—an excruciating, blood-soaked affair that made pants feel like a torture device. This one, though, was pure hell. There were stabbing cramps, painful bloating, diarrhea, massive clots—all the bells and whistles. At 4 a.m. the morning of the wedding, Lepage shook her partner awake. Drenched in a cold sweat, she begged him to go out and get her some drugs. "I was contemplating trying to go to a doctor in Chicago. I thought I was going to have to walk into the emergency room," she tells me. The only reason she didn't was the exorbitant cost of an ER visit at an American hospital. Instead, she holed up in the bathroom feeling like she was on the edge of death. The day of the wedding, she emerged from her porcelain prison for just one hour to show her face, as if she was giving the newly married couple the gift of a proof of life. What was meant to be a getaway had turned into a hostage situation, with Lepage's uterus acting as her captor.

As soon as Lepage returned to Toronto, she booked an appointment with her doctor. *Something* needed to change. Her doctor had a long history of brushing her period problems aside, but surely she could not ignore the Chicago incident's gravity—right?

Wrong. Lepage says her doctor looked completely uninterested as her patient complained of extreme pain and bleeding. Until, that is, Lepage dropped the bomb. "I'm also still unable to conceive," Lepage told the doctor. The GP snapped her head up, a gentle admonishment emanating from her lips: "Why didn't you come to me sooner?" Her hands became a flurry of action as she ordered rounds of testing.

On her way home, Lepage thought about the encounter. "The thing that stood out to me the most was like, unless I was trying to conceive, no one even cared about bleeding and pain," she tells me. "It's like, 'We don't care about anything that has to do with your daily life and quality of life. It's your job as a woman to procreate, and—oh my God, if you can't procreate, then it's a problem. Sure, we'll take that seriously. But otherwise, eh, who cares?'" She hated how easily the script was flipped, how those magic words—"I want a baby"— transformed her doctor.

In that moment, she became painfully aware of how the other side lives: how pregnancy and fertility care fast-track a patient through the system. It felt like a bizarro healthcare system where doctors actually help people with chronic illness. It was just so unfair, and yet here she was, benefiting from the same system that had kept a diagnosis and treatment away from her for so long. She clutched the life preserver thrown to her. Maybe now she would finally get some answers.

◆

The pharmaceutical industry has long had its tentacles wrapped around reproductive health. Almost as soon as the pill hit the American market, doctors and patients had reservations about its safety.[421] In 1957, Enovid had just been approved by the FDA to treat menstrual disorders, including endometriosis.[422] Of course, there was no fooling anybody about what the pills in the brown glass bottle were really for, and many doctors prescribed it off-label as a contraceptive.[423] By the time it was officially approved as a contraceptive in 1960, women around the country had already been taking it for some time.

It's well known that the pill was a key ingredient in women's liberation and that its ability to control reproduction changed lives practically and ideologically, transforming conversations about female sexuality, pleasure and economic equality. It challenged the very concept of personal freedom and who gets to be free in this world.

But that doesn't mean that it was a flawless invention.

The safety of contraceptives was investigated by the U.S. government a number of times, including during multiple government subcommittee hearings in which senators and members of Congress heard from a gamut of stakeholders on all sides of the issue.

At the same time that these concerns were being aired and debated, the pill remained on the market—not because it actually was safe, but because it had not been proven *unsafe*. Recall that Enovid's original formula was many times stronger than it needed to be to effectively thwart pregnancy—a dose that caused some women to die. The pill was a gold mine for the flourishing pharmaceutical sector, and no amount of subcommittee hearings could stop the birth control juggernaut.

Throughout the 1960s, the U.S. government convened meetings and committees, and commissioned reports to explore matters related to population and birth control. Most of them ended with some version of the same recommendations: 1) expand the scope and powers of the FDA to monitor drugs, and 2) more research is needed to make any significant conclusions about the safety of the pill. The mounting concern around the pill was transformative for the FDA, too, noted a veteran reporter in the *New York Times*: "Many of the steps that underlie modern drug approvals—extensive clinical trials, routine referrals to panels of outside experts, continuing assessments of a medicine's safety and direct communications between the FDA and patients—were pioneered to deal with evolving concerns about the pill's safety."[424]

In 1969, a book called *The Doctor's Case against the Pill* by feminist and activist Barbara Seaman was published, which used anecdotal stories to show that women faced massive potential harms by using birth control. Around the same time, Seaman also wrote a six-page letter to Democratic senator Gaylord Nelson asking him to seriously consider examining the consequences of the pill.[425] Nelson found Seaman's arguments curious and compelling, and early the following year, he convened Senate subcommittee hearings on the pill and on anti-competitiveness in the drug industry.[426, 427, 428]

The Nelson subcommittee members heard testimony from pill proponents and opponents alike. Some argued that contraceptives prevented maternal mortality and abortion-related deaths, and that "rapid multiplication of the human race" quashed the life-expectancy gains people in the developed world had earned—a nod to the ideologies of eugenics.[429] They also heard that drug companies generated profits from propaganda surrounding the pill, including claims that it was safer than pregnancy.[430] The efforts led the pill to become, as one doctor testified, "the most casually refilled prescription ever written."[431]

The hearings were highly publicized and politicized, and a Gallup poll[432] noted that a fifth of respondents who took the pill said they would "never use it again."[433] More alarming, two-thirds of poll respondents said their doctors had never told them about the hazards of the pill. Even after dosages were reduced, the synthetic hormones caused a number of side effects that made some women wary. (That said, Enovid's maker G.D. Searle made $201.5 million in sales the same year of the Nelson hearings.[434])

Planned Parenthood and the Population Crisis Committee decried the meetings, accusing Senator Nelson of creating a culture of fear around the birth control pill, and predicting that the hearings would scare so many Americans that 100,000 unwanted and unloved "Nelson babies" would be born that year.[435]

On the other side of the political aisle were people like Dr. Herbert Ratner. He told the panel that in the four years since hearings and a report in 1966,[436] more than fifty metabolic changes had been observed in people on the pill, and that it had been associated with, among other things, thromboembolism, depression, diabetes, migraine, sterility, libido loss, high cholesterol and hypertension.[437] Considering all this, Ratner continued, how could the FDA maintain that the risk-benefit ratio was such that the pill could continue being designated safe? This safe designation gave drug companies a green light to continue selling the drug with impunity. What would it take to stop them? "Even Aristotle knew that although effective drugs given to sick people may get them well, effective drugs given to the healthy are bound to lead to imbalance and disease," he implored.

In the 1970 book *The Pill: An Alarming Report, Washington Post* investigative journalist Morton Mintz wrote how the drug had been approved based on tests for efficacy but not for safety.[438] Once it was approved, physicians uncertain about the pill's effects relied on experts like Kistner and on the FDA for guidance, Mintz wrote. "Doctors assumed that it would not have been admitted to the market had its safety not been demonstrated in advance to the FDA. But for the most part they were not even faintly aware of the gross ineptitude that prevailed in the FDA."[439] The FDA, he continued, had for years mislabeled contraceptive drugs and provided contradictory warnings about drugs with the same formulations. Mintz's reporting echoed Ratner's concerns.

Although Ratner, who died in 1997,[440] was an active anti-abortionist who thought the pill should be taken off the market, many of the shots he fired over contraceptives went on to hit their targets. Scientific research has overwhelmingly confirmed that hormonal birth control does prompt metabolic changes, and that it does contribute to a variety of health problems including many of the ones identified by Ratner. His most prescient condemnation, however, was of the drug companies and the power they hold over both regulatory agencies and doctors themselves—relationships which are now central to the pharmaceutical-first treatment of endometriosis.[441]

♦

Lepage arrived at the ultrasound clinic looking for answers. She'd already run a gamut of testing to see why she couldn't conceive. Now here she was, about to get penetrated again by another x-ray dildo.

Lepage dutifully removed everything from the waist down and climbed onto the exam table. Her technician entered, a "little bit of a crusty, Eastern European hard-ass kind of woman," and began the ultrasound.

The ultrasound technician usually keeps mum, withholding the information they see on the screen and telling the patient their doctor will follow up with them. In Lepage's case, the technician glared at the monitor, then began asking a series of questions. Do you have a history of cysts? Do you have endometriosis?

Lepage said she'd had that one cyst that kept her from a good night's sleep for two years. "How big was it?" Two centimeters, Lepage answered. The technician clucked her tongue. "They really needed to keep following you," she stated firmly, hinting to Lepage that something was wrong—but not actually telling her, as per protocol. "I left there obviously knowing something was not right," Lepage tells me.

When she got in to see her doctor for the results a few weeks later, she learned the original cyst had not only doubled in size, but that it was now accompanied by two other cysts. Then the doctor paused. "Are you . . . a walk-in? Am I your GP?" she asked, perplexed. A few moments later, she asked Lepage to confirm her name. The doctor seemed to have no recollection of ever meeting Lepage. And she made no mention of endometriosis. Instead, she said she'd refer her to a fertility specialist. "I'm like, 'Okay, that's great for my fertility, but what about my pain? That's really why I came,'" recalls Lepage. The fertility specialist would figure it out, her doctor assured her.

By then Lepage assumed she had endometriosis, and her self-diagnosis was supported by the fertility specialist. However, the disease could only be officially confirmed with laparoscopic surgery—and that would only delay Lepage's efforts to conceive. By then, she was thirty-seven and running out of options. On top of the probable endometriosis—which is found in between 25 and 50 percent of infertility cases[442]—she also discovered she had a diminished ovarian reserve,[443] described to her as "the ovaries of a fifty-year-old." She was going to need in-vitro fertilization—a hefty out-of-pocket expense—and because of her age and limited supply of eggs, she would need to take extra drugs to improve her chances.

The first attempt was not great: just one embryo survived the fertilization process, meaning she had a single shot at pregnancy. It was a high-stakes moment, and these were very long odds. To improve her chances of successfully implanting the embryo, the specialist made a suggestion: let's treat your endometriosis. After more than twenty years of suffering, it was the first time anyone had offered to help beyond prescribing the pill.

◆

Synthetic progestin wasn't created with the intention of harming women.

Chemist Carl Djerassi—considered the father of the pill—originally meant his 1951 discovery of norethisterone to be used for menstrual disorders, cervical cancer and infertility, not contraception.[444] Population control was the furthest thing from Djerassi's mind. He was a Jewish refugee who had fled Austria for the United States in 1939 to escape the Nazis.[445] He just wanted to contribute to the realm of scientific discovery while making some money.

An equally pivotal person in the development of birth control was Margaret Sanger, the founder of Planned Parenthood. Sanger believed with every fiber of her being that motherhood should be voluntary. "Long has woman been called the gentler and weaker half of humankind; long has she borne the brunt of unwilling motherhood; long has she been the stepping-stone of oligarchies, kingdoms, and man-made democracies; too long have they thrived on her enslavement. The time has come at last when she demands her physical and spiritual freedom—and her liberty," she said in 1917.[446]

Five years later, Sanger's tone shifted. She wrote, "The least intelligent and the thoroughly degenerate classes in every community are the most prolific [. . .] Birth control has been accepted by the most clear thinking and far seeing of the eugenicists themselves as the most constructive and necessary of the means to racial health."[447] With this thinking, Sanger became a powerful figure in the eugenics movement of the early 1900s, which promoted the idea of selective breeding, as well as the belief that overpopulation posed a massive threat to humanity. Some American eugenicists believed the U.S. would have 100 million more people than it could support by 1980,[448] and advocated to reverse this trend through the attrition of the "unfit"—a label that included people of color, low-income individuals, as well as those with mental and physical disabilities. By preventing them from reproducing, the "mentally and physically fit, and therefore less fertile, parents of the educated, and well-to-do classes" could maintain their supremacy.[449]

Sanger is also controversial because, while her organization argues that she tried to promote a type of eugenics that didn't discriminate against race or religion,[450] she leaned on prevalent classist, racist and misogynist attitudes in society to guide the development, commercialization and policy-making around the pill. In her book *The Pivot of Civilization*, she wrote, "The lack of balance between the birth-rate of the 'unfit' and the 'fit,' admittedly the greatest present menace to civilization, can never be rectified by the inauguration of a cradle competition between these two classes. [. . .] Possibly drastic and Spartan methods may be forced upon American society if it continues complacently to encourage the chance and chaotic breeding that has resulted from our stupid, cruel sentimentalism."[451]

Sanger wielded an unusual amount of power for a woman in the early 1900s. In *The Birth of the Pill*,[452, 453] author Jonathan Eig writes how the pill was born almost single-handedly of the collaboration between Sanger, her friend and rich benefactor Katharine McCormick, scientist Gregory Pincus and OBGYN John Rock. Sanger met Pincus in 1950 and implored him to create a birth control pill, at the time seemingly unaware of Djerassi's work with progestins. She convinced her friend McCormick to bankroll Pincus's research. In turn, Pincus recruited Rock, an old acquaintance, to help test the drug in his fertility clinic.[454] Together, the group saw the completion of the first pill experiments on humans in 1953–54, which were secretly done out of Rock's Boston fertility office and at a mental asylum in a neighboring town, where sometimes they got patient consent, and sometimes they didn't.[455]

In early 1954, Pincus traveled to Puerto Rico and found a dense population with an existing network of birth control services—a perfect cohort for pill trials.[456] The first trial began in 1956, with G.D. Searle providing its experimental contraception drug—later to be named Enovid—for testing. Pincus's local team recruited candidates from a poor area of Puerto Rico: One hundred "suitable experimental subjects" who would receive the drug, and 125 non-users for the control group.[457, 458] They would later also run tests on Haitian women.[459]

Relevant to Pincus and Rock's decision to use Puerto Rico as the pill's testing ground is the fact that between the 1930s and 1970s, Puerto Rican women were sterilized in droves—many against their will. This was made possible by U.S. colonialism, which since the 1898 Spanish-American War invasion has dispossessed the majority of Puerto Ricans of their land, resulting in widespread poverty. According to the Eugenics Archive, "U.S. eugenicists seized on the resulting poverty, blaming overpopulation and targeting poor women for sterilization and pharmaceutical experimentation." By 1976, 37 percent of Puerto Rican women had been sterilized, most of them getting la operación while still in their twenties.[460]

The issue of informed consent surrounding these experiments emerged much, much later. The historical record suggests that, for the most part, the women participating in Pincus and Rock's work knew they were taking birth control. That said, standards and regulations for human experiments then were nowhere near as stringent as they are today, leaving many question marks around what the subjects knew about the drug and exactly how ethical this work was.[461]

By the mid-1950s, the demand for birth control in the U.S. was huge and getting bigger every day. The radio played rock 'n' rollers like Elvis Presley, Buddy Holly, Chuck Berry and Little Richard, harbingers of a massive culture shift. Middle-class housewives were beginning to get restless. The Sanger crew knew then that contraception was no longer an *if* but a *when*. So they bluffed, Eig told NPR radio host Terry Gross in 2014.[462] Although by then they'd experimented on fewer than a hundred Puerto Rican women, in September of 1956 Pincus deemed the trial a success while at a conference near Montreal. "I think it's one of the great bluffs in scientific history," said Eig. "[Pincus] knows that he's got the science. He's not sure that it's really ready. He hasn't tested it on nearly enough women. And his partner, John Rock, is saying, 'Don't you dare announce that we're ready to do this yet. If you do, I'm out.' He's furious with Pincus, but Pincus does it anyway. He realizes that they've got some momentum, and they need to keep it going because this whole thing could fall apart if too much opposition is raised." By 1957, doctors around the U.S. were prescribing Enovid.

Amid all of this excitement, a few of the less palatable elements have been lost to progress: the unapproved drug was overwhelmingly tested in higher than necessary doses on poor women of color and institutionalized people, with the initial intention of preventing exactly these kinds of people from procreating.

We should see the creation of the pill as part of a continuum in history, not as a standalone event. Mass sterilization campaigns were created shortly after the abolition of slavery in the U.S. Birth control's emergence came at a moment when mass sterilization was less palatable to the American public because of the Holocaust and the global witnessing of eugenics in action.

Many people have argued that Sanger's eugenicist stance was merely a reflection of the times and that it was in service of something—birth control and abortion—that was critical to the advancement of women. She was, however, undeniably a eugenicist who propped up the idea of controlling the proliferation of "unfit" people in order to gain support for the pill. She did it by framing the pill as a way to prevent overpopulation at a time when it was politically fashionable to do so. Because of this, we can't ignore that the pill was commercialized with violence against some women in mind. Even as early pill proponents used terms such as "maternal health," "child welfare," "reproductive choice" and "the war on poverty," it wasn't only about making motherhood voluntary, Johanna Schoen remarks in her book *Choice and Coercion*. Rather, as she writes, hormonal birth control "could extend reproductive control to some, or they could be used to control women's reproduction."[463]

The questionable evolution of the pill wasn't an anomaly. Rather, it showed the world how powerful contraceptive makers could be.

◆

In 1956, scientists discovered medroxyprogesterone acetate. By the time it was approved as a contraceptive by the FDA in 1992—after a multidecade delay owed to concerns of serious and irreversible side effects, including cancer and bone loss[464]—millions of people in the U.S. and in less developed countries were already taking it.[465]

The drug is better known as Depo-Provera.

In a field of controversial contraceptives, Depo-Provera stands tall as one of *the* most controversial. This long-acting injection contraceptive was forcibly administered to male sex offenders by court order and given to poor Black women sometimes without informed consent. Ultimately, it became an emblem of systemic medical violence.

William Green's book about Depo-Provera, *Contraceptive Risk*, details the protracted fight between drugmaker Upjohn and the FDA to get the contraceptive approved—a thirty-two-year battle to have the drug's side effects deemed "acceptable risk." Early drug testing saw beagles and rhesus monkeys suddenly develop breast or endometrial cancer.[466] Those results were eschewed by Upjohn because they didn't indicate how a *human* would react. But as early as 1971, researchers found that Depo-Provera users seemed to have a higher incidence of cervical cancer. There was also a long list of side effects ranging from weight gain to depression. By the time the animal trial results were made public, American women were already taking the drug off-label as a contraceptive. It had been approved in 1960 as a treatment for endometriosis and endometrial cancer and was greenlit in the early 1970s for use on people with mental disabilities—meaning that, in effect, human trials had preceded the animal ones. That also meant that it had been approved to treat people with endometriosis without solid scientific proof it would help them at all.[467]

Let's rewind to 1967. That's when a Depo-Provera "clinical trial" on human females began at an Atlanta clinic serving mostly lower-income Black women.[468] By the time it was shut down by the FDA in 1978 following a federal hearing, the clinic had already given Depo-Provera, also known as "the shot," to thousands of Black women—many of whom said later on they had no idea that the drug hadn't been approved as a contraceptive when they took it, that animal test subjects were developing cancer, and that they were part of a drug trial for an unapproved drug.[469] There's reason to believe some women at the Atlanta clinic were duped, or felt coerced, into getting long-acting contraceptives. A paper published in 1967 about that clinic's approach to IUDs noted that their overwhelmingly low-income Black clientele could better endure "minor complaints" than other populations—a comment that echoes the rationale for experimenting on enslaved Black women and immigrant Irish women.[470] The paper also said, "Negative aspects are presented [to patients], but not stressed because they are inhibitory to acceptance." Looking back on their unknowing participation in the Depo-Provera trial, some patients said their welfare case workers threatened to cut off their checks if they didn't get the shot.[471]

Testimony before a congressional subcommittee in 1987 tasked with examining the use of Depo-Provera by the Indian Health Service also detailed how hundreds of women had been outright lied to: they were told the shots contained vitamins or antibiotics, rather than a contraceptive. The testimony of Sybil Shainwald, an attorney focused on reproductive health reform, noted that the National Women's Health Network had been keeping a list of all Depo-Provera users. She said 90 percent of those who got the shot had *not* been informed that the drug hadn't yet been approved as a contraceptive.[472]

"Black women in the South and Native American women have been special targets," said Shainwald.[473] Women with mental disabilities, incarcerated women and drug users were also targeted, Shainwald continued, adding that the National Women's Health Network opposed Depo-Provera as a contraceptive "for any group because we are opposed to having different standards of safety for poor women and 'irresponsible women' and Native women."[474]

The drug was approved by the FDA as a contraceptive in 1992,[475] a decision preceded by a 1991 report co-authored by the World Health Organization (WHO) that stated that Depo-Provera posed only a slightly higher risk of certain cancers, and that the benefits posed by the drug outweighed those risks.[476] The drug's link to bone loss and osteoporosis received only a short mention. Later studies on this link led to Depo-Provera getting a black-box warning in 2004, which said patients should avoid taking the drug for longer than two years, unless other contraceptives were inadequate.[477] It was too little, too late. Twelve years after its FDA approval, millions of people around the world were already on Depo-Provera—some of them for much longer than two years.

Today, Depo-Provera—now manufactured by Pfizer—is on the WHO's list of essential medicines.[478]

The legacy of Depo-Provera is clear evidence that the dangers of hormonal contraceptives were known from the very beginning, and that safety came second to profits. Many inventors and companies saw dollar signs dancing in their eyes. In 1963, the FDA admitted to the conflicts of interest that defined the relationship between medicine and industry. When asked during hearings about why the FDA hadn't set up advisory panels to improve drug safety, commissioner George P. Larrick replied, "The conflict of interest rules under which we must operate have proved to be a problem. The real experts in the food, drug, therapeutic device and cosmetic fields have generally been associated in one way or another with the industries that we regulate."[479]

Seven years later during the Nelson hearings, Dr. Hugh Davis, a Johns Hopkins professor and research scientist, warned of the oral contraceptive pill: "Never in history have so many individuals taken such potent drugs with so little information as to actual and potential hazards."[480] During that same testimony, Davis was also questioned about a rumor that he held a patent on an IUD.[481] Davis denied any financial interest in such a device, then went on to highlight the dangers of the pill. A year later, Davis's invention—the Dalkon Shield IUD—hit the market and became an overnight success.[482]

Reading between the lines, it seems as though he chose to denigrate the pill so that his device would be considered a better option. However, as is now well known, the Dalkon Shield led to infections, blood poisoning, unintended pregnancies and other injuries, as well as eighteen deaths.[483] The Dalkon Shield scandal was exposed by

Washington Post journalist Mintz, who later wrote in a book about the Shield that it had not been adequately tested before its manufacturer, the A.H. Robins Company, began marketing it to doctors.[484] Mintz's revelations about the IUD ultimately led to heavy litigation against the company.[485] In the late 1980s, a judge announced that A.H. Robins's liability totaled $2.475 billion. By 2001, more than 218,000 people claimed compensation, totaling $1.5 billion in pro rata payouts.[486]

Untold numbers of other victims will never be known: after the Dalkon Shield was withdrawn from the U.S. market in 1974,[487] the company began dumping its supply of unsterilized IUDs—more than 700,000—onto poorer countries with the help of the U.S. Agency for International Development.[488, 489]

These are just some of the stories of how hormonal contraceptives came to dominate reproductive health. Across years of subcommittee testimony and other evidence, we can hear people struggling under the weight of the birth control pill. Yes, it gave them new pathways to economic independence, to education, to self-realization. It also came with medical abuse, unmanageable side effects and unanswered questions about long-term outcomes. It was the very definition of a double-edged sword: so much more opportunity, but also so many more consequences.

These were seen as necessary evils. The benefits, after all, outweighed the risks. The FDA not only kept most of the original contraceptives on the market, but over time also greenlit a number of other controversial hormonal drugs.

Today, 407 million people in the world use hormonal contraceptives.[490] That's just over 11 percent of the entire population assigned female at birth and nearly 22 percent of those in childbearing years (fifteen to forty-nine). Most of those people are using hormonal contraceptives that were developed decades ago, made by a self-stunted industry that doesn't have to innovate on birth control to profit.[491] It's deeply telling that the clotting risk of hormonal contraceptives remains at between three and nine per ten thousand,[492, 493] while the rare, one-in-a-million clotting risk caused by the AstraZeneca COVID-19 vaccine led to millions of doses going to waste at the height of a deadly global pandemic.[494]

It isn't only older brands of birth control that present greater-than-average risk. Take Bayer's Yaz and Yasmin, for instance. In 2013, Health Canada revealed that at least twenty-three women died from clots related to these two brands of birth control, both of which contain drospirenone, one of the newest progestins.[495] Deaths from these two drugs were also reported in the U.S. around the same time. Drospirenone carries a blood clot risk one-and-a-half to three times higher than other hormonal contraceptives made without it.[496, 497] Because of the clotting issue and the related risks of deep vein thrombosis, stroke, heart attack, pulmonary embolism and loss of gallbladder, Bayer has been sued or is actively being sued by countless people and class actions; already, more than 19,000 suits have been settled.[498] More than $1.6 billion had been paid out by 2013.[499]

Meanwhile, in 2020, Yaz, Yasmin and Yasminelle (another drospirenone-based pill) netted Bayer $670 million, making them the company's fifth bestselling group of pharmaceutical products that year.[500] The risks of drospirenone have not changed.

Shortly after the fatality data was made public in 2013, an article in the Canadian Medical Association's journal stated that the risks of blood clots were well known "and that the benefits of Yaz and Yasmin outweigh the potential dangers"[501]—a refrain that has echoed around birth control since it was first created, and which has over time worked to shift responsibility for risks onto patients and away from regulators, manufacturers and medical associations.

To be fair, Bayer isn't the only maker of drospirenone-based contraceptives, and these aren't the only hormonal contraceptives with problems. And not every user has side effects. Still, this is all pretty shocking if you sit down to think about it. Drugs meant to prevent pregnancy and/or reduce pain are being prescribed to millions of people with little discussion of potentially significant and maybe even fatal outcomes.

For some people—especially people in chronic pain—birth control may be worth the potential problems, and there are many good, trustworthy doctors. Even if you have the best doctor ever, though, we should probably still rethink how our culture gives doctors blanket trust and immunity from criticism. They are, after all, representatives and proxies of the medical and pharmaceutical systems we rely on. More transparency into that whole thing would be great. It's not likely, though—and that means it falls to us as individuals to take the initiative and read medical research to understand the real possible outcomes of prescriptions and to make informed decisions about whether the pill is worth those risks. Considering how unreadable a lot of scientific literature is, that's only possible for a portion of the population. That means a lot of us rely on what doctors tell us—and isn't it just so interesting how so many doctors conveniently downplay the psychiatric side effects of drugs, but also dismiss us as "crazy" when we challenge their opinions?

◆

When the fertility specialist told Lepage they would treat her endometriosis, she was hopeful that there would be some answer to her pain beyond going on another birth control pill.[502]

They prescribed Lupron instead.

Lupron Depot is a trade name for leuprolide acetate and belongs to a class of drugs called gonadotropin-releasing hormone (GnRH) agonists. Other brand names include Eligard, Leuplin and Enantone, but Lupron is by far the most popular name on the market and has become synonymous with the drug. It is an injection drug that essentially shuts down the pituitary gland; it reduces testosterone levels in testicles, and suppresses the pituitary gland-to-ovaries signal, lowering estrogen levels. The drug was first patented in 1973, and it was approved in 1985 for palliative treatment of advanced prostate cancer.[503] Since then, it's been repurposed at varying dosages for use in IVF,[504] chemical castration for male pedophiles and sex addicts,[505] gender transitions and puberty blocking.[506] For people with endometriosis, Lupron is used to temporarily stop menstruation by cutting off a patient's systemic estrogen and putting them into a state of fake menopause.

The FDA approved the monthly Lupron Depot shot for endometriosis in 1990; five years later, it was approved to improve the blood counts for anemia caused by fibroids. In 2001, the FDA approved combining Lupron with a progestin called norethindrone acetate as a way to prevent the diminished bone mineral density associated with the drug.[507] This is known as add-back therapy, where a progestin is added to counteract the bone loss caused by leuprolide acetate.

Although Lupron is not a contraceptive, it is becoming increasingly popular with doctors treating endometriosis. There is some evidence Lupron can help with endometriosis pain, and some people do benefit, but whether it's any better than contraceptives and NSAIDs is a subject of continuing debate in medical and scientific circles (including the American College of Obstetricians and Gynecologists[508]). That's partly because Lupron is only authorized for a maximum of six months of use across a person's entire life, or for twelve months with add-back therapy.[509] That means that a person with endometriosis is only supposed to take the drug for a year at most; after that year's up, their cramps and heavy bleeding return and it's back to the birth-control-and-naproxen grind.

We know that endometriosis creates its own supply of estrogen; if you took out someone's ovaries but left all their endometriosis behind, they would still likely grow more adhesions. This shows the premise of a drug like Lupron—that is, shutting off systemic estrogen to ostensibly prevent disease progression—is flawed from the jump. And yet it was the first thing suggested to me when I found myself in the office of Dr. Kapper (not her real name), the gynecologist from the sticky note that the stern red-haired doctor in the dog-poster office gave me.

I met Kapper when I was dangerously close to the end of my rope. I found myself in her office just a few months after the IUD incident and my morbid attempt at songwriting, and I was beyond desperate for someone—*anyone*—to operate on me. I didn't think I could handle another rejection. Cue the waterworks: as soon as she entered the office, tears of anxiety sprang to my eyes. I was overcome by a cocktail of emotions as cautious hope peeked through my anticipation of disappointment and the trauma of neglect. The more I fought to regain my composure, the more tears trickled down my cheeks. Kapper saw my bloodshot blue eyes and paused. I could see the doubt in her eyes. Perhaps, she ventured, I should try Lupron to see if I could "handle" menopause? After all, a hysterectomy without hormone therapy would throw me into a state of surgical menopause. Did I have the mental fortitude?

I paused. Lupron? I didn't know anything about any Lupron back then. What I did know was that natural menopause would come for me eventually, whether or not I tried it out first. It's not optional. Her proposal seemed asinine to me. I eyed her suspiciously and demurred. I would have to think about it, I told her.

Once home, I promptly consulted Dr. Google. The side effects of Lupron rolled out before me: long-lasting loss of memory and libido, insomnia, anxiety and joint pain. *Wow, sounds great.* Depression and suicidal thoughts, especially for those with a history of mental illness. *Cool, I just wrote a song about not caring if I died.* Bone mineral density loss . . . potentially irreversible? *Who needs bones, anyway?* I smirked at my screen as I thought about my former GP denying me a hysterectomy because of how it would erode my bones. And now here I was, with another doctor offering me a drug that would erode my bones. How interesting that bone loss was sanctioned in service of a drug I didn't want, but not the hysterectomy I desperately wanted.

I sat back in my office chair, my mind swirling with thoughts. How could Kapper think I was an appropriate candidate for this drug, when I was exactly the kind of person who shouldn't be taking it? My anxious brain went into spinning mode. Was this going to be like the time that the other gynecologist blackmailed me into getting an IUD? The spinning quickened. No! I would *not* be coerced. I had to stop it from happening again. I began pasting links and passages from research into my Notes app, evidence I would use to mount my defense.

The night before my second visit to Kapper's office, I reviewed my case and prepared for battle. But it was all for naught. Moments after I entered the exam room, I heard the news: that last ultrasound I'd done—the one that diagnosed my endo—showed I had too much disease for her surgical skills. I was a hot potato once again.

◆

Lepage, for her part, already knew about Lupron when her fertility specialist suggested it to her. She was a specialist in embryology and developmental biology, and she'd previously dealt with Lupron while working for oncology companies. She'd also taken it in tiny doses as part of her IVF protocol; it was part of the process of manipulating her hormones and ovaries into producing eggs. The Lupron hadn't been *so* bad then, she thought—like, maybe it wasn't exactly a walk in the park, but it also wasn't the worst thing she'd ever experienced. And besides, she'd come so far, having sunk so much time, heartache and $45,000 into IVF treatments. She'd had a miscarriage. She apparently had the ovaries of a fifty-year-old. She had just one single embryo to try, a one-shot deal. What's the worst that could happen? she said to herself. She brought the script to the pharmacy and forked over $400 for the drug's uninsured portion. Then she carried it to the fertility clinic, where a nurse injected it into her butt cheek.

Lupron is no joke for many of the endometriosis patients who take it.

Between 1984 and the start of 2022, the FDA recorded more than sixty thousand incidents of adverse reactions from people who took all available brands of leuprolide acetate for all reasons, and about half of those reactions were considered serious.[510] The FDA Adverse Event Reporting System (FAERS) database reveals that five people taking Lupron for endometriosis died by suicide, the most recently of whom was a thirty-seven-year-old woman in 2018. As well, at least seven others with some kind of menstruation-related disorder have attempted suicide to date.

FAERS data doesn't account for the pre-existing mental state of those who attempted or died by suicide, which makes it difficult to compare these figures to overall suicide statistics. However, an online search of "Lupron suicide" and "Lupron depression" show a number of anecdotal stories about the correlation. As well, consider the fact that 86 percent of women with chronic pelvic pain are depressed,[511] and that women are twice as likely as men to develop depression in their lifetimes.[512] Is enough being done by doctors to warn patients with histories or propensities for depression about the risks of certain drugs?

In my own experience, that answer is a resounding no.

The FAERS database has other limitations. First, submitting complaints is optional and can be done by anyone, including patients and their families. Keeping it open like this can improve transparency and accessibility, but it also introduces the potential for false or erroneous reporting. The reporting system doesn't account for those with an axe to grind, and it definitely doesn't demand proof that a medication directly caused an adverse reaction. As well, the way side effects are grouped and categorized in the dashboard leaves too much room for interpretation; the system doesn't easily distinguish whether a nervous system reaction is a headache or a seizure, whether a vascular reaction is a hot flush or an aneurysm. As for Lupron specifically, despite its many other uses, the drug is still primarily a cancer treatment and many of the adverse events reported are the deaths of cancer patients who may have died whether or not they took the drug. Simply put, there are too many caveats on FAERS data to use it as a standalone source of truth.

But it's still *a* source, and it points us in an important direction. Its data—in combination with outside research, medical opinions, patient testimonies, lawsuits and media stories—clearly shows that GnRH agonists are associated with serious consequences for a wide range of people. In addition to suicide risks, FAERS shows that some users of leuprolide acetate reported depression, anxiety, insomnia, panic attacks, hallucinations, intentional self-injury and a host of other psychiatric side effects. Meanwhile, a 2017 article from the Center for Investigative Reporting and Kaiser Health News reported that people in their twenties on Lupron suddenly began experiencing thinning of the bones and tooth enamel, osteoporosis, cracked spines and degenerative disc disease. A twenty-six-year-old needed a total hip replacement.[513] Additionally, the number of incidents reported in FAERS jumped by 28.4 percent between 2020 and 2021, suggesting more widespread prescribing of leuprolide acetate.

These side effects are life-altering, and yet none of the endometriosis patients who'd taken Lupron who spoke to me said they were fully informed of the physical and mental health risks at the time of prescription or administration. They were just told it would help with pain—and it did help some people. Kathryn Phillips, a thirty-eight-year-old cis woman of mixed race (Black and white), was on her second month of Lupron when we first spoke.[514] Hot flashes, nausea and vomiting followed the first dose, but after about two weeks it began to level off, and she felt pretty good. But she already knew that feeling good for a few months isn't a substitute for permanent relief. "I go back to my gynecologist in August. I'm going to push for a hysterectomy because I just want everything taken out. That's my end goal. She didn't say no, but I know you can't stay on Lupron for a long time," Phillips says.

When I follow up with her by email after that August meeting, Phillips says it was a no-go. "She shut it down right away because the Lupron has been successful in treating my symptoms," she says. "I want the hysterectomy. It's a shitty situation to be in."

Meanwhile, a newer drug called Orilissa—the same drug that Kellyn Pollard mentioned in the chapter Typical Girls—has been featuring heavily in endometriosis care since its 2018 entry onto North American markets. Orilissa is the trade name of a GnRH receptor antagonist called elagolix, which is expressly marketed as a solution for endometriosis pain.[515] (A second drug containing elagolix is Oriahnn, which also has estradiol and a progestin called norethindrone acetate; that drug is predominantly used on people with uterine fibroids.[516]) Elagolix works by binding to the pituitary gland's GnRH receptors and blocking normal GnRH signaling, which leads to lower production of estrogen and progesterone.[517]

For many patients actively taking it, Orilissa does reduce pain. It's reported that the 200-milligram dose helps every two or three people with painful periods who take it, and that the 150-milligram dose helps every four to six people.[518]

But it's a temporary solution with notable risks that include liver injury and bone loss, the latter of which is why elagolix is only approved for a maximum of twenty-four months at the once-daily 150 milligrams and six months at the twice-daily 200 milligrams.[519] The drug is also very expensive. In the U.S., the drug costs about $1,000 a month for the one-a-day, 150-milligram dose, and about $2,000 a month for the two-a-day 200-milligram dose.[520] A 2018 report on the drug's cost-benefit ratio noted just one-quarter of eligible patients would be able to afford the drug, and that elagolix was cost effective only when compared to no treatment at all.[521]

The drug carries a warning for suicidal ideation and behavior, because a clinical trial participant died by suicide while testing it.[522] Despite this, the drug was still approved by the FDA and Health Canada in 2018. Since then, FAERS notes another suicide took place in 2020, and that eight other people have attempted suicide. When I asked the FDA why they approved a drug linked to a clinical trial suicide, they responded that they take all reports of suicidal ideation and behavior seriously. In this particular case, they tell me, they couldn't determine whether the suicide was related to Orilissa or to other life stressors.[523]

◆

Soon after getting the Lupron shot injected into her butt cheek, Lepage's hormones began swinging like a pendulum on speed. She slept maybe one or two hours a night, three if she was lucky. She was debilitated by a pseudo period caused by the initial spikes in estrogen, one of the most painful experiences of her life. She desperately wanted the Lupron out of her system, but there was no way to reverse the injection. On the phone we morbidly laugh that it's like gobbling up a handful of potent THC edibles; you can't stop the train once it's in motion.

American endometriosis surgeon Dr. Jeff Arrington says stories like Lepage's highlight a key way misinformed consent propagates through endometriosis care. Hormonal contraceptives and GnRH modulators may mask some endometriosis pain, but they don't stop the spread of the disease as far as current research shows.[524]

Yet you would be hard-pressed to find a doctor who would admit this in a consultation; they either don't know it, or they don't care.

"Some may think, 'This [drug] can make my life easier, this can make my practice easier,'" explains Arrington. "They're going to jump all over it, really without even doing a lot of due diligence; they'll just hear the numbers presented [by] the drug company. But yet they don't kind of delve into them and find out what these numbers really say and what they really do."

All they hear is "endometriosis" and "drug" and they immediately interpret that to mean the drug treats the disease when in fact it only modulates pain, he continues. "They say, 'We're going to use this medicine to suppress the disease' or 'We're going to use this medicine to prevent the progression,'" says Arrington.

"Too many doctors don't actually define what 'suppress' means, and there is no data to support 'preventing progression,'" Arrington says, noting that the American College of Obstetricians and Gynecologists (ACOG) bulletin on endometriosis management supports his argument.[525] It's mentioned in passing on the seventh of the bulletin's nine pages, easy enough for a quick or careless reader to miss. But there it is, in black and white: "There are no data to support use of medical treatment to prevent progression of the disease."[526]

The endometriosis specialist says that because of that fact's lack of prominence in the ACOG bulletin, many doctors aren't even aware that drugs like hormonal contraceptives, as well as GnRH agonists and antagonists, don't stop the spread of endometriosis. "People just read through that and say, 'This hormone will keep your endo from progressing' and it doesn't," says Arrington.[527]

Strangely, even ACOG's director of clinical practice, Dr. Christopher Zahn, tells me that GnRH agents can stop progression by "burning lesions out"—causing them to die through hormonal manipulation.[528] He maintains this even after I read that line back to him: "There are no data to support use of medical treatment to prevent progression of the disease."

"Well, again," he replies, "There's not large-scale data, but certainly there is data to support that patients may . . ." He trails off. "I mean, look at it this way: if there wasn't data to support that, why would we use it?"

Why, indeed.

◆

Because drugs form the first line of endo treatment, patients who want kids end up spending five, ten, fifteen years on contraceptives and other hormonal drugs thinking they're stopping the spread, only to realize when trying to conceive that their disease has progressed to such an extent that their fertility is totally compromised. Patients who don't want children often become sicker and sicker through medical inaction until their case is so advanced that hours of surgical work are required, commonly involving the removal of some or all of their reproductive organs.

At various stages of her life, Lepage has been on all sides of that issue, and then some.

Her Lupron-and-implantation ordeal was momentarily fruitful: she got pregnant. Not long after, though, Lepage miscarried again— except it wasn't a normal miscarriage. It was a *missed* miscarriage, meaning the embryo had died but her uterus had not expelled it.[529]

Heartbroken, she had a D&C at the end of November to remove the tissue, a procedure meant to spare her the trauma of passing it at home. By January, though, her HCG pregnancy hormone hadn't gone back down to zero as it should have. The doctors shrugged it off, telling her she was probably fine. Then she got a period unlike any other, in which big "chunks of tissue" slipped out. Lepage thought back to another recent trip to the bathroom and put it all together.

Before the period, she had spotted what could have been an embryo in her toilet. "Like, it could have been another piece of tissue that just looked very much like, you know, an eight-week embryo.

But also, embryology and developmental biology is my specialty. I have a PhD in that. I have seen many, many embryos. This was totally an embryo," says Lepage. She took a picture just in case, but when she explained what happened and showed her doctors the picture, they denied it, saying it was simply impossible.

Given her training, Lepage would know as well as any fertility specialist what a human embryo looks like—and yet, in the sick role, her expert-level knowledge was totally written off, even when she brought photographic evidence to support her discovery. "I felt like I was crazy, like I was being told that I was making it up," she says.

While reeling from the experience, she received an unexpected call. She could have her endometriosis excision surgery in six weeks, her surgeon told her. She'd only just been placed on his waitlist a month earlier, and expected a long wait because elective surgeries had been put on hold due to COVID-19. His call came at a time of major sadness and frustration; she'd miscarried in such a traumatic way, and she was running out of options to get pregnant.

Feeling unlucky about her prospects for conceiving, her mind shifted back to her pain. Even if she never birthed a baby, at least the surgery could help ease her suffering, she thought. "I was willing to basically try anything to get my pain to stop, and the fact that I'm likely not going to get pregnant and the fact that I'm going to poten-tially have periods for the next ten years at least . . . I can't do this. I need some options to help reduce the pain. But I also didn't want to close the door on trying to conceive. So that's why I didn't want to go the hormonal route," she tells me.

"I spoke to a surgeon about getting the surgery done, and he seemed pretty optimistic about the whole thing. I felt like it was my only shot."

None of the patients I spoke to for *BLEED* had an ending to their stories. Their fights aren't over. Maybe they'll never be over. As a potentially lifelong disease, there may be years of inactivity, followed by short intense periods where *everything* happens. This disease forces us to face many, many crossroads over time, often leaving us to choose between the lesser of two (or more) evils.

I followed up with Lepage by email a couple of months after we first spoke. She had her excision surgery in the late winter, with the hopes it could improve her chances of conceiving. Or, at the very least, her chances of being pain-free. The surgeon removed the big cyst, as well as the adhesions down the back of her uterus and one that had glued her uterus and an ovary together. She most definitely had endometriosis, he told her. At the very least, after all this, she finally had a diagnosis. But that realization only gave her short-term relief. As she told me in an email:

> Just six months after surgery, and I already have new suspected endo cysts and lesions, including in places it never was before. I learned that my uterus is anteverted-retroflexed, which is quite common for people with endo, and probably explains a lot of my symptoms. Not sure if this is new, but it's the first I've heard of it. I also learned for the first time that there's evidence of adenomyosis and possible bladder involvement. Basically, I'm a huge mess.
>
> The surgeon presented these options:
>
> 1. Do nothing (if I want to keep trying to conceive)
>
> 2. Three months of GnRH agonist/antagonist, then reassess
>
> 3. Another surgery
>
> I could probably deal with the pain for a bit longer, honestly, but I'm worried about my urinary tract symptoms. I've recently had recurring UTIs and UTI-like

symptoms that I didn't think much of until my ultra-sound revealed mild bladder dysfunction. Not 100 percent sure it's endo-related, but I don't want to risk this getting worse.

Surgery seems pointless to me since my endo came back so fast after the first. My surgeon agrees this is the least desirable option.

So that leaves me with drugs. This scares me—Lupron was a nightmare. Instead, he prescribed Orilissa, so that I can easily adjust the dose or stop taking it if the side effects are too much to handle. After three months, if things have improved, I'll take one last try at getting pregnant. If no improvement, I'm going to cut my losses and seek a hysterectomy. I will be starting Orilissa with my next period, so sometime next week. Can't say I'm looking forward to it.[530]

◆

In 2018, Orilissa became the first drug approved for endometriosis in twenty-eight years.[531] The one that preceded it was Lupron.

Both drugs are made by the same company: AbbVie.

AbbVie didn't discover elagolix. It was discovered in the late 1990s by a pharmaceutical development company called Neurocrine Biosciences.[532] In 2010, that company entered into an agreement with Abbott Laboratories to develop and commercialize elagolix; when AbbVie spun off from Abbott, it inherited the partnership. At the time of signing, the partnership was estimated to be worth US$575 million.[533] According to annual SEC filings from 2010 to 2021, Neurocrine has already collected more than $355 million from

AbbVie for activities related to Orilissa and Oriahnn, including $57.4 million in sales royalties.[534]

Since elagolix's 2018 FDA approval until the end of 2021, the drug has so far netted AbbVie $374 million, according to its SEC filings.[535] Perhaps even more interestingly, it is one of the drugs AbbVie pays the most to promote. In 2018, the year that Orilissa entered the market, manufacturer AbbVie spent $767,000 on payments to 12,202 physicians.[536] The drug was only approved in late July, leaving just five months left in the year. The company has also paid celebrity influencers like professional dancer Julianne Hough to promote the drug. As now-defunct media outlet *The Outline* reported, "AbbVie [. . .] orchestrated awareness campaigns to drive media coverage of endometriosis as part of the launch of its own endometriosis drug, Orilissa, the 'first and only' treatment of its kind, in that it treats endometriosis-related pain. With an estimated 200 million worldwide potential patients, many of whom are undiagnosed or without access to available treatments, AbbVie has engaged this kind of advertising to expand the 'top of the funnel' for the sale of Orilissa."[537]

To endometriosis patients, this cash grab doesn't necessarily signal relief. In fact, for many patients the medical process of solving their pain—which is already front-loaded with pharmaceuticals—probably won't improve at all. As the Neurocrine Biosciences SEC filings note, elagolix is in direct competition with hysterectomies and ablations—and, one presumes, excisions.[538]

AbbVie also pays a considerable amount annually to promote Lupron to doctors. In 2018, the company spent $4.32 million on Lupron-related payments to 11,680 physicians. The top ten recipients were obstetricians, gynecologists and reproductive endocrinologists, each of whom accepted between $72,000 and $95,000 of Lupron money.[539] In 2021, AbbVie made $783 million from Lupron worldwide.[540]

AbbVie hasn't always been Lupron's manufacturer. It originated under the wing of TAP Pharmaceutical Products, a joint venture between Takeda Pharmaceutical Company and Abbott Laboratories— a company that was subject to a federal investigation following a whistleblower complaint over how TAP marketed Lupron. The case centered on an accusation that TAP sales reps colluded with doctors to double-dip the Medicare system by getting government reimbursements for free samples provided by TAP. In 2001, the company was ordered to pay $875 million for committing Medicare fraud and illegal marketing around Lupron.[541, 542]

In 2008, the company split; Takeda took over the TAP brand and Lupron went to Abbott.[543] Three years later, another Takeda whistleblower tried to sound an alarm, this time about the company allegedly hiding side effects of several of its drugs. Although it was a different sort of allegation than the double-dipping scheme, court records revealed a compelling conversation between the whistleblower and a colleague: "Dr. Chapman asked Dr. Ge [the whistleblower] why TAP never learned its lesson from Lupron, and Dr. Ge told him that it was because the Lupron fine was not big enough, and they both believed that to be true."[544]

The reality is, both Lupron and Orilissa are part of an industry-wide practice that in the U.S. sees billions in pharma money handed out to hundreds of thousands of doctors, either in direct payments, research grants or in-kind gifts. According to the publicly accessible federal reporting system Open Payments, in 2021 533,056 physicians and 1,237 teaching hospitals received a collective sum of US$10.9 billion in disclosed payments from 1,721 pharmaceutical and medical device companies.[545] Of that total, $7.09 billion was earmarked for research and $1.26 billion was derived from ownership stakes and investment interest. The remainder, $2.55 billion, is classified as "general payments"—speaking and consulting fees, free samples, coffees and dinners, travel and lodging and so on. Doctors across all areas of medicine benefit from this system.

That said, the database shows that in 2020 more than 165,000 payments ranging from one cent to $9,975 were made to 33,905 doctors in the field of obstetrics and gynecology. Some practitioners received multiple payments; for example, in 2020, one gynecologist collected a total of $90,739 over sixty-five payments from AbbVie—which, in addition to Lupron and Orilissa, is a major maker of hormonal contraceptives. That same doctor's global take in 2020 from all her pharma suitors amounted to just over $148,000, of which just $13,750 was earmarked for research.[546]

While most doctors would probably say that they are independent, ethical thinkers who aren't swayed by drug marketing, extensive reporting proves that isn't quite true. Dollars for Docs, a years-long reporting effort by nonprofit investigative journalism outlet ProPublica, shows that even a free lunch out with a drug company rep can lead doctors to prescribe more of that company's drugs—and drug companies spend billions on lunches, coffees, travel, lodging, conference speakers' fees, consulting fees and grants.[547] See it for yourself: if you have a doctor in the U.S., look up how much money and in-kind gifts they have received from drug and medical device companies on OpenPaymentsData.cms.gov.

If your country doesn't have a database like Open Payments, it's not because doctors don't take cash; it's because there's no legal obligation or effort to disclose it to the public. For instance, Canada doesn't currently have laws that compel doctors or companies to disclose payments. That said, ten pharmaceutical companies agreed in 2017 to annually report aggregated sums of money paid to Canadian doctors and institutions[548]—except that this information isn't in any central repository, and the information that is available doesn't clearly show who received how much for what reason. It is also unclear who, if anyone, holds these companies accountable for disclosing accurate information. Nonetheless, in 2019, AbbVie said it paid Canadian doctors and institutions $8.1 million in fees for healthcare professional services, $4.1 million to healthcare organizations and $475,149 in healthcare professionals' travel fees.[549]

There's a lot we don't know about this problem. What we do know, however, is that the entire point of drug company marketing and schmoozing is to influence doctors to prescribe a company's drugs and devices, and it is incredibly effective. A research team at Memorial Sloan Kettering Cancer Center in 2020 found that receiving industry money increases brand-name prescribing over generics, and that contributes to ballooning healthcare costs for everyone.[550]

The issue of physician payments is so pervasive that the American College of Obstetricians and Gynecologists (ACOG) itself took a position on it. In 2012, it published a committee opinion, which it reaffirmed in 2020: "Evidence has accumulated that gifts from industry often misdirect physicians from their primary responsibility, which is to act consistently in the best interests of their patients. Several studies have demonstrated that the prescribing practices of physicians are influenced by both subtle and obvious marketing messages and gifts. Marketing influence on prescribing was found even when the gifts were of nominal value and delivered in an educational context. The physicians studied did not recognize or admit to any changes in their practice of medicine."[551]

Ironically, an analysis done by a group of gynecologists published in 2020 found that a number of agenda-setting members of ACOG received payments from drug and device makers.[552] Using Open Payments data from 2014 to 2016, they found that forty-four members of the OBGYN practice bulletin committees received a collective $60,403. About 10 percent of these payments were in the form of food and drink; the remainder were honoraria, consulting and speaking fees, and travel and lodging.

ACOG's conflict of interest policy says that board directors, committee chairs, task force chairs and executive staff are barred from accepting anything more than $50 at a time, to a maximum of

$250 a year, from any pharmaceutical or medical device company.[553] However, as the writers of the 2020 analysis point out, this policy is not inclusive of every single person sitting on practice bulletin committees, and committees may have more than thirty people on each of them.[554] Committee members are asked to avoid conflicts of interest and have to submit disclosures of all business dealings above $100 for review by ACOG staff.[555]

However, ACOG also does not publish the names of its committee members, and declined to provide me with their names—meaning I could not look them up in Open Payments.

Even though the analysis writers found three physicians who were noncompliant with the conflict of interest policy, they said they found no evidence of bias within practice bulletins and "only minimal" conflicts about those involved in developing ACOG's clinical practice guidelines.

Even with this policy in place, though, some people working in endometriosis believe that conflicts have swayed ACOG's stance on treating the disease.

Heather Guidone of the Center for Endometriosis Care suggests ACOG has clearly been influenced to favor pharmaceutical interventions over surgery in its endometriosis guidelines. "ACOG is well funded by pharma, and their endometriosis stance reflects that," she says.[556]

Indeed, various people working in endometriosis care and education have alleged that excision has gotten the shaft in favor of pharmaceutical interventions—and that money and industry ties have a lot to do with it.

Zahn at ACOG says it isn't so.[557] When he and I speak in July 2022—under the watchful eye of a press officer—I point out that after having sifted through Open Payments records, the practice of OBGYNs accepting pharma money seemed fairly widespread.

"I think that is incorrect and too simplified an assumption," he answers. "Our conflict of interest policy specifies [that] our board of directors and committee members and committee leadership cannot have a financial arrangement [with pharmaceutical companies]." As for clinicians in general accepting cash and gifts, Zahn says the days of pharma companies springing for ski trips are long gone, the PhRMA Code having ostensibly put the kibosh on them back in 2002 when it was created. Standing for the Pharmaceutical Research and Manufacturers of America, PhRMA is a group of pharmaceutical and biotech companies. Their code—which offers guidance on navigating financial relationships between clinicians and companies—is entirely voluntary. Still, Zahn maintains that "funding that is received and what industry is allowed to do is much different currently than what it used to be a number of years ago," and that change is largely attributable to self-regulation in the pharma industry. Now, he adds, "Anything that you're doing with an individual clinician has to be tied to education."

But of course, with more than 62,000 members, ACOG is not in a position to enforce any guidelines on accepting cash for people beyond institutional and committee leadership. With its voluntary adherence, the PhRMA Code is clearly not an enforcement mechanism either.

By law, clinicians have to disclose any pharma money they get—hence, the existence of Open Payments. Open Payments puts hard numbers on soft enforcement. Even if companies promise their money is going toward strictly educational purposes, allowing the industry to self-regulate on this practice leaves a lot of room for creative accountability.

Also ironic is that the Open Payments database shows that some of the writers on the conflict of interest analysis have also collected money from drug companies, though they were comparatively tiny amounts. Still, I think, their criticism holds water—and, if anything, shows just how pervasive and systemic the practice is.

A little bit of pharma money can go an awful long way. Guidone tells me that she and a group of other advocates trying to modernize

ACOG's endometriosis guidelines provided more than 60 citations as to why surgical excision should become the gold standard of care, only to be told there was not enough compelling evidence to promote excision. Meanwhile, she says, the committee accepted comparatively scant evidence from pharma that their drugs work.

Put another way, most money looking at endometriosis comes from—and goes to—pharma. The proof is in the pudding: right now, endometriosis patients are overwhelmingly treated with what specialist surgeon Arrington says is "palliative care"—pharmaceutical interventions that may take the edge off the pain and bleeding but which do not meaningfully address the disease.[558] Many doctors treat endometriosis patients this way because that's what they're taught, and because that's what ACOG's guidelines say they should do.

In our call, Zahn tries to play down ACOG's responsibility. "I think one of the things I need to probably set straight, is I think you're interpreting the guidance as this is the bible. It's not. Guidance is guidance. These are guidelines on how you can treat patients and diagnose patients," he says. "But all of those have to be taken into the individualization approach. There is no, like, 'Here's the checklist, go through every step on the list.'"[559]

It's true that ACOG does not have rule-setting authority in the ways that medical boards and colleges do. It's also true that ACOG's guidelines are used to guide the treatment of endometriosis by OBGYNs—and sometimes other clinicians—across the U.S. Arrington says that while ACOG might argue its bulletin is not an attempt to define standards of care, it's very much used that way on the ground.

"That is not the reality of what it's used for in residency training," he says. "It's opening the door for OBGYNs to follow what they are taught from those documents, or follow the main points of the documents and then they get a patient where they've been on hormones for five years and then find out their fertility is shot and she's upset. If that patient comes back with an informed consent problem to the doctor, I mean, ACOG is leaving them hanging out to dry."

From secretive drug trials to mass-sterilization campaigns to uteruses perforated by IUDs to whistleblower complaints to billions in drug-company payments to doctors and hospitals, the pharmaceutical industry has its claws buried deep inside female reproductive health—and really it's only the beginning. A market research firm said in early 2022 that the endometriosis drug market is expected to grow from $1.1 billion in 2020 to $2.98 by 2030—buoyed by additional GnRH antagonists coming onto the market and greater awareness of endometriosis.[560]

With this seventy-year legacy and future market outlook weighing on their care, how can endometriosis patients ever possibly win?

◆

Talking about the forces that make hormonal contraceptives a steady, reliable cash cow for doctors' offices and pharmaceutical companies might make me seem like I have a desk drawer full of shiny aluminum-foil hats. I don't mean to imply that we should throw away all our pills, rip out our IUDs and never trust another doctor ever again. What I'm saying is that the trouble with all these drugs is that it's hard to know their troubles.

If we assume patients primarily learn of potential side effects from reading the package insert, that means they will only know these risks once they've already paid for their prescription. For Depo-Provera, that could run them anywhere from $0 to $150 every three months. Lupron, meanwhile, costs anywhere from a few hundred dollars to almost $1,900 out of pocket, depending on insurance coverage.

And that's if they get to read the warnings at all. Lupron and Depo-Provera are administered by injection, which means nurses and pharmacists are typically the ones who unseal the packaging and inject the drug. Assuming the package isn't tossed into the trash, a patient might only get their first real opportunity to read the insert once the drug has already been injected into them. Even if they do read it beforehand, though, is metaphorically clicking "agree" on this impossibly long terms-and-conditions agreement really considered informed consent?

Lepage, for her part, did know about the side effects of these drugs before taking them. She took them anyway because she was desperate for pain relief and wanted to have a baby.

Her experience with healthcare is representative of how we are all failed, and harmed, by the system in our own unique ways, be it through laziness, willful gaslighting or sheer incompetence: The GP who couldn't find Lepage's cervix. The doctor who didn't investigate fourteen-year-old Lepage's pain. The one who forgot her name in the middle of the appointment. All the doctors who didn't take her pain seriously, until she wanted to conceive—and even then, there was the fertility specialist who failed her when she denied that the post-miscarriage D&C was incomplete. Lepage spent years of her life not even bothering with doctors because she didn't think they would help. But she went back eventually, because she was suffering. And that's the rub, isn't it? We always go back. After trying painkillers and hormones and vitamins and yoga and carb-free diets and weight-lifting and psychologists and CBD oil and just getting out in nature, the pain is still there.

So, what else can we do, but go to the doctor?

And then those doctors tell us having kids will get rid of the pain. That losing weight will cure our disease. That the hormones only work locally, with no systemic effects. That they ration painkillers to make sure some of us don't become addicts, while giving drugs freely to others. That a hysterectomy is a cure, except they won't excise the disease outside of our uteruses.

I ask Lepage what she wants doctors to know.

"It's hard to advocate for yourself," she answers. "And, really, should you have to advocate for yourself? How much do you have to complain that you're in pain before somebody listens? And then in terms of which options are available to you—as somebody who's dealing with gynecological problems, it's just 'slap some hormones on it.' That seems to always be the solution, with very little follow-up. Let's talk about long-term plans. And let's talk about what the source of your pain is, versus 'Oh, it just has to do with your uterus.'"

After her excision surgery in mid-March 2021, she hoped she would be able to close the chapter on one of the most difficult parts of her story. But when we speak three months later, she tells me her period just ended: "It was in my top five of the worst ones I've ever had."

7. I WANNA BE WELL

the pain scale and other lies

In retrospect, I probably shouldn't have gone to the bachelorette party.

I'd woken up that morning with terrible cramps. It was day two or three of my period, but so what? I'd pushed through my pain so many times before. Surely, I could high-function my way into having a good time. I hoped a few drinks and some laughs with friends would distract me enough to make the best of a shitty situation.

If I'm being honest, though, I was tired—really, really tired.

Six weeks before the party, on September 6, 2019—the day I frantically called Kapper from the airport—I'd traveled to New Orleans to catch up with my old roommate Diana; once she returned home, I stayed on alone to attend a journalism conference. Then I flew directly to Chicago to visit one of my BFFs, Kat, and attend the Riot Fest punk rock festival. I was home for a week before hitting the road again, this time flying off to Oslo, Norway, for a tech conference whose organizers had graciously paid my way to be there. I took advantage of my Scandinavian jaunt, tacking on thirty-six hours in Copenhagen before heading home—a day and a half where I biked all over the city, through an open-air hash market to a friend's hair salon to chat, drink rosé and get a bang trim.

In between that flurry of activity, I got my period. It always ran like clockwork, every twenty-two-ish days, and I'd become so attuned to its warning signs I could usually predict within a few hours when it would start. Before taking off for Oslo, I stuffed my menstrual cup, fistfuls of pads and tampons, extra underwear, my wearable TENS machine and my bottle of prescription naproxen into my suitcase. (A TENS machine is an electrical device that reduces pain signals in the body and helps generate more endorphins, which are natural painkillers.)

But no amount of supplies could have prepared me for just how awful this period would be. It arrived during my twenty-hour overnight trip. As usual, the first day was pretty bearable: some pain, some bleeding, lots of exhaustion. The second and third days were always the worst; on those days, I'd have to empty my menstrual cup seven to ten times a day to prevent it from capsizing inside me. And the pain—oh, the pain. My 550-milligram tablets of naproxen at the start and end of the day, plus two Tylenol every four hours in between, barely took the edge off. The agony hit me from all sides: I always felt it in my pelvic floor, in my rectum, in my lower abdomen, plus headaches and shoulder pain from near-constant bracing and teeth grinding.

More recently, though, I'd also developed a new, seemingly random pain: intense charley horses that contorted my calf muscles and ankle tendons, locking my feet into ninety-degree angles. They always happened at night, jolting me out of a deep sleep. In the dark, I would silently pace around my room, kneading my leg, trying to get my ankle to rotate so I could free my foot. That summer they happened a few times a month, and no matter what I did, they still rocked me out of my sleep without any apparent schedule.

When I got off the plane in Oslo, my abdomen was so swollen that my skin ached to the touch. Still, I had a long list of things to get done, and it was only early afternoon. After dropping my bag off at the hotel, I walked fifteen minutes to pick up my conference badge.

Stretching my legs and breathing in the crisp Nordic air felt good after such a long flight. I met the media liaison at the café serving as a venue for a panel that evening, and she offered me free pizza and salad. I hung around until the sun began to set. It was still the first day of my period, so it wasn't awful yet. I took advantage by stopping in on a bartender friend whom I'd met the previous year while attending the same conference. I sat at the bar and had a few drinks while we chatted over rock 'n' roll and the loud laughter of a pair of American patrons. Ah, *this*—this is why traveling alone is the best, I thought as I walked back to the hotel. I took my makeup off, washed my face, brushed my teeth, took a naproxen and went to sleep.

Around 3 a.m., a leg cramp shook me out of bed. My calf was rock-hard and unmoving, so seized I couldn't put my foot flat on the floor. I lunged forward and bore down on the joint, trying to free these wicked calf demons, but they refused to be cast out. After an hour of pacing, massaging, stretching and crying, I laid down and began Googling in the dark: *recurring leg cramps at night. Potassium. Potassium-rich foods. How do I know if I'm getting enough potassium?* None of the results made sense in my situation. I thought for a minute, then started a new search: *Naproxen leg cramps.*

I was surprised to read the results that rolled out before me. In rare cases, naproxen can be associated with leg cramps, the *American Family Physician*[561] journal told me; in fact, up to 3 percent of patients experience this side effect. I was thirty-five then and had been on prescription naproxen since the age of twelve or thirteen, yet this was the first time I'd ever heard of such a link. I thought back to my summertime charley horses. They *did* seem to coincide with my cycle, I thought. I put my phone down on the duvet, my vertiginous thoughts dancing around the inside of my skull. While the drug hadn't been helping much for a long time, I felt married to it because it was the only painkiller doctors would prescribe me. Now that I'd connected it to my leg cramps, I felt backed into a corner: nothing works. Alone in the dark Norwegian hotel room, 3,500 miles away from home, I wept.

I returned home at the end of September and hit the ground running. Four medical appointments happened in quick succession: the first, the ultrasound that diagnosed my stage-four endo and adenomyosis; the second, an explosive appointment during which I fired my GP (more on that later); the third, the one with Kapper in which she said my endo was too complex for her surgery skills; and the fourth, my first consultation with the surgeon to whom I brought my hysterectomy permission slip. Three days after that last one was the bachelorette party.

It was a humid mid-October night, and I'd driven myself the two and a half hours to my hometown of Montreal to partake in the festivities. My period joined me—and worse, it was day three. I'd resolved to stop taking naproxen for a while to test my charley horse theory. That meant I was toughing it out with off-the-shelf Advil and Tylenol and my TENS machine. Surely I could do this, I thought. I was tough. I was high-functioning. I was *used to it*. And, if I'm being completely honest, I was afraid to be excluded from the group, my fear of abandonment magnified by my plummeting hormones and spiking emotions. I arrived in town a couple hours early to get ready, and in a friend's guest bedroom, I styled my hair and put on eyeliner, eyeshadow and mascara; on my lips, my favorite magenta lipstick. I dressed in my go-to pair of high-waisted stretchy black jeans and a black T-shirt emblazoned with the name of an Italian glam rock band written in big pink bubble letters. I tucked Advil, pads and tampons into my purse, and away we went.

Little did I know I was running head-on into a breaking point.

My friend and I arrived at the hotel suite which we'd pitched in to rent for the bride-to-be's party and found our pals sitting around, eating snacks and sipping fancy cocktails made by our tiki-enthusiast friend who'd been recruited to tend bar. Punk rock and '80s hits wafted out of a Bluetooth speaker as people circulated, greeting each other with the double-cheek kiss customary in Quebec. I grabbed a cocktail and took a seat on the couch. The party organizer handed us an assortment of funny homemade tiaras with various words glued to them. I plucked the one spelling "badass" out of the pile and put it on my head.

I thought I looked pretty cute, all things considered. But when I look back at the selfies I took that night, my eyes are so obviously heavy with exhaustion and pain. I'd always thought no one else could see it, but I suppose I wasn't good at hiding my pain anymore.

A couple of drinks into the night, sharp, nauseating pains began stabbing me in my guts. I fished a couple of Advil out of my bag and quickly downed them, hoping they would lessen the blow. Then I felt it: a panic attack rising in my chest. I didn't get them often, but when I did I usually opted to run home so I could hyperventilate by myself. But I didn't live down the street anymore; my bed was two and a half hours away. I was about to be *seen*.

I ducked into a bathroom, hoping no one would notice my absence or knock on the lockless door. Some solitude would help me calm down, I thought. I looked in the mirror and dabbed the corners of my bloodshot eyes with a tissue, trying to stop the tears from ruining my makeup. I admonished myself: *You shouldn't have come. They would have been better off without you.*

As time ticked on in the bathroom, the anxiety began to wane. I made a plan: just go outside to smoke some weed, get some crisp air on your face, come back more chill, have fun. But as I prepared to make my escape, the bathroom door flew open. A fellow partygoer whom I didn't know all that well saw my puffy face and demanded to know what was wrong. Her alarm summoned others to the bathroom, and people began crowding the door. A chorus of concern mounted. All I had wanted was to be invisible, to bring down my anxiety and blend into the background. Now, a spotlight shone directly over me. I grappled around in my pit of anxiety looking for an explanation, but the words that tripped out of my mouth sounded like dumb excuses.

The thing about other uterus-havers is that they all think they know what periods and cramps are, and I felt judged for being such a weenie. I could almost hear them thinking, "How could you ruin this special day by making it about you?" Feeling cornered and deeply embarrassed, I could not overpower the intense urge to flee. I pushed my way out of the bathroom, grabbed my jacket and bolted.

Outside, I leaned against a wall on a secluded side street around the corner from the hotel, sucking on my weed vape and hoping the gentle, low-THC high would tamp down my pain and distract me from my panic. Staring into the fluorescent lights of a gas station across the street, I pondered how to return to the party gracefully. Could I summon a good joke out of this wreck?

A ding interrupted my thoughts. From inside the suite, a close friend texted that they were about to take off for their next destination. Could she get me anything? I asked for the purse I'd left inside the hotel suite.

As she joined me to deliver my bag, words came tumbling out of my head. It was my first period since my diagnosis. I couldn't take my painkillers anymore. The ultrasound proved I was right all along—I *was* sick. That means I spent two-thirds of my life being gaslit. How was it right? How was it fair? The tears once again breached my lower eyelid, streaming down my face. My friend rubbed my shoulder and listened empathetically, telling me that none of it should have happened to me. Then the stretch limo pulled up and the crew poured out of the hotel, ready to hit new wave night in the Gay Village. I watched them from the sidelines, too ashamed to be included. Everyone was in such good spirits, laughing and taking photos and it occurred to me that maybe I hadn't ruined the evening. Maybe I could still salvage my good time.

As the limo pulled away, I started walking the mile to the bar. I hoped some alone time and a slow, meandering stroll through my old neighborhood would let me shake off my nerves. I arrived before the others, who were no doubt partying it up in the limo somewhere. So I decided to wait outside. As I perched myself on a shallow cement ledge, a drunk creeper tried to hit me up for conversation. Then two strangers began yelling on the sidewalk. My cortisol spiked again. Fearful this scene would ruin my progress, I retreated inside and took a seat on a shabby Victorian-style sofa. Soon, my friends eventually sauntered into the bar in a chorus of happy, tipsy chatter.

I looked at them but felt incapable of controlling my legs. That's when I knew it was over. The pain and anxiety had won. I waited for the end of the night, glued to the couch at the back of the room, mired in a dissociative state as my friends danced under a disco ball to Billy Idol and Depeche Mode.

◆

Pain is so complicated.

Most people experience pain when they stub a toe, do too many lunges, cut their finger slicing cucumbers, fall down some stairs or get a headache from drinking too many margaritas. The pain they feel is the consequence of an action, deliberate or not. Some people get predictable pain, like a killer migraine or an achy knee on a rainy day. And sometimes we do things that we know will cause pain, like getting a tattoo or forgoing an epidural during childbirth.

These pains are nothing like chronic pelvic pain.

It's true that not everyone with endometriosis has chronic pelvic pain, and not everyone with chronic pelvic pain has endometriosis. A range of research studies have shown us that one out of every three to five AFAB people regularly experience painful sex, a condition scientifically known as dyspareunia, regardless of any other health conditions.[562] It's so prevalent that some are shocked to discover that sex *isn't* supposed to hurt. If you put on a brave face and have sex anyway, sometimes even orgasms can hurt. Talk about a thankless task.

Among endometriosis patients, two-thirds of us experience sexual dysfunction including painful sex, and about half that figure experiences deep dyspareunia.[563, 564] It's exactly what it sounds like: deep vaginal pain, sometimes accompanied by pain near where nodules and adhesions are present, or loss of tissue elasticity due to the disease. An adhesion in the colon can make the pressure and rubbing from vaginal penetration downright excruciating. Sometimes all the lube in the world can't stop sex from feeling like you're copulating with sentient sandpaper. These instances are commonly classified as deep infiltrating endometriosis—unironically shortened to DIE—which affects up to 37 percent of those with the disease.[565]

There's little opportunity for reprieve.

In many situations, people avoid the source of their pain. You don't get burned, then immediately put your hand back on the stove. Fool me once, right? In that way, vaginal and pelvic pain are unlike anything else. We are expected to continue having sex despite our pain, because we want it, because they want it, because we've been socialized to believe it's supposed to hurt, because we are afraid of losing our relationships if we don't have it often enough. The tightness of internal pelvic pain can't be softened by Advil or naproxen, or fixed through vigorous exercise or a "clean" diet. Pelvic floor physiotherapy can help relax tightened pelvic muscles and promote healing, but it is expensive, invasive and a frustratingly well-kept secret among GPs. (Hot tip: if you have insurance, you can usually claim it under general physiotherapy. Also, look up pelvic wands.)

Chronic pelvic pain interlaces with our brains to create crossover experiences of mind-body suffering. It routinely triggers loops of depression, anxiety and pain catastrophizing—that is, ruminating and magnifying pain, and feeling helpless and hopeless about being able to control it.[566] This is common across all kinds of chronic pain, with a team of Brazilian researchers finding that 85 percent of chronic pain sufferers are depressed, as are 86 percent of chronic pelvic pain sufferers.[567]

Concerning endometriosis specifically, a 2019 study done by the BBC in partnership with Endometriosis UK showed half of the 13,500 respondents said they'd contemplated suicide.[568] The BBC study flagged a lack of support as the main reason, but chronic pain is another major precursor to taking one's own life.[569] That's what happened to Trinity Lillian Graves, and to many, many others. Sometimes people accidentally die from taking too many painkillers. In the winter of 2021, a twenty-six-year-old British woman with an excruciating case of endometriosis died alone at home of an overdose of morphine and Tramadol, both of which had been prescribed to her for her pain. A coroner's inquest deemed her death accidental, the result of "combined drug toxicity"—itself a danger endometriosis patients face.[570]

In addition to its psychosocial dimensions, pain can also trigger neurobiological changes. One experiment on mice showed that endometriosis changed brain gene expression and the heart's electrical activity, which researchers said led to pain sensitization, anxiety and depression.[571] Other work has shown that chronic pain and depression share many regions of the brain, and that the neural mechanisms of people with both conditions saw increased pain signal transmission, turning the two conditions into co-conspirators.[572] People with chronic pelvic pain have decreased gray matter in the left thalamus, the "relay station" of our brains that passes along sensory elements like color, sound and touch to the cerebral cortex on the outer surface of the brain—a key part of our consciousness.[573] The left thalamus is also involved in alertness, learning, memory and emotion.[574]

Ultimately, all this evidence amounts to a compelling case: being depressed or anxious about pain can make us more sensitive to it, which makes us more depressed, which increases our sensitivity, and around and around we go.[575] All this in a world where a tenth of all women[576] have experience with depression, and where 70 percent of chronic pain patients are women.[577] It is a snake eating its own tail, a vicious ouroboros endlessly spinning into oblivion.

All this isn't good news for sufferers of endometriosis, an incurable disease that many people rate as worse than unmedicated labor. At least, Lara Wellman would certainly say so. In an interview, she described how one period landed her in the ER.[578]

"I had my period and I wasn't feeling well. The best way I could describe it is, it was like a charley horse in my uterus that lasted, like, half an hour. I've had three babies. I've had a tooth infection. I've *had* pain, right? And I was just brought to tears by it," says Wellman, who is a white forty-five-year-old cis woman. After three of these charley horses on one summer's day, she dragged herself to the ER. "I remember thinking, 'It would be stupid if I died.'"

Until her early forties, Wellman hadn't ever considered the possibility that her pain was somehow bigger than other people's pain, nor that her intense periods were abnormal. It wasn't until after that first ER visit that she discovered she had endometriosis—a diagnosis she only discovered because she took the initiative to read her file on her health network's e-records app. It was confirmed in a follow-up with an obstetrician. After a couple more ER visits that summer, Wellman got the full picture: her uterus was adhered to her bladder and intestines. She also had one endometrioma on each of her ovaries, one measuring eight centimeters and the other ten centimeters. Her lesions ate her appendix, and her organs were so inflamed the doctor called them "unrecognizable." She had a total hysterectomy in late 2019, with the surgeon emerging later to tell her, "In case you need reassurance, it was bad in there."

It's stunning to me that Wellman didn't seek out care sooner for her pain, but I suppose it's further testament to the idea that women are socialized to believe pain is part of life. I'm curious, though—was her endometriosis pain really worse than her birthing labors?

"A hundred percent," she answers without a moment's hesitation. "I remember one friend who had a baby saying to me, 'You didn't scream at all?' No, I didn't scream. It was never more painful than a bad period cramp. I think people who don't have period cramps like that, labor might be very shocking. But if you've had that your whole life you're like, 'Yeah, yeah.' It hurt, but lots of things hurt. I was never in tears in labor. But there were times, like the second time I went to the ER, where I just spent the whole time crying."

◆

How bad is your pain on a scale of zero to ten, with zero being no pain at all and ten being the worst pain imaginable?

This is the pain scale, and it is tragically flawed. As we've already seen, pain is impossible to diagnose objectively, and because of that, doctors often refer to a chart of emoticons to understand how their patient is feeling. At the bottom of the chart is the frowniest of frowny faces: pure, unadulterated agony. At the top is a carefree and happy smiley face: no pain at all. This self-reporting tool is otherwise known as the Numeric Rating Scale, which dates back to the origins of the opioid epidemic, when OxyContin was first approved in the mid-1990s and the American Pain Society developed the Pain as the Fifth Vital Sign initiative. In *Empire of Pain*, Patrick Radden Keefe explains how OxyContin's maker, Purdue Pharma, along with other pharmaceutical companies, "subsidized" the American Pain Society and the American Pain Foundation[579] (both of which have been shut down[580, 581] for taking pharma money to push opioids[582]). Because the pain scale failed to improve pain outcomes and helped drive the opioid epidemic, a movement has been born in the U.S. to abandon the scale altogether.[583] But it is just that: a movement—not policy. The pain scale is still widely used across medicine.

The less commonly used visual analogue scale is an older pain-rating tool. It's mostly used to measure pain associated with chronic conditions such as endometriosis. It consists of a straight horizontal line; both ends are capped with a short vertical line to mark the extremes of pain. Then the patient is instructed to mark an X to approximate how much they are suffering.

Whichever scale a doctor uses, the use of a scale at all brings up an important question: how does your doctor know what your ten feels like?

Because there are endless flavors of pain, your doctor can only really compare your pain to their own personal experiences. Your doctor might know what it's like to have a broken toe or a sore back, but have they ever felt like an alien was about to burst through their abdomen wielding knives in each of its slithery tentacles? Maybe they have, maybe they haven't.

If they compare you to other patients, just exactly who are they comparing you to? Is it other people with your problem, or other people in general? Are they comparing you predominantly to people of your own gender, or to a mix of genders? If you're trans or non-binary, how do you get categorized or compared? How can they know the difference between my worst pain and your worst pain? Suddenly the pain scale becomes a tug of war, a battle of who suffers most convincingly. If the doctor's ten is the guy who caught on fire during a multi-car pileup on an icy highway, where does my puny little endometriosis pain fall on the scale?

The subjectivity of experiencing and judging pain is nowhere near an exact science, and that leaves a lot of room for bias to bloom—especially because most of the world's chronic pain patients are women.[584]

Before I go any further, a caveat: the overwhelming majority of research on sex differences in pain focuses on differences between men and women, without any definition of gender nor mention of trans, non-binary or other gender non-conforming people. Because many researchers tend to refer to sex as innately biological, we can assume that unless it is otherwise specified, most studies fold all AFAB people into "female" or "women" categories. However, as mentioned earlier, some research suggests trans women have pain levels similar to or greater than those of cis women. As well, testosterone usage can increase pain in some trans men and reduce pain in others. For instance, testosterone can generate pain linked to vaginal atrophy and inflammatory conditions such as vaginitis, and may also be responsible for cramping in the lower abdomen, below the belly button.[585, 586] On the flip side, some studies show that androgens such as testosterone can reduce chronic pain in trans men.[587, 588]

Pain is not a purely physical phenomenon. Instead, it has important psychosocial factors that may increase pain sensations—and research demonstrates that trans individuals are more likely than cis ones to report depression, anxiety and other mental health problems.[589] And as Princeton University anthropology professor Agustín Fuentes argues in a 2022 article titled "Biological Science Rejects the Sex Binary, and That's Good for Humanity": "Genitals, hormone levels and chromosomes are not reliable determinants of sex. There are, for example, people with XY chromosomes who have female character-istics, people with ambiguous genitalia and women with testosterone levels outside the typical 'female' range. Biologically, there is no simple dichotomy between male and female."[590]

Trans and non-binary pain research is still a young field, so less is known about how it fits into the existing body of science surrounding sex and gender differences in pain. As you read this chapter, consider cis and non-cis interpretations of pain differentials.

Dr. Jeffrey Mogil is a neuroscientist at McGill University who has studied sex differences in pain for thirty years. When we speak, he's also the Canada research chair in the genetics of pain and the E.P. Taylor Chair in Pain Studies.

He says women make up the majority of chronic pain patients due to a confluence of factors: one, that women are more sensitive to pain; two, that women are more susceptible than men to get painful diseases; and three, that women are more likely to go to the doctor, which transforms them from chronic pain sufferers into chronic pain patients.[591]

To throw another wrench into all this, Mogil says different genders may not even be operating with the same pain scale. "When you're talking about sex differences, the problem is, well, what if women have a bigger range than men do? What if they can imagine more pain? And why would they be able to imagine more pain? Well, if they've given birth, they've been in more pain than most men ever have. I mean, unless the man in question had a particularly bad injury, or some sort of gunshot wound, or a kidney stone, the woman's probably been in more pain. So maybe her scale is bigger," says Mogil. "If she gives you a five and the man gives a five, it looks like they're giving the same pain rating, but actually the woman's five is bigger than the man's five." Of course, the opposite is usually how that information is interpreted: women's pain is considered less intense or serious than that of men. If I say my pain is a ten, and a doctor understands that to be a five, maybe I'll go home with antidepressants instead of pain meds.

This breakdown in belief and understanding is a defining feature of a medical model founded on patriarchy and paternalism. But that wasn't what was on Mogil's mind at the pivotal moment he realized there were genuine differences in how men and women experience pain.

As the story goes, the lab where Mogil worked as a grad student in the early 1990s bred its own mice on which to experiment. It was a cheaper option than buying them, but there was just one problem: half the mice were female. At the time, the scientific community overwhelmingly used only male subjects regardless of who the drugs' target markets were. Part of this was because of the usual paternalistic "protection" of women's fertility, but a second reason for this exclusion was the strong belief that female-specific variables such as sex hormones would skew lab results. The rationale wasn't exactly rational: human females take many of the same medications that males do. Wouldn't drug companies want to make sure a drug worked equally well in both?

Beyond the flawed logic, they were also flat-out wrong. In reality, each sex has its own set of hormonal and biological variables, and neither skews results any more than the other.[592] Although this has been proven multiple times, and despite newer rules requiring health researchers to include female subjects in testing, even in 2021 female rodents and humans alike were still excluded from a lot of preclinical and clinical research.[593]

Back in his grad lab, instead of killing all the females, Mogil and his labmates simply used them alongside the males. One day, he decided to check out the sex differences on an experiment testing mice for stress response. The mice had heat applied to their feet; the time it took for them to recoil was counted as pain response. After that, the mice were injected with the painkiller being tested. When the team looked at the results the first time, they had determined the drug had a moderate effect. But when Mogil looked at the data again, he found that while both sexes responded to the stress the same way, only the males benefited from the painkiller. It only appeared as though the drug had a moderate effect because the team had averaged the response across all subjects.

The next day he told the study's lead researcher of his discovery. The supervisor told him, "Sex differences are to enjoy, not to study," he recounts with a chuckle.

Mogil ignored that advice.

Nine years later, in 2001, the Institute of Medicine published a report sponsored by multiple arms of the U.S. government.[594] That report made the definitive case for why the scientific community needed to evaluate sex differences in their research, with the authors arguing that sex hormones aren't the only things that make females and males different from each other. There is a vast array of genetic, physiological and experiential disparities that define our biological sex (and gender, for that matter). In truth, they explained, males and females have partially different genomes, which can be detected at the cellular level. Because of all this variability programmed into us, there are notable differences in the way males and females respond to drugs, food, vitamins, preservatives, pollutants and microorganisms. When we generalize findings in males to females, we run a massive risk of errors, some of which can be highly dangerous and even fatal. The report hammered home the desperate need to create policies that required evaluating sex differences in research: "Until the question of sex [. . .] is routinely asked and the results—positive or negative—are routinely reported, many opportunities to obtain a better understanding of the pathogenesis of disease and to advance human health will surely be missed."[595]

In the years that followed, the European Union and Canada, followed in 2016 by the United States, introduced policies referred to as sex as a biological variable for research and preclinical studies.[596, 597] Typically, under these policies, researchers applying for funding are asked to explain how they've factored sex into their research designs and analyses. If they use only cis male subjects, they have to justify it. As a consequence, accounting for sex has grown considerably. Actual integration into the finished product and circulating this information to the public have been stumbling blocks, though. Researchers often fail to include their definitions of sex or gender, and often exclude trans and non-binary people from their studies. Scientific and medical journals aren't obligated to verify if the authors have considered sex as a biological variable.[598] And, as Mogil explains, it's common even today that studies only mention that females were included in the research, without accounting for the data differentials between female and male subjects. "If they never tell the reader whether there was or wasn't a sex difference, there's really no point in disclosing it in the first place," he says.

There's a failure of leadership on the issue. While science-informed policy is seen as a gold standard, applying scientific definitions of gender to more nuanced conversations spells significant consequences around how healthcare is delivered. For instance, the language of science has been weaponized in political contexts to create gender-segregation policies and laws. As a 2022 paper in *Science* notes, "Using biological definitions in the law may sound like responsible governance, but it can result in harmful or illogical outcomes. This can occur through a variety of means, including taking biological sex categories out of context and applying them to cases of human legal rights where they are not relevant; uncritical use of binary sex categories in science; and ignoring bioscientific evidence about the complexity, mutability, context specificity and plurality of sex and gender."

The paper continues: "When scientific uses of biological sex concepts lack clarity, precision and rigor, this increases the risk that legal advocates will misunderstand misrepresent scientific research on biological sex."[599]

So a lack of firm policy guidelines and a lack of punishments for noncompliance—compounded by a lack of understanding of gender plurality—have opened up a lot of loopholes. Since these policies were introduced, the percentage of published neuroscience studies using only male rodents has actually grown.[600] And, of course, sex as a biological variable is a string attached to publicly funded research; private researchers, like drug companies, aren't obligated to account for sex at all.

Considering all the ways non-cis males are habitually excluded from research, I guess we can make a few guesses as to why there isn't more evidence on endometriosis. In earnestness, though, getting the concept of sex as a biological variable right could really revolutionize how people in pain get help. If we knew a common painkiller worked 20 percent better in males, we could give females higher doses to give them the same relief. We could create new medications that help certain types of pain better than current market catchalls, and we would know what works and what doesn't in people with female biology. This is a critical puzzle to solve, considering not only that the majority of the world's chronic pain patients are women, but also that AFAB people are more prone to suffer from diseases where pain is a major symptom.

Even if a cure for endometriosis was discovered in a lab tomorrow, though, we may not see it in use for a long, long time. Overall, it takes an average of seventeen years for research evidence to be introduced and integrated into clinical practice—and that's just an average.[601] If a cure for cancer took two years, and a cure for endometriosis took thirty-two years, the average would still be seventeen.[602]

In short, we have no reason to believe endometriosis relief will be swift and effective.

◆

Endometriosis is a disease that turns star athletes into pill-poppers, straight-A students into high school dropouts, people with rich social lives into recluses.

We don't lose our quality of life. We are robbed of it by a system that refuses to understand, believe and treat us.[603]

A big part of why this happens is pain. I'm not talking about a slam-your-finger-in-the-car-door or a twist-your-ankle-while-walking-the-dog kind of pain. I'm talking about severe chronic pain that unpredictably alternates between radiating nerve pain, dull aching and sharp stabbing. These sensations leave a person drained of all energy and emotion, and they happen for at least a few days every single month, twelve months a year, for an average of forty years.[604, 605] Worse, some people suffer beyond their so-called reproductive years, the disease having been found in fetuses[606] and septuagenarians alike.[607] All pharmaceutical treatments currently available are palliative, meaning they do not reduce or cure the disease but rather work to make the patient more comfortable.[608] For many people, prescription drugs have little effect. The most helpful intervention is excision surgery, as it physically removes diseased tissue from the body.[609] Unfortunately, surgery is typically reserved for exceptional cases, which means patients are left to take ineffective drugs until their disease *becomes* exceptional. Meanwhile, new research suggests the average age at diagnosis in the U.S. is twenty-nine for white people, thirty-one for Black people and thirty-three for Hispanic people.[610]

I was diagnosed at thirty-five, after waiting twenty-four years. Being robbed of that time is probably the greatest injustice of my life.

Routinely encountering these kinds of pain changes our relationships, our goals in life, our bodies and our brains. It compromises our ability to love being alive, to enjoy sex, to make and keep friends, to live up to our fullest potential. We try to make the best of things, only to have our resilience held against us by the people around us. If things are as bad as you say they are, then how can you possibly work, go to school, travel, make art? But when we complain, we are dramatic attention-seekers or self-absorbed narcissists. For so many people and for so many reasons, chronic pain becomes a part of how we are perceived by others and even how we perceive ourselves.

Still, many endo patients reject being viewed as disabled, and do our best to act normal despite having legitimate reasons to ask for accommodations. This tracks with disability theory, notably Tobin Siebers's vision of it. In the book *Disability Theory*, he writes that our society treats disabled people as if they are narcissistic when in fact it is systemic and institutional hyperindividualization that forces them to look out for number one. "The disability of individuals is always represented as their personal misfortune," writes Siebers, explaining that "containing the effects of disability" allows society to curtail disabled folks' ability to organize and demand better as a group. "It isolates them in their individuality, making a common purpose difficult to recognize and advance as a political agenda."[611]

There's some special hell in suffering, feeling completely alone in suffering and then being made to feel as though you cannot talk about or even acknowledge said suffering. That has made openly acknowledging and describing pain an act of rebellion—and that's exactly why I asked the people I interviewed to describe their pain as if explaining it to someone who'd never felt it.

Below is a cross-section of what people told me about their pain. I've included people's ethnicities and genders for context and transparency, but I'd like to reiterate that age, socioeconomic status, sexuality, body size, mental illness, disability and sometimes chronic pain itself are other factors by which people experience medical discrimination.

Jax, twenty-one, white trans man: "It feels like someone has put barbed wire into an ovary or has put hot coals into each one of them. The ones I actually hate the most are very sudden vaginal pains, like someone stabbed me with a knife up there."[612]

Marit Stiles, fifty-one, white cis woman: "Stabbing is a good way to think about it, although it was just constant. It was my abdomen, mostly, but it also went into my back. It made me nauseous. It was the kind of pain that meant that when I was seated, like in school, I was basically meditating. I learned how to focus on an object or thing and bring my breathing down to just to a point where I could just bear it."[613]

Catherine Reisch, forty-one, white cis woman: "For the most part, it feels like I'm walking around with a, like, hundred-pound brick sitting in my uterus that's putting pressure on the vaginal canal. There's also as if your ovaries are popping like fireworks—like a popping, searing, burning kind of pain. I mean, I have contractions."[614]

Sally Zori, thirty-six, trans Iraqi: "It felt like someone had gone into my ovaries and my lower abdomen and grabbed them with two big hands and was just squeezing so, so hard. It also felt like there was something in there that was trying to inflate and burst out of me, like this feeling of compression and inflation that felt like my insides were trying to explode and implode at the same time."[615]

Celia, thirty-eight, white, genderfluid: "When I was ten years old, my dad ended up taking me to the emergency room with what I know was my period because I remember seeing large clumps of tissue. Sometimes I'll get my whole uterus shape come out. They were like, 'Oh, you're really constipated, and you're really emotional.' I wasn't really emotional, I was just in so much unbelievable pain. [. . .] They did tests on me for about a week and a half and then determined I had psychosomatic pain. I was put in psychiatric care."[616]

Jasmine Galang, twenty-seven, Filipino/white mixed ethnicity, cis woman: "I got my period at ten, and then after that I was constantly forever in pain. They were always super heavy and so irregular, and I would always get [from doctors], 'Oh, that's normal, you're a teenage girl, you're young.' By the time I was sexually active, which was thirteen, fourteen-ish, I was diagnosed with pelvic inflammatory disease. Sex was always so painful. I always thought it was due to maybe an ovarian cyst rupturing, but by the time I would get to the hospital, we wouldn't be able to find anything. I think [the reason doctors treated me poorly] was just mostly age, low socioeconomic status and the fact that I'm female, to be honest."[617]

Donna, forty-three, Black cis woman: "It felt like muscle contractions to me, like really intense contractions of the uterus that would come in waves. The waves were constant, so even though it would let up for a minute or two, it would come back. And it would be lower back pain as well, and sometimes I could feel it in the top of my legs.

So, low back pain, upper leg pain and diarrhea the first three days of my period, like clockwork."[618]

Ted Combs, thirty-nine, white trans non-binary person: "With my PCOS, particularly my left ovary—it looked like a golf ball in ultrasounds because it had so many cysts all over it. And they'd occasionally pop, and that is the worst pain ever. You feel like somebody has stabbed and twisted your gut. Whenever I'd have one pop, I couldn't get up and walk on my own, really. I would just be doubled over in such bad pain, curled up in a ball and crying. For a while, my spouse would have to help me to the restroom if I needed to pee."[619]

Lana Krupey, forty, white cis woman: "It destroyed me growing up. I went from a happy, vibrant, athletic popular kid to being ostracized because I was the sick girl. My mental state was horrible. Being that my parents were apathetic and every doctor I ever talked to wanted to refer me to psych care, I rebelled. I just went, 'Well, fine, if no one's gonna treat me'—I started doing drugs. I didn't care about my life. I didn't care if I overdosed; I didn't care if I drank myself and died in a ditch. I felt like nothing. I felt like I was worse than nothing. I was a throwaway."[620]

Nancy Petersen, eighty-one, white cis woman: "I spent from age eleven to age forty-nine in pain. At twenty-seven, I had a complete hysterectomy with removal of ovaries, and six weeks later a laminectomy [back surgery] and fusion for white-hot leg pain and back pain. And none of those things helped. For the next twenty-two years, I slept two hours a night in twenty-minute parcels. It made me so mad that I had spent thirty-eight years in pain from endometriosis that had been unrecognized, dismissed as neurotic, treated with other tools, that [managing the Nancy's Nook endo education Facebook group] sort of became a second career for me. This is ridiculous, that women should have to live like this."[621]

Eileen Mary Holowka, twenty-seven, white non-binary person: "It's debilitating. When things are really bad, I'm just on the toilet shitting and vomiting at the same time. And shaking. You aren't a person, at a certain point. You're just a body that is trying to survive. [. . .] I had diagnostic surgery in 2017 and came out of surgery with really horrible pain, and the doctor just said, 'You're probably one of those people that are in pain all the time.'"[622] (As it turns out, Holowka and I shared a doctor—the one who coerced me into getting the IUD.)

If I had to describe my period pain to someone who didn't have endometriosis, I'd say that the heights of my pain felt like a dull knife being dragged across the lowest part of my abdomen, sawing back and forth to slice me open. Sometimes, sitting down on the toilet felt like a dagger being twisted inside my colon, cutting into my perineum. When that happened, the blood would drain from my face, my forehead growing damp with cold sweat, bile rising in my esophagus. I would gasp, trying not to vomit or faint, digging my fingernails into my thighs. And then, after the moment passed, I usually just went back to work.

Trying to explain any of this to a person who doesn't know it firsthand feels useless. Has a doctor or partner ever really experienced a pain like having their testicles pushed into their rectum, then stapled into their intestines—not just once but several times a month, every month, for most of their lives? Has your BFF ever been stabbed directly in the butthole with a serrated bread knife? Has a teacher or employer ever missed a day because their vaginas were full of red-hot shrapnel?

At the same time, we need to bear witness because this kind of chronic pain can rule every aspect of a person's life. Throughout this book, we've met people whose disease has triggered life-altering consequences—not only because of the severity of symptoms, but also because many of them are marginalized to begin with.

Take Shelia Ivany, for instance.[623] The thirty-five-year-old Indigenous cis woman from Haida Nation calls herself a "big baby" and "drama queen" when it comes to pain. She thinks she's got a lower tolerance for pain, despite the fact that she's probably experienced more pain than most people. To doctors, though, her supposed low tolerance looks like exaggeration or manipulation. It doesn't matter that there are scientifically proven connections between pain, trauma and depression, and other evidence that women are more sensitive to pain. To most of the doctors she's come across, Ivany has just been a dramatic drug-seeker haunting the ER. They even put that label—"drug-seeking"—in her file. Black, Indigenous and low-income people often run up against such prejudice, even when they have acute and obvious injuries. Frustrated by their abdication of care, she began answering doctors' accusations by saying, "If I was looking for an easy high, it's a small town—I can go find drugs, and I can just pay for them. It would be easier than coming in here and asking for free [drugs] from you."

In reality, Ivany had stage-four endometriosis. After undergoing a hysterectomy, she learned the disease covered her rectum, bowels, ovaries and uterus, and like me, she also had adenomyosis. However, the surgeons chose to leave her ovaries behind during excision because she was "too young for menopause"—and because of that, her pain came back less than three months later, her endo having almost completely regrown. Her gynecologist shrugged it off at the time. "Oh, that happens sometimes," she told her. Now, to get her through her day-to-day life, Ivany depends on oxycodone, hydromorphone and Tylenol T3s, which are a mixture of codeine and acetaminophen, plus antidepressants and anti-anxiety drugs. When we first speak, she's also on Lupron, which she hates (she discontinued it after four shots). Even after a second excision surgery in January 2022, her pain keeps pulling her away from work, interferes with her ability to care for her three children and prevents her from doing some of the most basic things people take for granted. "I shouldn't need to call one of my daughters to get down on the floor and hold the dustpan for me [while I sweep]," she says. "That's where a lot of my depression comes in. You feel like a failure."

Since we first spoke in 2021, Ivany has been diagnosed with two other inflammatory diseases: acrodermatitis continua of Hallopeau (which causes painful pustules on the hands) and an autoimmune disease that is a combination of psoriasis and arthritis. In the face of these additional painful conditions, she says she's had to "toughen up" the past year.

Being in physical pain is hard enough. The psychosocial experience of pain combined with all those little instances of discrimination, though—that's what really cuts a person in half. And often doctors don't even realize that what they say and do make things so much worse for their patients.

One particular conversation with a doctor stands out in the memory of Brandi LaPerle.[624]

LaPerle is a thirty-nine-year-old Red River Métis comedian and public speaker who, while on tour across Canada, made a point of speaking with endometriosis patients and gynecologists in almost every town she visited. I ask her what the main themes were of what she discovered. "I think a lot of patients and medical professionals actually have many of the same concerns. Pain is a huge one because of how pain is treated, or mistreated," LaPerle answers. She tells me she sought out one particular doctor because so many of his patients had told her just how awful he was at dealing with their pain.

When their conversation over lunch turned to pain, the doctor complained that he found it just so frustrating dealing with patients with chronic pain, for whom you can do very little. "That's just not my area," the doctor told her.

"Yeah, I get that," LaPerle replied. "But here's the issue: it's not your area, it's not the ER's job, it's not the gynecologist's job, it's not the family doctor's job. Whose job is it? It has to be somebody's job. But it's nobody's job, and the patient suffers for that."

LaPerle says many of the doctors she spoke to on that tour think pain clinics are a partial solution to this problem. The thing is, there aren't enough of them. That means long waiting lists for people who live close enough to a pain clinic, and for others who live in more remote areas, it's a long waiting list *and* a long round-trip journey. Additionally, she explains, many doctors are unaware of existing inter-provincial agreements that allow them to send patients to pain clinics in other jurisdictions—meaning patients languish on a local list when they could be getting care elsewhere. And, of course, your mileage may vary even if you do get into a pain clinic; after all, the doctor who made me get the IUD did so within the confines of a hospital pain clinic. LaPerle thinks multidisciplinary centers treating pain *and* disease are a better use of resources.

These are simply too many caveats for someone living in constant excruciating pain. The gaps in the system that this pervasive pass-the-buck mentality creates are harmful to almost every chronic pain patient. Endometriosis patients are particularly harmed because we live in a misogynist society with a disease that is viewed exclusively as a women's problem—a fact that can be doubly brutal for trans and non-binary people. These harms are not only physical; they are also deeply emotional and spiritual, chipping away at our entire bodies and minds.

LaPerle knows this reality all too intimately. "I was a competitive athlete until I was sixteen. I was expected to perform in every area of my life, but as things were progressing, I was falling further and further behind," she says. "There's a point where you mourn the person you used to be. Like, I've lost a lot of people in my life to death, and the grieving is the same—except you're grieving for yourself, the person you used to be or the person that you could be. People judge you."

It was only at age thirty-one that she was finally diagnosed with endometriosis. By then, she'd had years of intense pain, some of which sent her to the ER with mysterious symptoms. She describes her pain as "giving birth and then you have a migraine on top of that, and you just stubbed your toe, and somebody has a gun to your head yelling at you to solve math equations and if you get the answer wrong, they're gonna shoot you." The Lupron they eventually put her on made it even worse; one day she left home for work at a legal office without realizing she didn't have pants on.

She's had three surgeries so far, including a hysterectomy and excision, but those have been a fight. One particularly dramatic encounter with a surgeon saw LaPerle getting vaginally biopsied not in an operating room but in a dingy doctor's office, without freezing or local anesthetic. And when she refused to see that doctor again, word got around because the surgeon was well connected in LaPerle's community. Another gynecologist she later consulted excoriated her for "doctor shopping," accusing LaPerle of abusing the healthcare system for forty-five minutes. Because of her local blacklisting, she had to get her next surgery in another city three hours away.

Throughout her journey, LaPerle has used her career as a comedian to raise awareness about the disease. In her routine, she often tells the story of the time she was on stage when her rectum prolapsed. At first, she didn't realize what had happened. "I thought it was a turd," she recounts. But as the standup crew went off to a Denny's after the show to get some late-night food, she realized she couldn't sit down. "I realized it wasn't a peek-a-boo. It was attached to me. This was part of my anatomy sticking out," she tells me. But at the hospital, she overheard a doctor tell a colleague, "She's just here for drugs. There's nothing wrong with this one."

Incensed, she told the doctor she could hear him, then called him back into her room. When he returned, she dropped her pants, bent over, spread her cheeks and demanded, "What is this?"

Despite the seriousness of this disease, a lot of people with endometriosis have excellent, if morbid, senses of humor, and many try to remain optimistic and positive and hold onto life as best they can. In an endless dark tunnel, we learn to be our own lights.

◆

In 2020, the U.S. government said it would put $26 million toward endometriosis research after hearing the personal story of Abby Finkenauer, a (now former) congresswoman with the disease. The funding increase doubled the previous year's allocation for endometriosis and was supposed to take effect at the dawn of the new fiscal year on October 1, 2020.[625] The increase was proclaimed in news headlines and celebrated by endometriosis foundations.

Twenty-six million bucks may seem like a lot, but consider that the U.S. National Institutes of Health (NIH) spends about $42 billion a year on medical research.[626] In 2020, the NIH allocated $7 million for hay fever, $10 million on Tourette's syndrome, $73 million on food allergies, $101 million on underage drinking, $161 million on infertility and $788 million on research related to breast cancer.[627] That year, endometriosis got $14 million of NIH research money. Of that cash, a $1.1 million grant went toward a project studying the use of elagolix (Orilissa) before IVF to improve rates of pregnancy.[628] That same project collected grants in 2019 and 2021 as well, meaning it has received $3.2 million of NIH funding to date.[629] Tangentially, Open Payments shows that elagolix's manufacturer, AbbVie, paid one of the project's leads almost $115,000 in non-research money between 2014 and 2018.[630]

When I checked to see how the NIH spent its influx of endo cash, I couldn't find anything. The column that should have said $26 million said $14 million. That was just one million dollars more than 2019's allocation, not double. Perplexed, I wrote to the NIH asking about the discrepancy. They told me that although the amendment was passed in the House, it never made it further than that:

"This language was not included in the final bill, and therefore, was never enacted."[631]

That $26 million—as small as it was—never even existed. Like so much in endo, it was merely an illusion.

I should mention that after the NIH answered my media request, the agency's funding database was updated to show that it had allocated $20 million to endo in 2021. It *is* more than $14 million—but it isn't $26 million, and it's certainly not enough considering the devastation this disease wreaks.

In any case, there's still something weird about the whole thing. After doing some digging, though, it seems this dog-and-pony show for endo funding is a matter of routine. In early 2022, the Endometriosis Foundation of America (EFA)—which has worked to become the face for endo advocacy in the U.S.—posted a blog titled "Endometriosis Research Funding Bill Passed in Congress."[632] In that post, spokeswoman Padma Lakshmi, the *Top Chef* host who co-founded the EFA with her celebrity endo excision surgeon, was quoted as saying: "What a bright spot in an otherwise dark period. I'm over the moon that Congress is continuing to take this devastating disease seriously."

Except I could not find an endometriosis funding bill. Looking at the Appropriations bill, I couldn't find any dedicated endo funding. Only in writing to the foundation was I informed that the real news was that two agencies responsible for allocating money for endometriosis research got additional funding. But that money is for *all* of their programs, not only endo—and they have a lot of programs. When I asked the foundation if there were promises made about how much of those agencies' new money would go to endo research, the answer in so many words was no.[633] There's no actual guarantee that any of that new money will go toward endometriosis research.

I can appreciate the PR tactic of spinning this to keep endo in the headlines, but why play it off as a win? To me, it smacks of the kind of one-dimensional gladhanding that greases the wheels of private foundation fundraising.

So I looked at EFA's money and did some math. IRS records show the EFA has grossed a cumulative $7.6 million in funding over its fifteen-year existence. Some of that money has gone to research grants, but a substantial portion of it typically goes to holding events to fundraise more money.[634] Even before deductions, $7.6 million over fifteen years is astoundingly little considering how many rich and famous people have endo, including Amy Schumer, Chrissy Teigen, Lena Dunham, Whoopi Goldberg, Dolly Parton and Susan Sarandon.

I don't mean that people who suffer from the disease are responsible for funding research on it. It may be that they donated money to other foundations or research on endo. But when the leading advocacy group in the U.S. isn't raking in huge donations from endo's most famous sufferers, the optics are kind of perplexing.

I can't pretend to know all the inside baseball of private endo funding—but I don't need to know to be able to say that endometriosis research funding is tiny compared to how prevalent and destructive it is. Consider there are about 168 million AFAB people in the U.S.[635] If we use the stat that 10 percent of them have endo, that means there are potentially 16.8 million endometriosis sufferers in the U.S. However, it seems only 7.6 million cases have been diagnosed,[636] so let's just use that number for the sake of this argument. At $20 million in NIH funding, that is $2.63 of funding per confirmed case for one of the most painful human conditions that exists.[637] If the $26 million had actually materialized, it would have been $3.42 per sufferer.

To really drive this home, let's look at how another predominantly female disease gets funded. In the U.S., breast cancer research is earmarked to receive $771 million in grants from the NIH in 2022, and the philanthropic sector typically raises an additional $460 million or so per year.[638, 639] The American Cancer Society estimates that 287,850 new cases of invasive breast cancer will develop in 2022, along with 51,400 cases of ductal carcinoma in situ, an early stage form of breast cancer that is generally not invasive.[640] All told, 43,250 people in the U.S. will die of breast cancer in 2022.[641] There are also 3.8 million living survivors of the disease.[642] The average five-year survival rate for breast cancer is 90 percent.[643] (Women of color have lower survival rates.)

Between the NIH and the philanthropic sector, the breast cancer cause receives gross funding to the tune of $3,628.59 per new case. That is 1,380 times more than per-capita endo funding when we only consider diagnosed cases.

I know: I'm comparing a "benign" disease to cancer. I'm not trying to say endometriosis is worse than, or even equal to, cancer. But you'd think that a lifelong chronic pain condition that erodes infertility would get a little more action. People love babies almost as much as they love boobies! What are we missing here?

In 2021, the *Journal of Women's Health* published an analysis that looked at funding for female-dominant diseases versus funding for male-dominant diseases. It named endometriosis as one of the most underfunded diseases considering its massive burden,[644] and suggested that at least part of the reason why it receives so little money is because some people wrongly believe it's a consequence of sufferers' lifestyle choices. This tracks with research that shows that diseases associated with smoking (lung cancer), drinking (liver disease and cancer) and sex (cervical cancer) also receive less funding than their equally fatal counterparts.[645]

This on its own is a damning display of how institutional and philanthropic funders choose to punish certain individuals for their behavior—except that endometriosis is not even caused by any "derelict" behaviors. Male-predominant diseases, meanwhile, rarely suffer declines in funding even when they are connected to lifestyle factors, including HIV/AIDS, alcoholism, substance abuse and hepatitis; in fact, many male-dominant causes are *overfunded*.[646] Unsurprisingly, the research team reached this conclusion: "NIH applies a dispropor-tionate share of its resources to diseases that affect primarily men, at the expense of those that affect primarily women."[647]

Pharma has in many respects taken ownership of endo in the absence of public and nonprofit prioritization, and whatever invest-ment it puts in comes back to them many times over because of endo's incurable nature. Pharma companies aren't sinking cash into endo for altruistic or humanitarian reasons, and as businesses they don't have to. Between birth control, painkillers and GnRH modulators, drug companies are making hundreds of millions dollars off the backs of endometriosis patients every single year.

We can gauge how much a society cares about a health problem or illness by the amount of money invested into curing it. By that token, hardly anyone cares about endo.

Why would they? The enigma surrounding endometriosis is a neutralizing force. There's no definitive scientific answer that explains this disease or proposes a cure for it, and that prevents patients and doctors from pursuing anything other than conventional therapies. If status quo interventions are seen as good enough, there's less interest and pressure to study and make it better. The fact that it's about chronic, non-fatal "lady problems" further drives down interest; there's no glory in studying menstruation. Meanwhile, because it's shrouded in mystery, misunderstandings and misrepresentations of endometriosis are rampant in the public sphere. That makes it a black box to potential research funders, who would probably rather park their money somewhere more likely to get results in their lifetimes.

Plus it's not like it's fatal, right?

This cycle of deprioritization is a major reason why endometriosis progress remains stalled. A 2021 *New York Times* article about MIT professor Linda Griffith, who both has the disease and is studying it, hits the nail on the head. As journalist Rachel E. Gross writes, "[Endometriosis] suffers from a branding problem: It falls into the abyss of 'women's diseases' (overlooked), diseases that don't kill you (unimportant) and menstrual problems (taboo). Researchers often call endometriosis 'benign,' as in noncancerous—but doing so, Dr. Griffith believes, lessens the seriousness of a common, painful disease."[648]

This speaks to an understated part of the endometriosis equation. Our societal and research-backed obsession with avoiding mortality means we don't look at morbidity—the act of suffering—which is the defining experience of endometriosis. That's a critical piece of why endo isn't treated with the same urgency as diseases that are fatal, but it doesn't fully explain it. After all, as we saw earlier, tons of research and money is poured into all kinds of benign problems accompanied by some kind of suffering, ranging from erectile dysfunction to seasonal allergies. We can't say fatal disease is the only kind that matters to public and private funders. We could blame the failure to fund on the fact that people don't understand endo or that it's a complicated disease, but that would imply there is no interest in studying endometriosis, and that's simply not true. There are amazing researchers out there toiling away for mere peanuts in underfunded labs, trying to stop people like us from needlessly suffering.

So, what are we really left with here?

I think of this funding ignorance as an invasive weed that's impossible to rip out and which never dies, not even in the dead of the coldest Canadian winters. This weed looks a lot like the lack of political and institutional will to change outcomes for women and others with marginalized genders. This invasive species is the lack of concern for our pain, even less concern for our pleasure and a complete lack of empathy for entire lives being destroyed.

This weed is misogyny, and until we band together to kill it, funding for endometriosis will always look like a rusty collection plate with a hole in it.

8. NOTICE OF EVICTION

2 legit 2 quit (the system)

On a dismal, overcast October day, I woke up early to prepare for my meeting with the surgeon. It was seventeen days after I returned from Scandinavia, two weeks after the ultrasound that diagnosed my endo, one day after I asked my boyfriend to write my permission slip. In three days' time, I'd be in Montreal for the fateful bachelorette party.

I'd decided on my strategy ahead of time: I would be a flawless patient.

That morning, I spent a couple of hours washing and styling my hair and applying just enough makeup to look respectable. I put on a modest black denim dress, with long sleeves and a high buttoned collar, pairing it with opaque leggings to hide as many of my tattoos as possible. I stood by the door and bent down to zip up my heeled leather booties. I *never* wear heels. I folded the permission slip and slid it between the pages of my little black notebook. On its pages were the questions I knew I'd forget to ask.

I'd found this surgeon on RateMDs.com, where he had a 4.8-star rating. "Excellent bedside manner," one reviewer noted. That was good enough for me. It's not like I had much of a choice, anyway; he was one of two surgeons in this city, and one of a small handful in the entire country qualified to do excision. A couple years back, the other local surgeon—one known for taking more of the "prestige" cases—had already declined to accept me as a patient because my imaging at the time didn't show that I was egregiously sick.

After finding my surgeon online in May 2019, I asked my then-GP to send a referral to his office. Then I raced home from the appointment and wrote a letter to the surgeon desperately pleading for him to see me, detailing all the interventions I'd tried over the years, emphasizing how deeply my quality of life had declined. I faxed it to him using a free online fax service, hoping it would be reunited with its referral companion. If my previous testing didn't show real problems, the testing was flawed, I reasoned. I *knew* I was sick. I just hadn't had the right care to find and treat it.

And then his assistant called: he would see me!

In ten months.

I deflated. The notion of waiting just one second longer than I had to sucked all the air out of my lungs, but I accepted the appointment anyway and asked to be put on the cancellation list. At that point, though, the sixteen years of experience I had as a journalist had taught me the craft of being a pain in the ass. I called every week inquiring about cancellations, making sure to be polite to the receptionist. Five months into my wait, she rang me up to give me a last-minute opening.

It was time to prepare. This doctor was part of a clinic specializing in maternal and newborn health. How would he treat a stranger pleading to have her reproductive system completely removed? I researched strategies for talking to doctors in ways that politely defer to their egos while standing firm in my own needs. On message boards, I read that doctors treat women better when a husband or boyfriend is in the room. Hmm, I thought. My partner had an important work meeting. Would a letter be enough?

I wrote down my talking points in my notebook and rehearsed what I wanted to say to him. I needed to be on the ball. The tenuous pact I'd made with myself to stay alive probably couldn't bear the strain of another crushing disappointment. If I heard just one more "you'll change your mind" about kids, I was going to lose it. I didn't want to hear about how pregnancy, or weight loss, or another kind of birth control could help me. I needed him to be different.

After primping and putting on my ankle boots, I set out to meet the man to whom I'd addressed my desperate, deranged fax missive. I left home early so I wouldn't be flustered by traffic between my downtown apartment and his office deep in the sprawling suburbs. I pumped upbeat music through the speakers of my red hatchback, trying to get myself into the frame of mind where I'm the most confident, charming version of myself. I had to play the game.

I pulled into the parking lot, doing my best to leave my emotional baggage in the car. You can't cry, I told myself. I gathered my purse and my courage and exited the car, feigning assurance as I walked to the door, then down the hall and to his office. I entered through a windowless wood door, checked in with the receptionist and dutifully filled out the forms she handed me.

The time of my appointment came and went. He was late. I felt that familiar sense of anxiety creep up into my chest. I watched every second of the clock tick away. He was an hour late. I begged my lungs to allow deep steady breaths. I couldn't let his tardiness affect my performance. I had to keep my morale and confidence up. I needed to be stoic but personable, funny but serious.

I looked around the waiting room from my perch against the corner back wall. In waiting rooms, I always sit with my back to the wall, feeling most at ease on the periphery. Most of the patients were pregnant, wanted to be pregnant or had recently been pregnant. Some were alone, but many had companions—mothers, sisters, friends, partners. Children's toys were piled up in the corner, and the animated movie *Ice Age* played on the television hanging in the corner. This was an office shared by several doctors dealing with matters of fertility and lack thereof. The injustice struck me. Some of these people desperately wanted children. Why couldn't I have been given a burlap sack for a uterus and let these people have a viable one? That was, of course, assuming I had a viable one. I had never actually been pregnant, even if I hadn't always been as careful as I should have been. The thought turned like gears in my mind. *Imagine after all this, after being denied surgery for so long because you "might change your mind about kids," you couldn't even conceive if you wanted to?*

Someone called my name and snapped me back to Earth. It was my turn. I scurried into the surgeon's office and took a seat across from him. Papers littered his desk. His ground-floor office overlooked a suburban parking lot, its grayness the only source of light in the room. It was nice, actually; overhead fluorescent lights have always bothered my eyes. He was handsome, with a generous head of hair. The top two buttons of his collared shirt were undone, letting some chest hair peek out. He seemed relaxed, like he had time for me.

He had my diagnostic ultrasound results. The endometriosis had spread to my bowel, gluing it and my uterus together, twisting the uterus backwards, he explained. He could also see adenomyosis. There it was in black and white—cold, hard evidence that proved I hadn't imagined the past twenty-four years.

I smiled my best confident smile and began talking. He listened, nodding and typing into the computer as I spoke. He asked questions. We had an actual conversation. And then I made my request: I want a total hysterectomy.

By then I was in my mid-thirties, almost too old to have children, but still young enough to have my period for another ten or twenty years. I emphasized my unwavering desire to be child-free. It was always at this point that my appointments usually stalled, with the doctor asking that dreaded question: What if you change your mind? The question became more annoying each time I heard it. These people barely knew me but acted as though they knew something about me that I didn't know myself, as if being child-free hadn't been a fundamental part of my identity and life. And, anyway, what if I did change my mind—so what? In almost every other circumstance, people have to reckon with the choices they make. People get laser eye surgery knowing they could go blind. People go skydiving knowing their parachute could fail. People get breast augmentations knowing the silicone may leak. I was never permitted to make my own choice. Instead, the choice was always made for me when doctors declined to help.

The surgeon asked how certain I was about not having children. I told him I had never been as certain about anything as I was about that. Then I gestured to my bag: "I have a letter from my boyfriend. He couldn't be here today, but he also really doesn't want children, so—"

The surgeon held up his hand as if to say stop.

"I don't need to see the letter," he told me. "It's your body. It's your choice."

It was my body, and my choice. My *choice*. *My* choice.

No doctor had ever given me a choice before. They'd always just made it for me, sometimes through direct denials but most often by questioning my rationale, my commitment, my sanity.

The surgeon asked me what I wanted to do.

"I want you to gut me like a fish," I said with a laugh, full of adrenaline.

He playfully admonished me for being gross, then pulled out a pad of tear-off sheets illustrating the uterus, fallopian tubes, ovaries, cervix and vagina and began drawing on it. Did I want the uterus gone or the ovaries too? What about the cervix? I wanted it all gone, to give me the best chance of not having the endometriosis recur. The best chance of finally closing the chapter on twenty-four years of medical trauma.

"I've never met a patient who knew what she wanted with such certainty," he told me. I thanked him and stood to leave, trembling with the jittery excitement of a dozen espressos. I floated to the reception desk, where I scheduled my surgery: June 2020. It was another nine months' time, but this was *finally* it! And when I got a call a few weeks later moving my date up three months, I was even more thrilled. March 26, 2020, would be the fateful day. I was beyond elated.

As the date neared, I told my freelance clients about my surgery and made scheduling arrangements so I wouldn't miss deadlines. Friends offered to bring me food so I wouldn't have to cook post-surgery. I went on one last trip before the eight-week recovery period to Lima, Peru. There, I ate ceviche and drank coffee and Peruvian beer and dipped my toes in the Pacific while thinking about how my life was about to change.

Sitting on the tarmac on our return flight home on March 8, my boyfriend and I noticed the passengers in front of us were wearing N95 respirator masks. We glanced at each other and rolled our eyes. We'd heard something about a flu on the news, but we'd just spent a week in a busy city where we'd crammed into packed buses, shopped in busy markets, met up with friends in loud bars, probably eaten with more than a few microbes on our hands, and we felt totally fine.

And then the world changed. A virus was decimating cities the world over. People began dying in droves. Hospitals were readying their ER departments for a massive influx of direly ill people. It felt like I was watching a zombie apocalypse movie. I refreshed the news every few hours, hoping not to see the news I feared most.

The call came just a few days before my March 26 surgery date: all elective surgeries were canceled, effective immediately. I would probably have to wait until this coronavirus thing was over, I was told; it might take a few months.

My heart sank, filling my chest with dread. The thing I had wanted so desperately for so long, that I finally had within my grasp, was taken from me without a single shred of empathy.

I cried.

◆

Surgery is both an art and a barbaric act. Cutting, hacking, burning, stitching into the unconscious bodies of patients sent home less than twenty-four hours later, or maybe forty-eight. We're discharged and wished all the best.

The concept of hysterectomies is as old as Greco-Roman history, but the first recorded instance of a uterus being pulled out of a vagina was in Bologna, Italy, in 1507.[649] From then on, history has recorded ligatures and lacerations and hemorrhages, scissors and speculums and forceps and scalpels and chisels. The procedures are anything but pretty. The reasons for operating were numerous: uterine prolapse, inversion, tumors, carcinomas. Probably endometriosis, too, since it was frequently conflated with endometrial cancer in medical literature.

In 1813, German surgeon Konrad Johann Martin Langenbeck performed what is often referred to as the first elective vaginal hysterectomy.[650] The patient, a fifty-year-old woman, had pain and a burning sensation in her uterus that caused her such agony she "begged" for an operation.[651] Langenbeck performed the surgery unassisted, and the patient soon began hemorrhaging. The surgeon grasped the bleeding part in one hand and tied a ligature using his other hand and his teeth. He inserted his entire hand inside her vagina and inserted a sponge to reduce pressure on her intestines. This procedure was done without anesthetic. The patient lived.[652]

Some of Langenbeck's peers celebrated him, and others were bitter; they had hoped to get the glory for themselves and cast doubt that he had successfully removed the uterus. He was, after all, the only witness to his supposed success, his assistant having died shortly after the operation. When the patient died twenty-six years later, four physicians performed an autopsy on her to determine whether Langenbeck had been honest.[653]

Apparently, he had been. But this initial success was not a guarantee of future successes. Many more women were sacrificed in the years that followed as he and his peers continued perfecting their craft. Still, Langenbeck died a medical hero. In the Philadelphia Museum of Art hangs a portrait of him looking off to the side, his hand resting on a book positioned next to two skulls.[654]

In Canada, 41,000 hysterectomies are done each year.[655] In the U.S., that number is tenfold, proportional to the two countries' population difference.[656] The majority of them are done for noncancerous conditions such as endometriosis and PCOS, a situation seen as unfortunate by an overwhelming number of journal-published doctors.

Getting a total hysterectomy became a fixation of mine early on because I had a simplistic idea of how to solve endometriosis. Removing the source of the pain prevents future trips to the doctor— right? But many surgeons don't believe that hysterectomy is a cure for endometriosis. One school of thought is that removing the ovaries removes a primary source of estrogen, the hormone that causes lesions to grow. But then what do we do with the information that endometriosis creates its own supply of estrogen?[657] The disease has recurred in people without any reproductive organs at all.[658] And what do we do for people who want to keep their ovaries, which sharply increases the likelihood that the disease will come back?[659] Does all this uncertainty mean the pursuit of a total hysterectomy is futile?

Dr. Jeff Arrington, the Center for Endometriosis Care surgeon we heard from earlier, tells me that many patients who ask for hysterectomies or have the procedure offered to them aren't given the full picture about the potential shortcomings of the operation.[660] "What they're told is that it's the only option, that it's definitive, that that's how you take care of it. In no sense of the definition does it meet the criteria for definitive—[but] that word is used in the ACOG bulletin,[661] and then it directly goes on to talk about patients who continue to have endometriosis after hysterectomy," says Arrington.

Medical residents are taught that a hysterectomy cures endometriosis—and that if disease persists after a hysterectomy, well, then it can't possibly be endometriosis. Arrington says this compromises future care and future insurance coverage. He also says this lack of knowledge can give patients unreasonable expectations about what radical surgery can accomplish. "It just opens up a major, major can of worms," he tells me.

Most of the people who spoke to me who had hysterectomies experienced significant pain relief—but that doesn't mean the disease hasn't recurred or never will. These gray zones are part of why the medical research community continues to favor hormonal contraceptives and GnRH modulators in place of surgery. Those therapies are seen as ways to help preserve patients' fertility (whether the patient wants it or not) while avoiding the costs and risks of surgery. If surgery is suggested, GPs and even some gynecologists may suggest ablation first, a well-known procedure in which endo cells are burned off. Arrington says that this approach often leaves deeper and less obvious lesions behind. "Also, in patients where the endometriosis is deeper, you really don't know how deep you need to burn, and how deep you *can* burn and how long you need to apply the cautery to fully destroy the depth of those cells," he tells me. "That comes into play when you have endometriosis, say, over a ureter or on the surface of the bowel or over the bladder."

He much prefers to dissect and excise cells and lesions because it is more precise and delivers a lower chance of disease recurrence. "I can treat it more like a dermatologist would a mole, where I can be more sure to get margins that are clear to fully remove the width and the depth of the lesion."

Despite its greater precision, though, excision is not considered a first-line treatment for endo. It's not even second or third line in many people's situations, according to ACOG guidelines. Zahn, ACOG's director of clinical practice, tells me that "following a stepwise approach is appropriate."[662] Patients' trajectories through the system may start with anti-inflammatories like naproxen before graduating to oral contraceptives. After that, maybe the doctor tries Depo-Provera or an IUD, then a GnRH agent like Lupron or Orilissa. Maybe an exploratory laparoscopy without excision is next, followed by ablation, then maybe excision—and maybe, one day, a hysterectomy. "Surgery has its place, but surgery should not be used willy-nilly," Zahn tells me, reiterating his point that patient care should be individualized based on how well lesser, non-surgical interventions are tolerated.

Even when they're not all that well-tolerated, though, surgery may still be discouraged. "Nothing is free in medicine," Zahn tells me. Rather, it's a game of balancing risks and benefits, and measuring the value of surgery against the side effects of medication.

I can appreciate that especially in a place as litigious as the United States, that doctors want to avoid needless surgeries. But hearing Zahn speak of this step-by-step process with no mention of the financial, physical and emotional costs of *living* through these layers of experimentation is disheartening. Who, ultimately, decides if a cost is worth paying? Zahn tells me the doctor and patient agree together—but we know by now that patients do not hold equal agency or decision-making power in this realm. The reluctance to be more inclusive of excision strikes me as off, especially when endometriosis specialists concur that excision is the most reliable way of helping patients.

But when I ask Zahn why ACOG hasn't got specific guidelines for endometriosis excision, or a committee that looks specifically at chronic pelvic pain conditions such as endometriosis, or recognition of endometriosis excision as a subspecialty, I think I see a faint scowl unfold across his lips. He and his press officer-slash-overseer are visibly uncomfortable when I point out that this seems like an obvious oversight considering how prevalent endo, PCOS and other pain conditions are. The overseer steps in: "I think all of the topics that we address are equally important at ACOG."

In looking at the list of committees on ACOG's website, though, I can't help but notice some glaring omissions—chiefly, that the committee responsible for developing endometriosis guidelines does not seem to require any endometriosis specialists to sit on the committee.[663] When I ask Zahn if any endo specialists sit the committee, he tightly nods his head. But of course, without knowing the names of commissioners—and without being allowed to see the draft of the new, forthcoming endo guidelines—I am not able to check to see if that's true.

With this line of questioning, I feel like I've just hammered a thorn into ACOG's side. As Guidone and Arrington of the Center for Endometriosis Care alluded to earlier, there appears to be a fundamental disagreement on endo—a widening gap between The Establishment (ACOG) and the new school (endo specialists) on how to diagnose it, how to treat it and how to give people back their lives with as little hurdle-jumping as possible. When I ask Zahn why endo specialists aren't recognized in current guidelines, he tells me that, "In women's health, the only place where we talk about referral is referral to a GYN oncologist for endometrial cancer," explaining that data has shown better outcomes when these kinds of patients get sent to a specialist. But, Zahn continues, ACOG doesn't see utility in referring patients specifically to endometriosis specialists. Instead, he warns me to be wary of "marketing."

"There are people that claim that they're super-duper specialized in certain aspects. It's a marketing ploy," he says.

Clearly, though, something is foundationally broken in the system if patients languish in agony for years—and sometimes even decades—before finally getting to see a doctor who takes them seriously, one who doesn't just shrug their shoulders and prescribe yet another pill. When even generalist gynecologists are unaware of excision's success in alleviating pain, the entire system suffers.

It's really a shame, says Nancy Petersen, the retired nurse and endo educator we met earlier.[664] Keeping patients in the dark on excision also keeps the status quo chugging along. "Endometriosis surgery done well is one of the more complex surgeries that have been developed to help patients, and not many are trained in its fine points. Which may be why ablation is commonly done, as it is quick and easy, however ineffective. Ablation keeps the OR door revolving," says Petersen.

Through her nursing experience and her role as an educator to desperate people, she has seen firsthand how the system operates—and for the vast majority of endo patients, it isn't good. She says patients have told her about their doctors "rationing" healthcare by telling them, "Look, you can limp along with this, it's not really a big deal." She says many patients have also reported that their insurers are the ones demanding lesser interventions before getting better surgery. "I think in some ways that the systems are containing costs on the backs of patients by not sending them on to specialty care. [In the U.S.] we do have insurance companies as gatekeepers, who will not let patients go to specialists or have a surgery, and insurance companies are actually even prescribing what should happen next—you need to take Lupron, you need to do this, you need to do that. And yet they're not really using evidence-based material to make their decisions. They're protecting their bottom line, is what I think is going on," she continues.

When I ask Arrington to comment on the role of insurance companies, he says that in his experience it's pretty easy for him to justify excision over ablation to insurers. Instead, he says, it's often GPs and gynecologists themselves who are telling patients to try birth control, Lupron, Orilissa and ablation first, sometimes giving patients the impression that the order is coming from insurers or some other overseeing force, and that the doctors' hands are tied. Adding to the confusion is that insurance policies are often complicated and require considerable administrative work on the part of the patient—an onerous process they trust their doctors to understand and explain to them. Unfortunately, what often gets lost as far as surgery goes is that past ablations can make future excision surgeries harder to do, because they can leave considerable scar tissue and lesions behind.

However insurance companies get involved, the idea of rationing healthcare and clearing lower hurdles first is prevalent in endometriosis, even in places with supposed universal healthcare. In Canada, every attempt to get specialized healthcare feels like an exercise in rationing, as if the healthcare system wins by making it harder for people with complicated health problems. I suppose the system does lose some of us through attrition—people who give up, people who travel out of country for care, people who die—but this approach is shortsighted. Wouldn't it ultimately be cheaper for the healthcare system to send an endo patient to an excision specialist sooner, rather than have them "drain" the system by seeing a GP a couple dozen times, then get multiple ultrasounds, then have one ineffective surgery, followed by another more effective surgery—all on the taxpayers' dime? Remember that, on average, it takes a person seven to ten years to be diagnosed with endometriosis from the first time they go to the doctor. A 2007 study in the U.K. showed that even back then, a third of women saw their GP at least six times before being diagnosed, and that although those GPs frequently requested their patients do ultrasounds, said ultrasounds only helped diagnose endo 10.6 percent of the time.[665] Given that, it would seem that GPs themselves are the real drains on universal healthcare systems when it comes to diagnosing and treating complex or chronic illness.

Amidst all this, we've also seen how endo care can work better. Sally Zori, a transgender Iraqi musician based in Vancouver, British Columbia, told me that they found it easier to get specialized care by going through trans community healthcare resources.[666] Before Zori had their hysterectomy or had even seriously considered getting one, their doctor referred them to an endometriosis specialist who noticed Zori was also on the waitlist for top surgery.

"She asked me, 'Are you planning on transitioning and taking hormone replacement therapy? Because if you are going to do that, part of that experience would be to have a hysterectomy, because there have been some studies that [say] taking testosterone can wither away those reproductive organs and can potentially cause cancer in the future,'" the specialist told Zori. "If you're not going to use them, and you don't want to have kids, you might as well take it all out." Two years later, Zori decided to go for it, and within twelve months got their reproductive system taken out. In that way, their endo helped them to step into their identity as a trans person.

With a tinge of jealousy in my voice, I tell Zori that their story is so unlike my own, and those of other patients who wait years and years to get referred to a specialist. "I'm very privileged to have had a really easy experience when it comes to this, and I'm really grateful for it," they reply.

Zori got lucky by meeting a doctor who was in a position to help expedite their surgeries, but a lot of trans and non-binary patients struggle to get compassionate, inclusive healthcare. Sunshine, a twenty-two-year-old non-binary intersex person, tells me that when they investigated getting a hysterectomy for their endo through transitioning healthcare services, they were told the only surgery a trans-positive surgeon would do was a hysterectomy, without excising any endo. Meanwhile, an endo specialist said the opposite: only excision, no hysterectomy.[667] It was one or the other, but not both.

Still, when delivered well, trans-positive healthcare has shown what advocacy in medicine can do to improve marginalized people's care.

That isn't to say all trans individuals are dialing a hysterectomy hotline to get preferential treatment. More often than not, interactions with the healthcare system are unkind, dehumanizing and trauma-tizing experiences for trans and other gender non-conforming people. From blissful ignorance to intentional maliciousness, many health-care providers don't know how to care for trans people, which means patients end up spending years trying to get basic, non-discriminatory healthcare services.

There are, however, small pockets of medical professionals who take an activist approach to their practice by providing gender-affirming, trauma-informed care. The blending of the medical and the political creates a kind of doctor-driven allyship that should be normalized, encouraged and extended to other groups.

From that perspective, I feel annoyed with myself for having been jealous of people who'd had an easier time than me getting a hysterectomy. Instead of dragging standards down to the level I'd languished at for years because of systematic denial, it makes so much more sense to raise the bar.

◆

It was the month before my surgery date, before I learned about COVID-19. In February 2020, I decided to record some voice memos documenting what I thought would be my very last period. In the first, I sound light, even happy, as I explain my morning covering Canadian news for *The Guardian*. As I shift into describing my period, though, my voice drops down, as if I can no longer hold up this facade. Between a week of PMS, an eight-day period, and a twenty-two to twenty-five day cycle, I only really get about ten days a month not defined by my period. "I'm very tired, and this is just kind of my normal. That all changes next month. This is my second to last period ever, and that's amazing to me," I croak into my phone mic.

My next dispatch comes a few weeks later, after my surgery was canceled but before I had any idea of the gravity of COVID-19. My voice is deflated and angry as I demand to know how this could be considered elective surgery. It's not like I'm getting a boob job or tummy tuck. To me, it is life-saving surgery.

I pause, my shoulders heaving as I exhale a big breath. The heartbreak in my voice is audible. "I guess I've lived with this pain for so long. What's another couple months?" I say, defeated. "I feel like I had it, and now it's slipping away from me. It just feels like it's never gonna happen, and that's pretty stressful because I just want it to be over with. I was . . . I was really ready, you know?"

March 26 comes and goes. I call the doctor's office almost every week between March and June, asking for information—*anything* they could tell me about what I could expect. Every week, the receptionist gives me a polite "I don't know." It becomes a part of my routine, dots of hope and dashes of disappointment stuffed between work and meetings and the rest of my life.

The first week of June, the receptionist is the one to call me. With excitement in her voice, she asks me what I'm doing next Thursday. The summer's dip in coronavirus infections meant some elective surgeries were back on, and they can squeeze me in. I'm in the parking lot of a suburban shopping mall when I get the call. I immediately sit up, adrenaline coursing through me as I sit alone in my car with my engine off.

I know it could still get canceled at the very last second, but even so tears of hope and joy flood my eyes. Maybe, just maybe, it will soon be all over.

♦

June 11, 2020: surgery day.

Before leaving home, my boyfriend gently pulls out my nose ring. They've promised to cut it off if he doesn't. I'm not allowed to have nail polish on, either—something about not getting a good blood oxygen reading.

I arrive at the hospital and make my way to the holding area, a room where the surgery cases of the day wait their turn. They give me a baby-blue gown and tell me to lay down and wait. After a while— twenty minutes? two hours?—a porter comes for me and wheels me down to the hall just outside of the operating room. An anesthesiologist meets me there and introduces herself, then taps a vein in my right hand for an IV port. Another member of the operating team comes out, a man this time, and explains things to me which I instantly forget.

They push the door open to the OR, and I walk in. Suddenly all eyes are on me.

"I feel like I'm about to have an alien autopsy," I nervously joke as I enter the operating room. A faint chuckle escapes my team of doctors, the seven or eight people—several of them residents—gathered here today to remove my uterus and any other sources of evil. In the era of COVID-19, they dress extra-cautiously, wrapped in layers of face masks, face shields, hair nets, paper coveralls.

It is just another day in the office for them. It is a life-changing moment for me.

The IV port installed in my right hand aches already. The anesthesiologist taped it too tightly to my hand, and I could feel the thin needle pressing into me. My blue paper slippers pad the floor as I gingerly step toward the operating table, a tiny metal bed covered in paper and sterile pads to catch my blood. They invite me to climb on top and lay down, then watch me as I do it.

Once I'm horizontal, the team springs into action. They're all over me. The anesthesiologist stands behind me, cradling my hairnet-wrapped head. Someone grabs my left arm and envelops it in a blood-pressure monitoring cuff that squeezes tighter than any other machine I'd previously met. Is this going to keep squeezing so hard throughout the whole surgery? I ask. Yes, they say, but you won't feel it when you're asleep.

A nurse on my right side starts talking to me, but her voice is just washing over me. I'm fixated on the overhead lights. They are like the ones at the dentist's office, except three, four times bigger. They're turned off for now, but I imagine the blinding glare, thinking of my vagina and insides on display to this room of strangers. I wonder what they'll say about me while I'm unconscious.

I make nervous small talk. "Have you ever been operated on?" I ask the anesthesiologist. Yes, once, when she was sixteen. The room is a refrigerator. Everything is so bright, so sterile, so white. They place a rubber mask over my mouth and nose and ask me to breathe deeply. I take four deep breaths.

I wake up seven hours later in a different bed, in a different room, with different people around me. It's time to take my medication. They put pills in a small cup and bring a straw to my lips. The ice water feels good. I am thirstier than I've ever been, my throat coated in unswallowable sawdust. More water please, I weakly plead in my medicated haze. I feel a stinging need to urinate, and they tell me to just let it go—I have a catheter in. The nurse picks up a bag of my urine to show me I've been going all along. But now that I'm awake, how can I just let it go? I feel a pad between my legs, but I'm not wearing any underwear. It's just there, held in place by my large thighs.

And then I feel it. The pain. How to describe it? It is all encompassing. The headache, like a caffeine withdrawal migraine except a hundred times worse. The ache deep inside my belly, which I can only imagine looks like a bloody piece of raw meat butchered into an unrecognizable tartare. The pain of the constant urge to pee. The gas pressure from all the carbon dioxide they pumped into me to be able to see my insides more clearly through the tiny incisions. Worst of all, my right shoulder feels like it's been repeatedly slammed into a concrete wall; it's the consequence of compression on my right phrenic nerve, which reaches from the vertebrae in my neck down to my diaphragm. It is unlike any shoulder pain I have ever experienced.

I hate the catheter and my body refuses to use it. Around midnight, I ask the nurse to escort me to the bathroom so I can pee. Standing is nauseating and makes my head spin, and the twenty feet to the toilet feel like two hundred. Upon my return, she helps me gently maneuver back into bed. The nurse sees my pain-wracked face and tells me there's no reason to tough it out, to be vocal about my pain so she can adjust my meds. One milligram of Dilaudid does nothing. Two, please. I can't sleep.

I scroll through my phone and find my airplane music, a compilation of Trojan Records ska and rocksteady songs from the 1960s and early '70s. Its repetitive, calming beats always lull me into a state of half-sleep hypnosis. But the snoring from the man with sleep apnea beside me keeps interrupting Alton Ellis and Desmond Dekker, and suddenly it's all I can hear. I flip to a true crime podcast and turn the volume up, letting the host's soothing Australian accent tell me about the Canadian boy who died after his parents tried to cure his meningitis with vitamins. I sleep in fits and starts.

The next morning, I go home, sore but thankful this is all over.

◆

Except it isn't over.

I start bleeding early on a Saturday evening, just sixteen days after my hysterectomy. Bright red blood gushes out of my vagina in volumes I have never seen. My boyfriend drives me to the ER but, because of COVID-19, can't accompany me inside. The ER is mostly empty, and I am triaged almost immediately. Soon, I am inside an exam room being tended to by nurses. I faint briefly while having blood drawn because my blood pressure is so low. I lay down, the horizontal position helping to staunch the bleeding. I'll just wait here for a doctor, I think.

Soon, though, a young nurse enters to evict me from the exam room. She needs it for other patients, she tells me, but the ER looks as empty as when I arrived. Exhausted and scared, I protest. "The bleeding slows when I lie down. I don't want to be bleeding all over the place," I tell her.

"I'll give you a couple of pads," she replies coolly and condescendingly. It appears I do not have a choice. She evicts me not only from the room, but also through the doors and into the hospital's main hallway, a major thoroughfare for patients and staff. I take the only seat available, a single plastic chair stationed diagonally across from the nurses' station, hoping I will see the gynecologist soon.

Instead, I wait, and wait, and wait. I watch as some people get called into the ER, and others get to leave. Doctors, patients, nurses all walk past me as I sit alone in the hallway, invisible in my single chair. Have they forgotten me? I wonder. I look at the other patients coming and going; none of them seem to have a situation as urgent as mine. I am bleeding profusely out of my vagina just two weeks after a major operation. Is that not urgent?

The anxiety rises in my throat; all my abandonment fears come home to roost. The people who are supposed to care don't care. They can't even see me. They think I'm crazy, that I'm hysterical. The tears begin to trickle down my cheeks, wetting the edges of the paper mask covering my nose and mouth. I try to hide my tears by looking down at my phone; I've always hated crying in public. Like I'm back at the bachelorette party, I hold a tissue to the corners of my eyes, dabbing my tears, hoping to get them under control, as if doing so would snap me out of the looming panic attack.

The dam breaks. Now I am openly weeping, just ten feet from the nurses' station in full view of the woman sitting behind the glass. She keeps glancing at me but never once asks me if I'm all right. Soon, my mask is soaked with tears and snot and I can't breathe, so I take it off. No one tells me to put it back on. No one in this busy hallway can even see me. And then an obviously intoxicated man stumbles past me, heading for the exit. Two security guards run after him, handcuffing the man and dragging him back behind the swinging doors that lead to the rest of the hospital. The man is kicking and screaming in protest. Stunned by the violence, I cry even harder.

The nurse who evicted me from the exam room casually chats with her colleagues in the nursing station. She's thinking about getting some coffee at Tim Hortons. And then the conversation turns to me. She mocks me to her fellow nurses, telling them how I had protested my removal by arguing that I "didn't want to bleed all over the hallway"—as if that was an irrational thing to say! The incredulity and meanness of jaded youth fills her voice as she continues talking. My face flushes hot. I am suddenly filled with rage. How could a nurse—especially an ER nurse—be saying these things, especially within earshot of patients? The more she talks, the more I can feel the anger swirling inside my head. Fight or flight, fight or flight . . . What should I do?

I suddenly hear myself yelling: "I CAN HEAR YOU."

The voices from the nursing station quiet and eyes turn toward me. I stand up, then they stand up. Now I'm in front of the glass-enclosed desk, words pouring out of me. "I have PTSD," I snap. "I am having a major anxiety attack. The receptionist can literally see me freaking out but hasn't thought to send anyone to check on me. I am bleeding two weeks after having major surgery, a surgery I waited to get for ten years. You don't know what I've been through, but if you don't think I need to be here, cut this bracelet off my wrist and let me leave. Making fun of patients is unprofessional. You are a nurse in an ER department. Where is your empathy?"

Their faces are frozen in shock. A younger me would've stewed in silence and wondered if maybe I was being a little crazy. Now I am vindicated. At thirty-five, I have no fucks left to give.

The ER resident in charge that night emerges from the treatment area claiming to have missed the entire episode, that she didn't know why I was upset but she would listen to my "side" of the story. She brings me into an abandoned area of the ER where I could be alone— why wasn't I put here in the first place?—and makes a show of listening empathetically as I retell the story. But when I ask for the nurse's name, she pretends she didn't hear the question. When I ask again and tell her I intend to file a complaint, she again fails to answer. A month or so later when I make the complaint, the ombuds office tells me they couldn't identify the nurse. When I get my medical records some time after that, I find the nurse's name almost immediately.

The resident leaves, and suddenly the gynecologist is ready to see me. By then, the bleeding has stopped. With a long Q-tip, she pokes at the stitches where my cervix used to be. She doesn't know why I bled.

Sometime after midnight, I return home.

The next day, a Sunday, I stay in bed streaming Netflix. My boyfriend brings me coffee and food so I don't have to manage the stairs and my two cats, sensing I am unwell, curl up beside me and purr. No bleeding so far. At midnight I decide to go to sleep. Moments after I close my eyes, *whoosh*. I scurry to the bathroom with blood pouring out of me twice as fast as it had the night before. It is cardinal red against the toilet paper, but in the toilet it grows darker and darker as it pools. I sit in silence, waiting for it to stop, but it just won't. Maybe it will stop again if I lie down, I think, so I stick an extra-thick, extra-long maxi pad to my underwear and prepare to return to bed—except, as I stand to wash the blood from my hands, nausea hits me like an ocean wave, doubling me over. My moans of distress wake my boyfriend and he finds me clutching the sink. Another wave hits, flooding me with nausea. Prepared to retch, I fold my body over the edge of the bathtub, my skin cool and clammy, my hair drenched with sweat. I fall in and out of consciousness as blood pours out of me and onto the floor.

He calls 911. The prospect of paramedics finding me naked pushes me out of unconsciousness, and I rush to put on the same outfit I'd worn to the ER the night before: sparkly rainbow leopard bike shorts and a striped tank top, no bra. Still alert when the paramedics arrive, I am gently coaxed down the stairs and into the ambulance on foot. At the hospital, I am being wheeled into the observation area of the ER when I see that callous nurse from the night before. "Not her! I don't want her touching me," I moan to the paramedics. They wheel me out of her section and into another. Overnight, my bleeding mostly stops again. Without the active bleeding, my case falls further and further down the priority list. I am the girl who cried hemorrhage.

I drift in and out of sleep for the next twelve hours, my head pounding from caffeine withdrawal. Again, I am poked with a long Q-tip, one spot so tender I gasp and curl all my fingers and toes. My red blood cells drop from 127 during my first ER visit to ninety; low, but if I take iron and am careful, I will recover, they tell me as I am discharged.

And what if I bleed again? I ask. Then you'll have to come back.

Desperate to avoid a repeat, I try my hardest to keep all of my blood inside me by getting up only when absolutely necessary. But it happens again that night, this time with the intensity of a garden hose on blast. At 4 a.m. I shuffle to the bathroom and sit on the toilet; within moments, I black out. I manage to summon my boyfriend, who was sleeping in the room closest to the bathroom. What would I have done if I lived alone? Massive clots the size of leeches slip out and clog the toilet. This whole experience feels like that scene in *The Shining*, the one where Wendy stands frozen, clutching her knife as blood comes crashing down the hallway. I can't stop the rolling blackouts, and this time the paramedics find me passed out in all my Elvis glory—on the toilet, naked except for the underwear around my ankles. "Oh boy," the paramedic says as he peers around the edge of the door at me. "Can you walk? Can you get into the hallway?" Extricating me from the tiny bathroom, with the toilet behind the door, would be a challenge. I say I'll try, but by the time I wake up again I'm lying down in the hallway with no recollection of how I got there. At least they'd draped a sheet over me, a kindness considering all four people standing over me were men.

The memories of how I went from sitting on the toilet to lying in the ER are snippets of images, like a broken movie reel. I remember being told that my red blood cells had dropped to seventy-six, and

I remember opening the calculator app on my phone. It told me that I had lost 40 percent of my red blood cells and about a fifth of my blood in seventy-two hours. I didn't know then that it was a life-threatening situation that can make the heart unable to pump blood to the organs. My surgeon later tells me that I could have had a heart attack if I'd lost any more blood. I get a transfusion a few hours later, and I absentmindedly watch as two bags of A-positive enter me through the IV port in my left hand. I wonder if I would have fought so hard for the hysterectomy if I had known this was going to happen.

Back at home, my boyfriend had heroically fished some of the massive chunks of tissue out of the toilet and took pictures of them beside a measuring tape. Some are five inches long and almost as wide, and they look like soft gelatinous pieces of liver. He texts them to me, evidence I can use to make the doctors understand what is happening to me. He is now in it with me. I feel loved.

By the time I left the hospital two days later, I had been operated on again. My surgeon sewed a few stitches into the loose seam of the vaginal cuff I had in place of a cervix. He told me a corner of the seam had a raw edge, and that was the source of all my blood loss. A tiny little fray in a hem was all it took.

In the days following my discharge, I swelled with anxiety. I read medical papers about vaginal cuff dehiscence, or cuff separation. These papers told me that this could happen years after a hysterectomy, and that it was in most cases provoked by sex. Oh my god, my mind gasped. Did that mean I could be eviscerated? I imagined my stitches ripping out of me like buttons popping off the shirt of a rapidly inflating Marshmallow Man. My surgeon corrected me some days later, after I called in a panic. It was *not* a dehiscence, he told me, assuring me the problem had been fixed.

As I write this, it is now mid-2022, and I am happy to report that I have considerably less pelvic pain and that I have not yet been eviscerated.

9. BAD REPUTATION

burning it down

It was
Forty days after my hysterectomy
And eighteen days since my hemorrhaging stopped
That my surgeon told me that maybe
I should consider losing weight
And that
Because he was vegan
I should be vegan
Just three weeks ago
I lost one-fifth of my blood

This situation deserves poetry, because every other sentence structure feels so inadequate. What else could I say? That it's supremely
fucked up that three weeks after being hospitalized for extreme blood
loss, my surgeon told me that as a gynecologist, and as a man who
had many close female family members around him, he couldn't
consent to cows being raped to make cheese? And that even after I
told him I had been a vegetarian for ten years, but started eating meat
again because it was impossible for me to lose weight otherwise, and
that after doing so I went on to lose eighty-five pounds, he suggested

I try intermittent fasting, even though I was at that time severely anemic from blood loss?

I recorded the online pathology appointment because I knew my memory would be unreliable given the anesthetic, the trauma and the pain meds, and I wanted his exact descriptions of what he found so I could Google them later. Listening back now, though, I realize that the parts of the conversation I remembered were only part of the story. My brain had discarded some of the wilder things he said to me.

I was incensed that he felt entitled to talk to me about my weight after everything I'd just endured. Even after I pushed back and told him that yes, I did have mirrors, and also that I had some kind of disordered eating thing, he persisted and went on to give me dieting advice. This was during the first year of the pandemic, when gyms oscillated between closed and open every other week. Not that I was even able to return to the gym in such a fragile postoperative state; my immune system was already taxed from healing my cut-up abdomen and the bladder infection that followed me home from surgery.

I'd asked my partner to attend the virtual appointment because I needed a witness, and I needed him to know just how sick I had truly been. With him sitting next to me at my desk, we listened as the doctor delivered dieting tips and ways to extend my lifespan. As he went on, the appointment shifted; the doctor was speaking to my athletic boyfriend, and I was the observer. I felt like the third wheel to my own pathology appointment. Of the thirty-nine minutes we were on video, just six minutes were spent discussing my surgical results and my next steps.

His callous weight-loss advice felt like an enormous betrayal. I was struck by how he seemed to have more empathy for cows than for the patient in front of him.

In retrospect, I hate that I even entertained this conversation, that to feel included I had detailed and defended all the work and energy and suffering I'd invested into feeling a little less awful about my body. I didn't owe him any explanations or promises. He wasn't even going to be following me as a patient. We would likely never see each other again.

That didn't change the fact that when I first met this man, I saw him as my savior, as the one and only person who would do the operation I had wanted for so long. He was the person who would finally put me out of my misery. I had noticed that, during our first meeting, he didn't mention my weight before my surgery. I thought he saw me as a *person*. I thought he was different. But I guess when he was forced to see my naked abdomen twice in three weeks, something in his brain told him he just had to say something.

I tossed the memory of this appointment on top of the heap of the other fucked-up things doctors have said to me. By then, I had accumulated quite the collection. Like other fat people, I'd had my size blamed for every health complaint I'd ever had. From cramps to back pain to migraines, the answer was always "lose weight."

When I really thought about it, I couldn't remember one single health professional who hadn't mentioned losing weight. There was the orthopedic surgeon I met in 2018, the first specialist I'd ever seen about my two slipped vertebrae in my lumbar spine. I believe I incurred the original injury back around 1998, when I bent down to pick up a volleyball in gym class, although the ER I visited then didn't bother to take any X-rays. It had become more and more painful over the years, no matter how much I weighed. It hurt when I was at my lowest adult weight as much as it hurt when I was at my heaviest. At that 2018 appointment, a resident checked my alignment as I lunged, squatted and walked, then watched as the surgeon told me I should consider losing weight. When those words tumbled out of his mouth, it felt like the connection between my brain and my vocal cords seized, like a helmet made of cement was pressing against my forehead. I shut down; it was clear he wouldn't be the one to help me. I sat on the exam table in stone-cold silence, eyes averted, unable to speak. He kept talking, but I wouldn't reply. Finally, my cerebellum propelled me off the table and out into the hall, then outside of the hospital and into my car, on the top floor of a parking garage. As I rounded the first curve in the spiral ramp, I fantasized about driving through the cement and crashing to my death.

Instead, I returned home, where I stewed over the appointment all day. I was immensely bothered that this stranger probably thought I was crazy. I needed him to know that he had hurt me in one of the ways that hurts me most. So I wrote him an email:

> I thought you should know why I was so upset by your comments.
>
> Instead of assuming that I haven't tried or considered losing weight, it would have been better to ask me what I've done so far. You didn't know, for instance, that I have struggled for more than ten years to lose weight. In that time, I actually lost eighty-five pounds, injured myself badly at the gym, then gained just over half of the weight back. I have literally thought about my weight every single day of my entire life. I have tried everything, including starving myself.
>
> You did know from my interview with the resident that I struggled with endometriosis, depression and anxiety. I think it would be obvious to almost anyone, especially people in the medical field, that there are distinct correlations between weight/self-image, chronic pain, depression and anxiety. Unfortunately, I was already at a low point yesterday for other reasons and your comments did a lot more emotional damage than they normally would have.
>
> To assume a patient is unaware of their body—that it is too big, and that they haven't made any efforts to

"fix" it—demonstrates such a massive lack of empathy and understanding. Weight loss is not a simple errand that can be crossed off a to-do list. Your repeated comments not only made me feel awful about myself, but they also minimized the very real pain I feel; as if, by some miracle, losing weight is the solution to all the problems I have with my back, and I'm just too lazy to help myself. But I have to tell you, these problems weren't fixed when I was eighty-five pounds lighter, and I sincerely doubt they will be fixed if/when I lose a significant amount of weight at some point in the future. Meanwhile, the pain I feel is happening right now. I truly do believe that if you had seen me at my thinnest, you would have taken me more seriously.

I have never written a note like this to a doctor and hope I never have to again, but I wanted to ensure no mystery remained as to why I was so upset. Hopefully it makes a difference in the future in the way you speak to people. However, I won't be returning to your office. In fact, my encounter with you has deeply discouraged me from seeking medical treatment for my back overall, from anyone.

His reply was fifty words long. He apologized that he "could not help" me and thanked me for my feedback.

I haven't seen him, or any orthopedic surgeon, since.

Then there was that early October day in 2019—just one day after the ultrasound that gave me my endo diagnosis—when I went to an appointment with my GP. I'd scheduled it to discuss my naproxen intolerance and ask for a referral to the local mental health hospital, which has a community program that dispenses mental health diagnoses in a one-and-done visit with a psychiatrist.

The hospital offers this service because of a profound shortage of psychiatrists in the community.

At the time, I knew I was depressed and anxious, but it felt so nebulous. My psychologist and I suspected PTSD was likely involved, and I trusted her judgment; she has more than thirty years of experience and teaches at one of Canada's top universities. But she had no prescribing power. For that, I needed a medical doctor.

For most of my life, I'd resisted when doctors pushed antidepressants. Like my weight, I saw the drugs as a personal failure—that I just hadn't tried hard enough or done the right things to cure myself. I'd tried a few in the years leading up to this GP appointment, though, but hadn't had great results. And so I decided I wanted to be properly diagnosed by a real psychiatrist, so I could stop trying random drugs to see if they stuck.

It didn't help matters that I disliked my GP and his condescending attitude. He'd only known me for a total of four appointments and acted like he knew everything about me. It irked me that he behaved like this when he was younger than me, having only become a licensed doctor one year earlier. Especially annoying was his office's fifteen-minute-max appointments, where patients were only allowed to discuss one problem at a time.

In my little black notebook, I wrote down my agenda for the day:

Oct. 3, 2019

Prescriptions for:

- Massage therapy
- Psychology
- Physiotherapy for back (spondylolisthesis)
- Naproxen causing leg cramps?

- Referral: [Hospital] mood and anxiety
  program? (has to complete form)

- Or psychiatrist

I sat down and opened my book as soon as the door closed and the fifteen-minute clock started ticking. He eyed me suspiciously as I nervously rattled off the things I wanted to address. He seemed both amused and offended that I was reading instead of looking at him. And then I got to the end of the list: psychiatrist.

In an instant, his face and tone transformed. No, he insisted—*he* should be the one to prescribe me medication. I protested, saying I would rather see a specialist so I could stop the disruptive trial-and-error process. He told me that if he referred everyone who asked, the wait time would be three or four years long.

By then he was standing across the room, arms firmly crossed across his chest, a look of contorted righteousness cast upon his face.

So, you're not going to refer me? I implored.

No, he sniped back.

Do you realize the consequence of not referring me is that I will remain unmedicated? I asked, astonished.

Yes, he sneered.

He dug in further, telling me that he didn't like that I came in here with my "little notebook" and started making "demands." Based on our previous visits, he spit at me, he thought I had borderline personality disorder.

I flashed back to that scene in the film *Girl, Interrupted* in which the asylum patients break into the resident psychiatrist's office at night to read their files. In the movie, set against the backdrop of 1960s social change, Winona Ryder's character discovers her diagnosis, which had been kept secret from her: borderline personality disorder. She plucks a textbook from the shelf and reads the description out loud: "An instability of self-image, relationships and mood.

Uncertainty about goals, impulsive in activities that are self-damaging such as casual sex. Social contrariness and a generally pessimistic attitude are often observed."

She looks up and tells the other patients, "Oh that's me."

"That's everybody," retorts Angelina Jolie's character.[668]

Indeed, borderline personality disorder (BPD) has long been wrongly diagnosed in women who don't actually have it, especially ones with severe trauma and histories of childhood abuse, as well as those with rebellious or antiauthoritarian streaks.[669] Over the years, evidence has mounted that overdiagnosis of this disorder is part of the history of pathologizing normal behavior in women. As one paper argues, "The diagnosis of BPD is the latest manifestation of historical attempts to explain away the strategies which some women use to survive and resist oppression and abuse, by describing these strategies as symptomatic of a disturbed personality/pathology."[670]

I sat there holding the emotional grenade the GP had just thrown at me, knowing that he expected me to use it to self-destruct. Instead, I told him that I disagreed and that my psychologist also didn't think I had BPD.

"Well, *she's* not an MD," he lashed back with all the vitriol he could muster.

I paused. *What. Is. Happening?* His response was a prime example of epistemic injustice and the idea that neither my therapist nor I had anything valuable to contribute because we were not doctors. But this guy had known me for a total of sixty minutes, while she'd known me for fourteen years. And I'd known my own body and brain for thirty-five years! Didn't that count for something?

And the sexism! I had a hard time imagining him ever talking to, or about, a man this way. My options flashed before me. I thought about storming out. I thought about slapping him. My amygdala screamed at me to pick one: fight or flight.

I fought.

"You are the most condescending, paternalistic doctor I have ever seen," I said firmly and evenly. "I know I am not the perfect patient, but you should consider what I've been through with all my health problems and trauma. I was just diagnosed *yesterday* with stage-four endometriosis. You should understand I have major anxiety about seeing doctors, especially you. You make me more anxious than any other doctor I have ever seen."

I paused. What did this doctor even do for me, I asked myself.

"You're not my doctor anymore," I informed him. "I would rather see a million walk-in doctors than ever see you again." I told him I wanted him to write the entire encounter down in my file and then I hurried out, through a waiting room stunned into silence. They had heard everything through the closed door.

A month later, a walk-in doctor I saw over video conferencing referred me to the mental health hospital. Two months later, a psychiatrist there diagnosed me with complex PTSD, a condition informed by both my childhood traumas and my medical traumas. I felt vindicated; I *knew* I was right. But even that victory was cruelly snatched away.

After the appointment, the psychiatrist walked me to the hospital's exit. As I turned to say goodbye, he told me, "You know, all this has probably stopped you from living up to your full potential."

With just one off-the-cuff remark, he equated everything I'd done thus far with failure; that if only I'd seen him sooner, I could have done more important things in life. That I had been weak by letting my pain hurt me. Even if there is a grain of truth in his comment, why had he *told* me? What good could it have possibly accomplished? I walked to my car in a disorienting mixture of validation and sadness, mourning the person I could have been and all the things I had missed out on.

I suppose I got what I came for: a diagnosis. I also left with a sense that I had signed myself up to be pathologized even more than I already had been.

As Dr. Jessica Taylor writes in the opening of her book *Sexy but Psycho*, "Psychiatry is the patriarchy with a prescription pad, and a pen full of ink."[67] She argues that the reason women and girls have been pathologized and dehumanized from time immemorial is because our societies do not want to be held accountable for the misogynistic harms they perpetrate and perpetuate. Of course, this line of thinking can be extended to LGBTQ+ people, as current and historical victims of patriarchy-driven pathologization.

After thirty-eight years on this planet, I am inclined to agree.

It's delusional to think that in a world full of abuses of power, that medicine is somehow exempt. Doctors are given enormous trust and power, by patients and by society at large, and some doctors abuse it at will.

Remember it wasn't always like this. As we saw in previous pages, it became this way through a mix of malevolence, masculinity and the idea that some people matter more than others.

In and outside of healthcare, so many people seem to have no trouble believing that women's anger or rebelliousness is a consequence of mental or moral delinquency, rather than a reaction to the systemic injustice and discrimination we endure. From "angry Black women" to "feminazis" to "fat cows" to "crazy bitches" to "stupid sluts," our communal vocabulary has so many vivid descriptions for defective women, yet almost none for cis men. Trans and non-binary people, too, experience incredibly specific insults about their bodies and genders and sexualities. Yet, if we speak out against these stereotypes, we "can't take a joke." If we remain quiet, we are viewed as dumb and deserving of our mistreatment.

As we learned earlier, uteruses have been blamed for defective females for at least as long as medicine's written record has existed. In a one-thousand-page, "field-defining" handbook on menstruation published in 2020, writer Sally King explains that when the concept of hysteria shifted from a physical condition to an emotional one in the 1600s, ill women came to be seen as "pathologically emotional and thus have a reduced capacity for reason."[672] Irrationality, irritability, anger and sadness became part of female illness, which neatly categorized womanhood into something doctors could treat. This coding became integral to the delivery of women's healthcare, to such an extent that even today physical illness is overwhelmingly viewed through an emotional lens, often leading to physical symptoms being brushed off or viewed as mental ones.

Even worse, this belief has trickled down to the general public because of our societal faith in medicine, and that has empowered our spouses, family, friends and colleagues to question whether our suffering is real or whether they're merely witnessing psychosis in action. Our periods in particular are blamed for every flash of anger or annoyance, every emotional moment.

The myth that our hormonal cycles make us unreliable and mentally unstable is so pervasive, but it is not an accurate depiction of reality. Rather, it smacks of a society-wide unwillingness to understand how female bodies work, and it supports the untrue notion that males aren't also influenced by their hormones. This obstinance is liberally sprinkled across our common cultural understandings and interpretations of the female. It even filters down to our own opinions of our behavior. Who hasn't blamed their period for at least one outburst, one meltdown or one depressive funk? "Sorry, I was having terrible PMS" is a universal bat signal that explains, with no further information necessary, that we were merely beholden to the blood goblins living inside of us.

In this way, women's emotions and illnesses are associated with incompetence—either the failure to control our bodies and minds, or the inability to override them when they malfunction. Worse, the more marginalized we are, the more accountable we're held for our perceived failures. "No excuses" is wielded against people facing enormous systemic barriers and socioeconomic inequalities. Our society condones meting out healthcare as if it were a meritocracy, and then it blames people for not "achieving" health.

This dynamic is fundamental to what nearly every single person I interviewed called "the game": appealing to doctors by trying to become the kinds of "perfect" patients they would want to care for. Beth Allan, from the chapter Typical Girls, told me that because of her weight, she felt she could never win the care she needed, because her doctors never saw her as a person. At the end of our interview, I asked her what she wanted doctors to know. "We need people to start recognizing that people are treated differently based on how they look and who they are and what resources they have available to them," Allan answered. "It doesn't seem fair that people have to play the game well to [get] treated. It would be really nice if everyone could just have someone be on their side and have someone believe them."[673]

In a doctor-patient relationship, we remove the intimacy aspect of gaslighting and replace it with paternalism. The gaslighter reminds us they are the ones who are trained professionals, not us, and that our concerns are frivolous or naive. When we challenge their knowledge or medical verdicts with the research and legwork we've done on our own to understand what is happening to us, we're told not to believe everything Dr. Google has to say. Our pain is constantly downgraded because there's simply no way we're suffering as much as we say we are. We're merely hysterical hypochondriacs who are making it worse by thinking about our suffering.

This chips away at our credibility and the legitimacy of our misgivings—and because we live in a misogynistic world, that's unfortunately very easy to do. And because we also still live in a deeply prejudicial world, it becomes even easier to discredit a person as intersections of "otherness" multiply along the fault lines of race and ethnicity, gender, sexuality, socioeconomic class, disabilities and body size.

This isn't mere discrimination. It is an act of violence.

This reminds me of a moment on *Good Morning America* in April 2022, when endometriosis and chronic illness advocate Jenneh Rishe went on national TV to discuss medical gaslighting in support of her book *Part of You, Not All of You*.[674] Rishe told her story of medical mistreatment to a reporter, who went on to discuss with another source how Black women are less likely than white women to be taken seriously by doctors. Then the camera cuts to host Robin Roberts speaking to the program's chief medical correspondent, Jennifer Ashton—a doctor who is also the only white woman involved in the story. Ashton begins by saying she shook her head throughout Rishe's story, then gets down to brass tacks. "Well, first, I think we have to start with the assumption that any physician actually wants to do the best by the patient—so unfortunately this does happen, but it is not the norm, number one," she says with a split-second grimace and a dismissive hand wave.

In a story about medical gaslighting, the correspondent gaslit Rishe live on TV with no one seeming to notice or give it a second thought. Then Ashton went on to say that patients should get a second or sometimes even third opinion, without registering the thought that perhaps the reason a patient might need two or three (or more) medical opinions is because the first doctors gaslit them.

Instances like this, along with my experience and the experiences of everyone else who spoke to me for *BLEED*, are part of an overwhelming body of evidence proving the general medical mistreatment of women, as well as trans and non-binary people, and the specific mistreatment of endo patients in particular. This abuse is egregious and yet is so deeply entrenched in the functioning of the whole medical machine that it's become almost completely invisible. As with the sick role, these scenarios arise so frequently and so naturally within doctor-patient dynamics that patients often don't even realize they're happening.

Worse, sometimes even doctors don't know they're gaslighting patients. An instruction to lose weight to cure your endometriosis might seem logical at the moment, but it's like being told to walk off a brain tumor. It's not a real solution, but that doesn't stop it from *feeling* real. And when it feels real, that's how you know the gaslighting has worked.

Against this fraught and complex backdrop, it's hard to imagine how anyone with a female-coded disease like endometriosis or PCOS can ever win the healthcare game.

◆

I admit that in my thirties I have become more adversarial, more doubtful of doctors' opinions and more willing to challenge them, and that doesn't particularly endear me to doctors. In their eyes, I am a "difficult" patient.

But I also know the consequences of deference. I have been given drugs that made me feel worse—if not physically, then mentally. But when I reported adverse reactions, doctors told me they'd never heard of *that* before. I was told that losing weight would solve all of my medical problems, with one walk-in clinic doctor in 2021 going so far as to try to trick me into giving him my height and weight so he could secretly calculate my BMI—a bullshit tool[675, 676, 677] used to measure "health" based on a person's height-to-weight ratio but which actually is used to stigmatize fatness. It took me years, and even decades, to get referrals to doctors who could have helped me in quicker, more meaningful ways—something that would have dramatically improved my quality of life and reduced my medical trauma. And yeah, maybe even increased my odds of reaching my full potential.

I suffered as a result, physically and mentally. The gaslighting made me doubt my sanity, made me hate my body, made me feel worthless, made me feel like I didn't deserve a good life. When my hope was taken away from me, I had to invent reasons and rewards for staying alive. Having to push, and push, and push just to be heard is exhausting, and it's so easy to give up and play along.

The sense of empowerment I've since gained has let me challenge my doctors on their cruel words and behavior, but only to a certain extent. I never did make any formal complaints against them, after being told by the medical college that it would trigger a process in which the doctor had a right to challenge it.

Why bother? I already knew what would happen. This retreat may feel familiar to those with endo, PCOS, adenomyosis and other chronic diseases. How do you assert yourself in situations where power is so unbalanced that doctors feel entitled to say the most hurtful, disrespectful things to you with no fear of being held accountable?

It is, after all, your word against theirs.

◆

I wish I could tell you that being an empowered patient gets me respect or better treatment, but it doesn't. Not really, anyway. Even if I mention that I wrote a literal book about endometriosis, showing my expertise often feels like showing Daddy what a good sandcastle I made.

But I've been trying to become more strategic, more specific and more insistent. I spent half of 2021 getting all of my medical records, from as far back as I could. I asked every hospital I'd ever been to and every clinic I could remember visiting for my blood test results, imaging, reports and notes, and then I compiled a massive spreadsheet with all the things I've ever been tested for, and what the results have been over time. I update it with every new result, and I make duplicates of the document whenever I want to share my results with practitioners. Keeping the integrity of the master copy also helps me keep my personal integrity intact.

Recently, my spreadsheet helped me to discover I have a severe vitamin D deficiency; the walk-in doctor I shared it with noticed I'd never been tested for it. Having this empirical data speaks doctors' languages. It's not a gut feeling or a fear. It's not a pain scale rating. It's cold, hard evidence that they cannot dispute.

This file-fetching exercise also gave me the opportunity to read doctors' impressions of me. Sometimes the words are difficult pills to swallow, because they serve to reinforce all the charges I've laid out here: that they really do pay attention to how you dress and how you look, that they notice when you get a little teary-eyed, that they think your doctors' office anxiety is indicative of some mental defect. One good thing to come out of the pandemic is the push to do remote consultations. I almost always choose a phone appointment instead of video because it takes away their ability to judge a book by its cover.

That I have to think about any of these things, though, is indicative of just how messed up this all really is. I shouldn't have to be strategic to get basic healthcare and respect.

◆

There is an extraordinary amount of gatekeeping in medicine, especially by primary care physicians. It makes me wonder: did doctors really go to school just to toe these lines?

"The thing is," Nancy Petersen tells me, "the system's against rebellious spirits, particularly in medical school and residency. If you start asking questions that are outside of the standard theory, or the standard approach, you put your career at risk. So you know, challenging the system isn't always a wise thing to do when you're a medical student or a resident."[678] That's not to say there is absolutely no bravery in medicine. Minimally invasive gynecologic surgery (MIGS) fellowships began as small acts of defiance, aimed at training gynecologists who can admit they haven't learned enough to treat diseases like endometriosis, PCOS and adenomyosis.[679] There is some momentum around MIGS, but the number of doctors with this specialized training are still scarce.

And of course, to get to those doctors, we have to run the gauntlet with all the others.

No single failure is responsible for the suffering of millions of people. Instead, we are deeply and repeatedly harmed by the failures of multiple systems and actors, and it leaves many of us feeling as though we have been thrown away. That's exactly why we need more rebels—practitioners who intentionally choose to help rebalance the power dynamics between them and their patients, people who believe in the ideas of patient-centered, inclusive, and trauma-informed care.

There are little glimpses of hope around the world that make it seem as though better care is coming.

Antonio Simone Laganà is an Italian gynecologist working at a Center of Excellence in Minimally Invasive Gynecology just north of Milan. He says Italy has an endometriosis hotline and that patients can access specialized care without a GP's referral.[680] Expanding this approach around the world would be game-changing for people with chronic pelvic pain conditions. Not only would it reduce misdiagnosis and improve outcomes, but it would also reduce patients' overall exposure to a system designed to discredit them.

This center in Italy is part of a small but growing movement toward multidisciplinary endometriosis care, a solution that can bring together the right specialists around each patient—urologists, colorectal surgeons, radiologists, pain specialists, psychologists and pelvic floor physiotherapists, among others—all different disciplines that work together to restore a person's quality of life much better than one single doctor can. Laganà also tells me that patients and expert doctors are working together to organize ultrasound training clinics for young doctors, so they can learn how to identify endometriosis in imaging—something untrained eyes can easily miss.

In Austria, Dr. Jörg Keckstein is building a new classification system for endometriosis called #Enzian, which is meant to be used pre-surgically to provide more information to both doctors and patients about the location, size and severity of disease, as well as its impact on surrounding organs.[681] "This is such a sophisticated disease," Keckstein tells me. He thinks using more advanced ultrasound techniques in combination with the #Enzian classification system would help clear backlogs of patients, because some people wouldn't need surgery to get diagnosed anymore. Plus, a more complete mapping means doctors can plan surgeries better, which optimizes OR time.

There are little sparks of progress in other parts of the world too. In 2018, Australia established a National Action Plan for endometriosis,[682] and in 2022 France said it would create one too.[683]

Maybe these are pieces of a revolution in endometriosis care. Still, there is so much more to do to create a better, more inclusive approach to medicine, and it makes me wonder if it's possible to make change from within a system so afflicted by misogyny, racism, ableism, ageism, fatphobia, homophobia, transphobia and all the other isms and phobias. How could we do it?

I'm not hopeful that doctors like my former GP can be reformed. It may be too late for people like him; they've already been dosed with the amphetamine of power. And I'm not hopeful the entire system can be reformed either. Look at how many cities increased police budgets after the Black Lives Matter movement rallied to defund the police. Even progressive professionals within the system are banging their heads against the wall. Trying to get excision recognized as the gold standard for treatment instead of hormonal drugs, or getting doctors paid according to length of surgery, are frustrating and seemingly futile exercises.

It's obvious that institutional and systemic power does not bend easily. Insurance companies, drug companies, medical associations and other healthcare stakeholders have too much at stake to relinquish their control.

What we need, more than anything, is courage.

Making change from the inside is only so effective. By now, we've all heard some version of Audre Lorde's famous quote delivered in an address on systemic sexism and racism: "The master's tools will never dismantle the master's house."[684] The before and after of that quote, so often missing from reproductions, is all the more relevant to us:

As women, we have been taught either to ignore our differences, or to view them as causes for separation and suspicion rather than as forces for change. Without community there is no liberation, only the most vulnerable and temporary armistice between an individual and her oppression. But community must not mean a shedding of our differences, nor the pathetic pretense that these differences do not exist.

Those of us who stand outside the circle of this society's definition of acceptable women; those of us who have been forged in the crucibles of difference—those of us who are poor, who are lesbians, who are Black, who are older—know that survival is not an academic skill. It is learning to stand alone, unpopular and sometimes reviled, and how to make common cause with those others identified as outside the structures in order to define and seek a world in which we can all flourish. It is learning how to take our differences and make them strengths. For the master's tools will never dismantle the master's house. They may allow us temporarily to beat him at his own game, but they will never enable us to bring about genuine change. And this fact is only threatening to those women who still define the master's house as their only source of support.

Where health is concerned, community, intersectionality and strategy are critical pieces of demanding and enacting change. No one group can do it alone.

We need researchers, medical students, professors and doctors to step up and empower each other to work outside the constraints of a deeply broken system. We need rebellious doctors who care more about healing people in their communities than they do about being invited to conferences or being celebrated in medical journals. We need more doctors to learn that their power was built off the backs of poor and marginalized people, and to recognize that healthcare inequalities not only still exist, but have proliferated because of that legacy. This medical system is the way it is because people did nothing when they could have done something.

Finally, we need more people—even those without these diseases—to hold defenders of the status quo accountable, to get angry at the rampant mistreatment of millions of people and to challenge the systems, in and outside of healthcare, that have so deeply failed us. We need both the least and the most marginalized people to come together in a movement strong enough to make a difference—if not by totally subverting dominant culture, then by at least carving out space for us to get care on our own terms.

We need to be united in the idea that we all deserve to thrive and not merely survive. Improving our prospects for a good life depends on eliminating systemic barriers that stand in the way of patient-focused and patient-led care for everyone who needs it, and we must insist that healthcare gatekeepers either adapt to this or get pushed out.

These big ideas start with one rebellious act: demanding better from every healthcare practitioner you meet. With this, we can each shine a light onto all the places where discrimination lives. That is the first step to better, fairer healthcare.

This is power. Know that we can use it.

EPILOGUE

born to lose, live to win

None of the sufferers I interviewed for *BLEED* have a nice, neat ending to their stories. Some people have found comfort in spirituality, community, alternative therapies, or Eastern medicine. Most people's struggles continue, pushing them through the endless meat grinder that is modern healthcare.

I had a hysterectomy that dramatically reduced my pain, yes. But it also put me into surgical menopause at the age of thirty-six. I don't take hormone replacement therapy because I am terrified that the estrogen will cause regrowth of lesions and adhesions. A couple of gynecologists told me that I'm probably right to be worried, especially since my surgeon didn't remove the endo on my bowel. A third gynecologist, who is a menopause specialist, said that if I used a hormonal vaginal cream, the hormones would only act locally—that there would be no systemic effects.

Surgical menopause hasn't been that awful, especially when compared with the alternatives: still having endo, or being dead. As it turns out, the antidepressant I was taking before surgery (Pristiq, a.k.a. desvenlafaxine) is frequently prescribed to menopausal people to help reduce hot flashes and other symptoms of "the change." That said, I was also essentially castrated when my ovaries were removed.

For most people, menopause brings with it some degree of sexual dysfunction, notably declines in libido and ability to respond to stimulation. It can also make sex more painful—which, when you already have endo, is hard to imagine. Instead of experiencing menopause gradually like most, I was plunged right into it in my mid-thirties. At least I'm not contending with that *and* cramps and bleeding.

Still, I don't know if before surgery, I fully appreciated the trade-offs of a hysterectomy, or how the procedure would change me in little ways. I don't sleep as deeply as I used to; my joints feel stiffer than before. Endometriosis was just such a massive monster under my bed, its shadows creeping up the walls of my life whenever I shut off the light, that I wasn't able to see beyond it. Through its many, many failures, the system forced me to become singularly focused on eliminating my endo-related suffering, determined to the point that I may have also stopped seeing myself as a whole person.

That said, the hysterectomy hasn't totally transformed me. I still feel like me—or, maybe, a version of me. I think I'm happier, not only because I'm not in persistent agony but also because I finally got some of the answers I spent years trying to find.

Like trying to bail out a sinking rowboat with a teaspoon, it's hard to heal from trauma when you're still stuck in the middle of it. Although I've done talk therapy for the better part of the past fifteen years, it felt impossible to make major progress while I was constantly being re-exposed to a traumatizing medical system.

I feel on the other side of it now, although recovering emotionally and physically during a pandemic has had its ups and downs, especially since my main sources of life enjoyment—traveling and going to music shows—were verboten. But through EMDR therapy with my longtime psychologist and the stability provided by the psychiatrist-prescribed antidepressant, I think I've done a considerable amount of healing over the past couple of years. As I write this, I am slowly weaning myself off the antidepressant because I want to test my unmedicated progress and see if therapy alone can work. I'm open to the possibility that I may have to go back on it. I may always need some help. But I can't deny that I am motivated by the idea of cutting one more dependence on the medical system, even if my new psychiatrist is a very nice man.

Writing BLEED has also been instrumental in my healing. Yeah, it dredged up some awful memories. But it also focused my anger and grief, allowing me to process the injustices I've faced while bringing me the hope that maybe I can help make the system fairer for other people.

It's hard to live a modern life totally untouched by medicine. It's impossible to guarantee you'll get the care you need and deserve, and it's even harder to find the agency required to commandeer medical bureaucracy. For instance, since my surgery, I've realized how the medical world is not built to care for youngish people in menopause. I recently called up the administrator for my community's breast cancer screening program to see if I qualified, given my menopausal state. No, they told me. Normally, they only start annual screenings at the age of fifty. When I asked why they chose the age of fifty as a starting point if not because of menopause, the administrator told me that's just the way it is. If I wanted one sooner, I'd have to get a referral from a GP.

It always comes back to the GP, doesn't it?

It's barriers like these that have had me Googling "med school admissions" and "can I be my own doctor?" Somehow, the idea of changing careers and going to med school feels more reasonable to me than asking a GP for anything ever again.

As it turns out, even without synthetic hormones, I have still grown a couple of new adhesions—but, as the gynecologist who did that laparoscopy told me, I'm still at stage zero. I was able to get that information because I went to another country and paid him to look inside me, no GP referral required. I'm extremely privileged to have been able to do that. Money bought me the luxury of being treated like a human with valid concerns. It bought me belief.

Fundamentally, the privilege of being believed is given to so few of us.

To have a feminized sickness that makes you invisible feels like the ultimate punishment in a world that hates women. I've spent so much time fighting for the basics that I'm not sure that I've ever fully mourned the other versions of myself that could have been, if only I had been seen. Have you mourned yours?

But then I think of what I have accomplished in my lifetime, how I made something from nothing. And maybe it hasn't been the biggest something—at least, not yet. Maybe I'll never live up to my full potential, like that psychiatrist said. It's too easy to let others make you feel worthless. Feeling worthy of more than what you are given is an act of rebellion, and I choose to be rebellious.

And so while I may never win a Pulitzer, I have still done some incredible things in my life. Amid the trash fire, I found joy in traveling, in music, in the art of creation. The photo album of my scattered mind is filled with pictures of sacred moments, pieces of history that make me who I am. Packed into a dark CBGB to witness Patti Smith take the stage. Talking to a woman with a therapy cat on a three-day bus trip across the USA. Sitting in a Oaxacan cemetery surrounded by the light of a thousand candles beckoning lost spirits home. Singing at the top of my lungs against walls of sound, propulsive music spinning people around like frenzied tornados. Floating in the perfect cerulean waters of the Adriatic Sea. Stumbling into the jubilant fan section at a Moscow hockey game, watching as fans drummed, danced and waved team flags. Getting swept into the St. Anne Parade on Mardi Gras Day, drifting into the Quarter on the notes of the brass band and too many Bloody Marys. Biking along the canals of Amsterdam, eating ceviche at a cantina in Lima, venturing to Tierra del Fuego at the ends of the Earth. I am worthy of the joy and the awesomeness these memories represent, just as I am worthy of the hopefully thousands more memories to come.

Yes, you and I have suffered enormously. But suffering doesn't have to be everything.

We can't forget to live.

ACKNOWLEDGMENTS

First and foremost, I owe an enormous debt of gratitude to all those who spoke to me for *BLEED*. I hope I have done your stories justice, and I hope I have brought you some element of peace and power.

To Jen Knoch at ECW Press and Marilyn Biderman at Transatlantic Agency, thanks for believing in the power of fury and for giving me the opportunity to set the system on fire. Thanks as well to Sarah Everts and Francine Darroch at Carleton University, whose insights were invaluable.

To sensitivity reader Rine Vieth and fact checker Emily Latimer, thank you for your precision and thoughtfulness—and for saving me from certain embarrassment.

I am massively grateful for my partner, who wishes to remain anonymous. Your support and patience have helped me to heal.

To my dear friends—most of all Jen, Julie and Kat—thanks for your love, kindness, empathy and cheerleading.

For more than seventeen years, my therapist Shawna has provided a safe space for me to process my many traumas. The existence of this book is testament that even deeply embedded pain can heal with time, work and encouragement.

This book was also made possible by a grant from the Ontario Arts Council.

Thanks to the medical professionals who read *BLEED* and use it to bring more compassion and activism to their practice. We need your rebellion.

Thanks also to all the researchers, scientists and journalists upon whose work I relied to weave together this shameful history of mistreatment and gaslighting.

To the sufferers out there: I see you. I believe you. You deserve so much better, and I hope you get it. And to the ones closest to them watching them suffer, remember that love and understanding are free. Being a partner in advocacy is one of the most powerful things you can do to help.

And finally, thanks to the cathartic force of punk rock. Music has taught me so much about values, friendship, love and how to live life in this world.

ENDNOTES

Prologue

1. "Endometriosis," World Health Organization, accessed February 16, 2022, https://www.who.int/news-room/fact-sheets/detail/endometriosis.
2. DataBank, "Population, Female," The World Bank, accessed February 16, 2022, https://data.worldbank.org/indicator/SP.POP.TOTL.FE.IN?end=2020 &start=1960&view=chart.
3. Giselle Hunt et al., "Endometriosis: An Update on Diagnosis and Medical Management," *BC Medical Journal* 63, no. 4 (May 2021): 158–63, https://bcmj.org/articles/endometriosis-update-diagnosis-and-medical-management.
4. Sukhbir Singh et al., "Prevalence, Symptomatic Burden, and Diagnosis of Endometriosis in Canada: Cross-Sectional Survey of 30,000 Women," *Journal of Obstetrics and Gynaecology Canada* 42, no. 7 (July 1, 2020): 829–38, https://doi.org/10.1016/j.jogc.2019.10.038.
5. "Introduction to Endometriosis," The Center for Endometriosis Care, accessed February 16, 2022, https://centerforendo.com/introduction-to-endometriosis.
6. Nikolaos Machairiotis et al., "Extrapelvic Endometriosis: A Rare Entity or an under Diagnosed Condition?," *Diagnostic Pathology* 8, no. 1 (December 2, 2013): 194, https://doi.org/10.1186/1746-1596-8-194.
7. Christina Rei, Thomas Williams, and Michael Feloney, "Endometriosis in a Man as a Rare Source of Abdominal Pain: A Case Report and Review of the Literature," *Case Reports in Obstetrics and Gynecology* 2018 (January 31, 2018), https://doi.org/10.1155/2018/2083121.
8. "What Is Epigenetics?," MedlinePlus, accessed February 16, 2022, https://medlineplus.gov/genetics/understanding/howgeneswork/epigenome/.

9.   Antonio Simone Laganà et al., "The Pathogenesis of Endometriosis: Molecular and Cell Biology Insights," *International Journal of Molecular Sciences* 20, no. 22 (2019), https://doi.org/10.3390/ijms20225615.

10.   John A. Sampson, "Inguinal Endometriosis (Often Reported as Endometrial Tissue in the Groin, Adenomyoma in the Groin, and Adenomyoma of the Round Ligament)," *American Journal of Obstetrics and Gynecology* 10, no. 4 (October 1, 1925): 462–503, https://doi.org/10.1016/S0002-9378(25)90591-1.

11.   John A. Sampson, "Heterotopic or Misplaced Endometrial Tissue," *American Journal of Obstetrics and Gynecology* 10, no. 5 (November 1, 1925): 649–64, https://doi.org/10.1016/S0002-9378(25)90629-1.

12.   Charles Ornstein, Mike Tigas, and Ryann Grochowski Jones, "Now There's Proof: Docs Who Get Company Cash Tend to Prescribe More Brand-Name Meds," *ProPublica*, March 17, 2016, https://www.propublica.org/article/doctors-who-take-company-cash-tend-to-prescribe-more-brand-name-drugs.

13.   "PCOS (Polycystic Ovary Syndrome) and Diabetes," Centers for Disease Control and Prevention, last updated March 24, 2020, https://www.cdc.gov/diabetes/basics/pcos.html.

14.   "Roughly One Quarter of U.S. Women Affected by Pelvic Floor Disorders," National Institutes of Health (NIH), September 27, 2015, https://www.nih.gov/news-events/news-releases/roughly-one-quarter-us-women-affected-pelvic-floor-disorders.

15.   Debby Herbenick et al., "Pain Experienced During Vaginal and Anal Intercourse with Other-Sex Partners: Findings from a Nationally Representative Probability Study in the United States," *The Journal of Sexual Medicine* 12, no. 4 (April 1, 2015): 1040–51, https://doi.org/10.1111/jsm.12841.

16.   "Cervical Cancer," World Health Organization, accessed March 5, 2022, https://www.who.int/news-room/fact-sheets/detail/cervical-cancer.

17.   "Cervical Cancer," World Health Organization.

18.   Hyuna Sung et al., "Global Cancer Statistics 2020: GLOBOCAN Estimates of Incidence and Mortality Worldwide for 36 Cancers in 185 Countries," *CA: A Cancer Journal for Clinicians* 71, no. 3 (2021): 231–34, https://doi.org/10.3322/caac.21660.

19.   "Cervical Cancer," World Health Organization.

20.   "Cervical Cancer—Statistics," American Society of Clinical Oncology, June 25, 2012, https://www.cancer.net/cancer-types/cervical-cancer/statistics.

21.   "'We Need Access': Ending Preventable Deaths from Cervical Cancer in Rural Georgia," Southern Rural Black Women's Initiative for Economic and Social Justice and Human Rights Watch, January 20, 2022, https://www.hrw.org/report/2022/01/20/we-need-access/ending-preventable-deaths-cervical-cancer-rural-georgia.

22. Cecile A. Ferrando, "Endometriosis in Transmasculine Individuals," *Reproduction and Fertility* 3, no. 2 (May 1, 2022): C7–10, https://doi.org /10.1530/RAF-21-0096.

23. Cecile A. Ferrando, Graham Chapman, and Robert Pollard, "Preoperative Pain Symptoms and the Incidence of Endometriosis in Transgender Men Undergoing Hysterectomy for Gender Affirmation," *Journal of Minimally Invasive Gynecology* 28, no. 9 (September 1, 2021), https://doi.org/10.1016/j. jmig.2021.01.018.

24. "Viagra Extended Patent Protection, Generic Wait until 2020," Intellectual Property Expert Group, accessed March 5, 2022, https://www.ipeg.com/ viagra-extended-patent-protection-generic-wait-until-2020/.

25. "Trans Journalists Association Style Guide," February 29, 2020, https:// transjournalists.org/style-guide/.

26. Robert W. Kistner, "Infertility with Endometriosis: A Plan of Therapy," *Fertility and Sterility* 13, no. 3 (May 1, 1962): 237–45. https://doi.org/10.1016 /S0015-0282(16)34503-4.

27. W. Glannon and L.F. Ross, "Are Doctors Altruistic?," *Journal of Medical Ethics* 28, no. 2 (April 1, 2002): 68, https://doi.org/10.1136/jme.28.2.68.

28. Audre Lorde, "The Uses of Anger: Women Responding to Racism," *Sister Outsider: Essays and Speeches* (Berkeley: Crossing Press, 1984), 124–33.

Chapter 1: What Do I Get?

29. Heather Vandenengel, "In Praise of Bagel Etc, Leonard Cohen's Montreal Breakfast Haunt—Eater Montreal," *Eater*, February 17, 2016, https:// montreal.eater.com/2016/2/17/11022286/bagel-etc-montreal-photos#0.

30. David Fleming, "March Madness Brings Increase in Number of Vasectomies," *ESPN*, March 18, 2021, https://www.espn.com/mens-college -basketball/tournament/2014/story/_/id/10675533/march-madness-brings -increase-number-vasectomies-espn-magazine.

31. "Vas Madness Information—It's That Time of Year Again!," Idaho Urologic Institute, February 15, 2018, https://www.idurology.com/its-that-time-of -year-again-vas-madness/.

32. Karen Stote, "Sterilization of Indigenous Women in Canada," The Canadian Encyclopedia, accessed February 16, 2022, https://www .thecanadianencyclopedia.ca/en/article/sterilization-of-indigenous-women -in-canada.

33. Samantha Allen, "It's Not Just Japan. Many U.S. States Require Transgender People Get Sterilized," *The Daily Beast*, March 22, 2019, https://www .thedailybeast.com/its-not-just-japan-many-us-states-require-transgender -people-get-sterilized.

34. Anne Lora Scagliusi, "Life without Children: Some by Chance, Some by Choice," *Vanity Fair*, August 30, 2021, https://www.vanityfair.com/london /2021/08/life-without-children-some-by-chance-some-by-choice.

35. Alanna Weissman, "How Doctors Fail Women Who Don't Want Children," *The New York Times*, December 1, 2017, https://www.nytimes.com/2017/11/30 /sunday-review/women-sterilization-children-doctors.html.

36. Committee Opinion, "Sterilization of Women: Ethical Issues and Considerations," American College of Obstetricians and Gynecologists, April 2017, https://www.acog.org/en/clinical/clinical-guidance/committee -opinion/articles/2017/04/sterilization-of-women-ethical-issues-and -considerations.

37. Moira Weigel, "The Foul Reign of the Biological Clock," *The Guardian*, May 10, 2016, https://www.theguardian.com/society/2016/may/10/foul-reign -of-the-biological-clock.

38. Kelly O'Shea, interview by Tracey Lindeman, June 28, 2021.

39. Elizabeth A. Hintz and Clinton L. Brown, "Childfree by Choice: Stigma in Medical Consultations for Voluntary Sterilization," *Women's Reproductive Health* 6, no. 1 (January 2, 2019): 62–75, https://doi.org/10.1080/23293691 .2018.1556427.

Chapter 2: Oh Bondage, Up Yours!

40. Denise (anonymous), interview by Tracey Lindeman, July 1, 2021.

41. Julie Brown et al., "Nonsteroidal Anti-inflammatory Drugs for Pain in Women with Endometriosis," *Cochrane Database of Systematic Reviews* 2017, no. 1 (January 23, 2017), https://doi.org/10.1002/14651858.CD004753.pub4.

42. "Aleve Caplets," Bayer, accessed February 16, 2022, https://www.livewell .bayer.com/document/2436.

43. "Is It Safe to Mix Naproxen and Acetaminophen?" Healthline, August 29, 2016, https://www.healthline.com/health/pain-relief/naproxen-acetaminophen.

44. Emily Sohn, "Why Autoimmunity Is Most Common in Women," *Nature* 595, no. 7867 (July 14, 2021): S51–53, https://doi.org/10.1038/d41586-021 -01836-9.

45. Meghan O'Rourke, "What's Wrong with Me?," *The New Yorker*, August 19, 2013, https://www.newyorker.com/magazine/2013/08/26/whats -wrong-with-me.

46. Talcott Parsons, *The Social System* (London: Routledge, 1991), 294–322.

47. Talcott Parsons, "The Sick Role and the Role of the Physician Reconsidered," *The Milbank Memorial Fund Quarterly. Health and Society* 53, no. 3 (1975): 257–78, https://doi.org/10.2307/3349493.

48. Parsons, "The Sick Role and the Role of the Physician Reconsidered."

49.　Michael Clemence, "Doctors Become the World's Most Trusted Profession," Ipsos, October 12, 2021, https://www.ipsos.com/en-uk/doctors-become -worlds-most-trusted-profession.

50.　W. Glannon and L.F. Ross, "Are Doctors Altruistic?," *Journal of Medical Ethics* 28, no. 2 (April 1, 2002): 68, https://doi.org/10.1136/jme.28.2.68.

51.　Mandi L. Pratt-Chapman et al., "'When the Pain Is so Acute or If I Think That I'm Going to Die': Health Care Seeking Behaviors and Experiences of Transgender and Gender Diverse People in an Urban Area," *PLOS ONE* 16, no. 2 (February 23, 2021): e0246883, https://doi.org/10.1371/journal.pone .0246883.

52.　Greta R. Bauer et al., "Reported Emergency Department Avoidance, Use, and Experiences of Transgender Persons in Ontario, Canada: Results From a Respondent-Driven Sampling Survey," *Annals of Emergency Medicine* 63, no. 6 (June 1, 2014): 713–720.e1, https://doi.org/10.1016/j.annemergmed .2013.09.027.

53.　Laura Colenbrander, Louise Causer, and Bridget Haire, "'If You Can't Make It, You're Not Tough Enough to Do Medicine': A Qualitative Study of Sydney-Based Medical Students' Experiences of Bullying and Harassment in Clinical Settings," *BMC Medical Education* 20, no. 1 (March 24, 2020): 86, https://doi.org/10.1186/s12909-020-02001-y.

54.　Christie Nwora, "Medical Schools Need to Do Much More to Protect Students of Color from Racism," AAMC (blog), July 14, 2020, https://www. aamc.org/news-insights/medical-schools-need-do-much-more-protect -students-color-racism.

55.　Nancy R. Angoff et al., "Power Day: Addressing the Use and Abuse of Power in Medical Training," *Journal of Bioethical Inquiry* 13, no. 2 (June 1, 2016): 203–13, https://doi.org/10.1007/s11673-016-9714-4.

56.　Clemence, "Doctors Become the World's Most Trusted Profession."

57.　Aviva Coopersmith, "How I Learned the Horrifying Truth about My Biological Father," *Toronto Life*, February 22, 2022, https://torontolife.com /memoir/the-horrifying-truth-about-my-biological-father/.

58.　"Dr. B. Norman Barwin, Inactive," RateMDs, accessed March 9, 2022, https://www.ratemds.com/doctor-ratings/72095/dr-b.+norman-barwin -ottawa-on.html/?page=2.

59.　Sharon Dixon et al., "Navigating Possible Endometriosis in Primary Care: A Qualitative Study of GP Perspectives," *British Journal of General Practice* 71, no. 710 (September 1, 2021): e668–76, https://doi.org/10.3399/BJGP.2021.0030.

60.　Moniek van der Zanden et al., "Strengths and Weaknesses in the Diagnostic Process of Endometriosis from the Patients' Perspective: A Focus Group Study," *Diagnosis* 8, no. 3 (August 1, 2021): 333–39, https://doi.org/10.1515 /dx-2021-0043.

61.　Marnie Goodfriend, "Reiki for Endometriosis: Healing Your Sacral Chakra,"

Endometriosis Foundation of America, January 17, 2019, https://www.endofound.org/reiki-for-endometriosis-healing-your-sacral-chakra.

62. Kate Seear, "'Nobody Really Knows What It Is or How to Treat It': Why Women with Endometriosis Do Not Comply with Healthcare Advice," *Health, Risk & Society* 11, no. 4 (August 2009): 367–85, https://doi.org/10.1080/13698570903013649.

63. Debra Carroll-Beight and Markus Larsson, "Exploring the Needs, Expectations, and Realities of Mental Healthcare for Transgender Adults: A Grounded Theory Study on Experiences in Sweden," *Transgender Health* 3, no. 1 (December 2018): 88–104, https://doi.org/10.1089/trgh.2017.0033.

64. John R. Blosnich et al., "Impact of Social Determinants of Health on Medical Conditions Among Transgender Veterans," *American Journal of Preventive Medicine* 52, no. 4 (April 2017): 491–98, https://doi.org/10.1016/j.amepre.2016.12.019.

65. Shanna K. Kattari et al., "Transgender and Nonbinary Experiences of Victimization in Health Care," *Journal of Interpersonal Violence* 36, no. 23–24 (December 2021): NP13054–76, https://doi.org/10.1177/0886260520905091.

66. "HIV Risk Among Persons Who Exchange Sex for Money or Nonmonetary Items," Centers for Disease Control and Prevention, January 12, 2022, https://www.cdc.gov/hiv/group/sexworkers.html.

67. Kate Young, Jane Fisher, and Maggie Kirkman, "'Do Mad People Get Endo or Does Endo Make You Mad?': Clinicians' Discursive Constructions of Medicine and Women with Endometriosis," *Feminism & Psychology* 29, no. 3 (August 1, 2019): 337–56, https://doi.org/10.1177/0959353518815704.

68. Barbara Ehrenreich and Deirdre English, *Witches, Midwives & Nurses: A History of Women Healers* (New York: The Feminist Press, 2010), 86–87.

69. Ehrenreich and English, 62–63.

70. Andrew Green, "The Activists Trying to 'Decolonize' Global Health," *Devex*, May 21, 2019, https://www.devex.com/news/sponsored/the-activists-trying-to-decolonize-global-health-94904.

71. Ijeoma Nnodim Opara, "It's Time to Decolonize the Decolonization Movement," *Speaking of Medicine and Health* (blog), July 29, 2021, https://speakingofmedicine.plos.org/2021/07/29/its-time-to-decolonize-the-decolonization-movement/.

72. Helen King, *Hippocrates' Woman: Reading the Female Body in Ancient Greece* (New York: Routledge, 1998), 1.

73. "Active Physicians by Sex and Specialty, 2019," Association of American Medical Colleges, https://www.aamc.org/data-reports/workforce/interactive-data/active-physicians-sex-and-specialty-2019.

74. Soumya Karlamangla, "Male Doctors Are Disappearing from Gynecology. Not Everybody Is Thrilled about It," *Los Angeles Times*, March 7, 2018, https://www.latimes.com/health/la-me-male-gynos-20180307-htmlstory.html.

75. Christine A. Heisler et al., "Has a Critical Mass of Women Resulted in Gender Equity in Gynecologic Surgery?," *American Journal of Obstetrics and Gynecology* 223, no. 5 (November 1, 2020): 665–73, https://doi.org/10.1016/j.ajog.2020.06.038.

76. Sara Babcock Gilbert, Amanda Allshouse, and Malgorzata E. Skaznik-Wikiel, "Gender Inequality in Salaries among Reproductive Endocrinology and Infertility Subspecialists in the United States," *Fertility and Sterility* 111, no. 6 (June 1, 2019): 1194–1200, https://doi.org/10.1016/j.fertnstert.2019.02.004.

77. Heisler et al., "Has a Critical Mass of Women Resulted in Gender Equity in Gynecologic Surgery?"

78. Linda-Dalal J. Shiber et al., "Current Trends in Compensation for Fellowship in Minimally Invasive Gynecologic Surgery Graduates: A 6-Year Follow-Up," *Journal of Minimally Invasive Gynecology* 28, no. 2 (February 1, 2021): 259–68, https://doi.org/10.1016/j.jmig.2020.05.008.

79. Heisler et al., "Has a Critical Mass of Women Resulted in Gender Equity in Gynecologic Surgery?"

80. Linda Marsa, "Labor Pains: The OB-GYN Shortage," *Association of American Medical Colleges*, November 15, 2018, https://www.aamc.org/news-insights/labor-pains-ob-gyn-shortage.

81. Reshma Jagsi et al., "The 'Gender Gap' in Authorship of Academic Medical Literature—A 35-Year Perspective," *New England Journal of Medicine* 355, no. 3 (July 20, 2006): 281–87, https://doi.org/10.1056/NEJMsa053910.

82. "Research Grants: Awards by Gender and Percentage to Women," National Institutes of Health Data Book, 2022, https://report.nih.gov/nihdatabook/report/171.

83. Anupam B. Jena, Andrew R. Olenski, and Daniel M. Blumenthal, "Sex Differences in Physician Salary in US Public Medical Schools," *JAMA Internal Medicine* 176, no. 9 (September 1, 2016): 1294–1304, https://doi.org/10.1001/jamainternmed.2016.3284.

84. Alexandra Dubinskaya et al., "Disparity in Medicare Payments by Gender and Training Track in Female Pelvic Medicine and Reconstructive Surgery," *American Journal of Obstetrics & Gynecology* 225, no. 5 (November 1, 2021): 566.e1–566.e5, https://doi.org/10.1016/j.ajog.2021.08.032.

85. Christopher M. Whaley et al., "Female Physicians Earn an Estimated $2 Million Less Than Male Physicians over a Simulated 40-Year Career," *Health Affairs* 40, no. 12 (December 2021): 1856–64, https://doi.org/10.1377/hlthaff.2021.00461.

86. Phyllis L. Carr et al., "Gender Differences in Academic Medicine: Retention, Rank, and Leadership Comparisons from the National Faculty Survey," *Academic Medicine* 93, no. 11 (November 2018): 1694–99, https://doi.org/10.1097/ACM.0000000000002146.

87. Anupam B. Jena et al., "Sex Differences in Academic Rank in US Medical

Schools in 2014," *JAMA* 314, no. 11 (September 15, 2015): 1149–58, https://doi .org/10.1001/jama.2015.10680.

88. Michael Mensah et al., "Sex Differences in Salaries of Department Chairs at Public Medical Schools," *JAMA Internal Medicine* 180, no. 5 (May 1, 2020): 789–92, https://doi.org/10.1001/jamainternmed.2019.7540.

89. Heisler et al., "Has a Critical Mass of Women Resulted in Gender Equity in Gynecologic Surgery?"

90. Heisler et al., "Has a Critical Mass of Women Resulted in Gender Equity in Gynecologic Surgery?"

91. Karlamangla, "Male Doctors Are Disappearing from Gynecology. Not Everybody Is Thrilled about It."

92. Brindha Bavan et al., "Leadership Aspirations among Residents in Obstetrics and Gynecology in the United States: A Cross-Sectional Analysis," *BMC Medical Education* 19, no. 1 (September 4, 2019): 332, https://doi.org/10.1186 /s12909-019-1757-x.

93. "ACOG Past Presidents," American College of Obstetricians and Gynecologists, accessed March 8, 2022, https://www.acog.org/en/about /leadership-and-governance/board-of-directors/past-presidents.

94. Ishani Ganguli et al., "Physician Work Hours and the Gender Pay Gap— Evidence from Primary Care," *New England Journal of Medicine* 383, no. 14 (October 1, 2020): 1349–57, https://doi.org/10.1056/NEJMsa2013804.

95. Christopher J.D. Wallis et al., "Association of Surgeon-Patient Sex Concordance with Postoperative Outcomes," *JAMA Surgery* 157, no. 2 (February 1, 2022): 146–56, https://doi.org/10.1001/jamasurg.2021.6339.

96. Steve Bearman, Neill Korobov, and Avril Thorne, "The Fabric of Internalized Sexism," *Journal of Integrated Social Sciences* 1, no. 1 (2009): 10–47, https//jiss .org/documents/volume_1/issue_1/JISS_2009_1-1_10-47_Fabric_of _Internalized_Sexism.pdf.

97. Caroline Medina et al., "Protecting and Advancing Health Care for Transgender Adult Communities" (Center for American Progress, August 2021), https://www.americanprogress.org/article/protecting-advancing-health -care-transgender-adult-communities/.

98. "Kahun Medical Papyrus," Digital Egypt for Universities, accessed February 17, 2022, https://www.ucl.ac.uk/museums-static/digitalegypt/med /birthpapyrus.html.

99. "Kahun Medical Papyrus."

100. Ann Ellis Hanson, "Hippocrates: 'Diseases of Women 1,'" *Signs* 1, no. 2 (1975): 567–84, https://www.jstor.org/stable/3173068.

101. King, *Hippocrates' Woman*, 93.

102. Hanson, "Hippocrates."

103. Hanson, "Hippocrates."

104. Hanson, "Hippocrates."

105. Hanson, "Hippocrates."
106. King, *Hippocrates' Woman*, 228–230.
107. King, *Hippocrates' Woman*, 228–230.
108. Terri Kapsalis, "Hysteria, Witches, and the Wandering Uterus: A Brief History," *Literary Hub* (blog), April 5, 2017, https://lithub.com/hysteria-witches-and-the-wandering-uterus-a-brief-history/.
109. Sander Gilman et al., *Hysteria beyond Freud* (Berkeley, CA: University of California Press, 1993), 21.
110. Gilman et al., *Hysteria beyond Freud*.
111. William Safire, "The Way We Live Now: The Vapors," *The New York Times*, March 24, 2002, https://www.nytimes.com/2002/03/24/magazine/the-way-we-live-now-3-24-02-on-language-the-vapors.html.
112. N. Senn, "The Early History of Vaginal Hysterectomy," *JAMA* XXV, no. 12 (September 21, 1895): 476–482, https://doi.org/10.1001/jama.1895.02430380006002.
113. Camran Nezhat, Farr Nezhat, and Ceana Nezhat, "Endometriosis: Ancient Disease, Ancient Treatments," *Fertility and Sterility* 98, no. 6 (December 1, 2012): S1–62, https://doi.org/10.1016/j.fertnstert.2012.08.001.
114. Deirdre Cooper Owens, *Medical Bondage: Race, Gender, and the Origins of American Gynecology* (Athens, GA: University of Georgia Press, 2017), 15.
115. Cooper Owens, *Medical Bondage*, 4.
116. Cooper Owens, *Medical Bondage*, 73–75.
117. James Marion Sims, *The Story of My Life* (New York: D. Appleton and Company, 1884), 231, http://archive.org/details/storyofmylifoosims.
118. Deborah Kuhn McGregor, "J. Marion Sims," Encyclopedia of Alabama, accessed February 17, 2022, http://encyclopediaofalabama.org/article/h-1099.
119. Sims, *The Story of My Life*, 226–28.
120. Sims, *The Story of My Life*, 230–39.
121. Sims, *The Story of My Life*, 236–37.
122. Cooper Owens, *Medical Bondage*, 2.
123. Sims, *The Story of My Life*, 454–55.
124. Sims, *The Story of My Life*, 298.
125. Rebecca Yamin, "Lurid Tales and Homely Stories of New York's Notorious Five Points," *Historical Archaeology* 32, no. 1 (1998): 74–85, http://www.jstor.org.proxy.library.carleton.ca/stable/25616594.
126. Cooper Owens, *Medical Bondage*, 94–95.
127. Thomas Addis Emmet, *A Memoir of James Marion Sims* (New York: D. Appleton and Company, 1884), 10.
128. Addis Emmet, *A Memoir of James Marion Sims*, 10.
129. Cooper Owens, *Medical Bondage*, 96.
130. Addis Emmet, *A Memoir of James Marion Sims*, 10.
131. Addis Emmet, *A Memoir of James Marion Sims*, 10.

132. Cooper Owens, *Medical Bondage*, 97.
133. Cooper Owens, *Medical Bondage*, 103.
134. Sims, *The Story of My Life*, 436–37.
135. "The Sims Statue Unveiled: A Heroic Figure in Memory of the Great Surgeon," *The New York Times*, October 21, 1894, https://www.nytimes.com /1894/10/21/archives/the-sims-statue-unveiled-a-heroic-figure-in-memory-of -the-great.html.
136. William Neuman, "City Orders Sims Statue Removed from Central Park," *The New York Times*, April 16, 2018, https://www.nytimes.com/2018/04/16/nyregion /nyc-sims-statue-central-park-monument.html.
137. Susan M. Reverby, "Memory and Medicine: A Historian's Perspective on Commemorating J. Marion Sims," *Perspectives on History*, September 17, 2017, https://www.historians.org/publications-and-directories/perspectives-on -history/september-2017/memory-and-medicine-a-historians-perspective-on -commemorating-j-marion-sims.
138. Safiya Charles, "Artist to Unveil 'Mothers of Gynecology' Tribute to Enslaved Black Women Operated on without Consent," *Montgomery Advertiser*, May 7, 2021, https://www.montgomeryadvertiser.com/story/news /2021/05/07/artist-unveil-mothers-gynecology-statue-honoring-enslaved-black -women-operated-without-consent/4937162001/.
139. "Anarcha Lucy Betsey Monument," The More Up Campus, accessed February 17, 2022, https://www.anarchalucybetsey.org.
140. S.E.D. Shortt, "Physicians, Science, and Status: Issues in the Professionalization of Anglo-American Medicine in the Nineteenth Century," *Medical History* 27, no. 1 (1983): 51–68, https://doi.org/10.1017 /S0025727300042265.
141. Leslie J. Reagan, *When Abortion Was a Crime: Women, Medicine and Law in the United States, 1867–1973* (Berkeley, CA: University of California Press, 1996), 93–94.
142. Dominique Tobbell, "Black Midwifery's Complex History," UVA School of Nursing (blog), accessed February 17, 2022, https://www.nursing.virginia.edu /news/bhm-black-midwives/.
143. Michele Goodwin, "The Racist History of Abortion and Midwifery Bans," American Civil Liberties Union (blog), accessed February 17, 2022, https://www.aclu.org/news/racial-justice/the-racist-history-of-abortion-and -midwifery-bans/.
144. Judith Walzer Leavitt, "'Science' Enters the Birthing Room: Obstetrics in America since the Eighteenth Century," *Journal of American History* 70, no. 2 (September 1, 1983): 281–304, https://doi.org/10.2307/1900205.
145. Reagan, *When Abortion Was a Crime*, 10–11.
146. Leavitt, "'Science' Enters the Birthing Room."
147. Reagan, *When Abortion Was a Crime*, 81–99.

148. Richa Venkatraman, "Horatio Robinson Storer (1830–1922)," The Embryo Project Encyclopedia (blog), September 21, 2020, https://embryo.asu.edu /pages/horatio-robinson-storer-1830-1922.

149. Reagan, *When Abortion Was a Crime*, 10–11.

150. Horatio Storer and Franklin Fiske Heard, *Criminal Abortion: Its Nature, Its Evidence, and Its Law* (Boston: Little, Brown, and Company, 1868).

151. Ryan Johnson, "A Movement for Change: Horatio Robinson Storer and Physicians' Crusade Against Abortion," *James Madison Undergraduate Research Journal (JMURJ)* 4, no. 1 (April 4, 2017), https://commons.lib.jmu .edu/jmurj/vol4/iss1/2.

152. Reagan, *When Abortion Was a Crime*, 13.

153. Angel Lopez, "Pope Pius IX (1792-1878)," The Embryo Project Encyclopedia, accessed June 30, 2022, https://embryo.asu.edu/pages/pope-pius-ix-1792-1878.

154. Abraham Flexner, "Medical Education in the United States and Canada: A Report to the Carnegie Foundation for the Advancement of Teaching," Carnegie Foundation (1910), 117.

155. Flexner, "Medical Education," 13.

156. Beverly Murphy, "Black History Month: A Medical Perspective: Education," Duke University Medical Center Library & Archives, accessed April 25, 2021, https://guides.mclibrary.duke.edu/blackhistorymonth/education.

157. Shortt, "Physicians, Science, and Status," 67.

158. "Figure 13. Percentage of U.S. Medical School Graduates by Race/Ethnicity (Alone), Academic Year 2018–2019," Association of American Medical Colleges, accessed February 17, 2022, https://www.aamc.org/data-reports /workforce/interactive-data/figure-13-percentage-us-medical-school -graduates-race/ethnicity-alone-academic-year-2018-2019.

159. "U.S. Census Bureau QuickFacts: United States," United States Census Bureau, accessed February 17, 2022, https://www.census.gov/quickfacts/fact /table/US/RHI125219.

160. "Social Determinants and Inequities in Health for Black Canadians: A Snapshot," Public Health Agency of Canada, accessed February 17, 2022, https://www.canada.ca/en/public-health/services/health-promotion /population-health/what-determines-health/social-determinants-inequities -black-canadians-snapshot.html.

161. John L. Powell, "Powell's Pearls: John Albertson Sampson, MD (1873–1946)," *Female Pelvic Medicine & Reconstructive Surgery* 14, no. 3 (2008), https:// journals.lww.com/fpmrs/Fulltext/2008/06000/Powell_s_Pearls__John _Albertson_Sampson,_MD.11.aspx.

162. John L. Yovich, "The History of Endometriosis Preceding Sampson," *Medical Journal of Obstetrics and Gynecology* 8, no. 1 (May 9, 2020), https:// www.researchgate.net/publication/341606942_The_History_of_Endometriosis _Preceding_Sampson.

163. Yovich, "The History of Endometriosis Preceding Sampson."

164. John A. Sampson, "Perforating Hemorrhagic (Chocolate) Cysts of the Ovary: Their Importance and Especially Their Relation to Pelvic Adenomas of Endometrial Type ('Adenomyoma' of the Uterus, Rectovaginal Septum, Sigmoid, Etc.)," *Archives of Surgery* 3, no. 2 (1921): 245–323, https://doi.org /10.1001/archsurg.1921.01110080003001.

165. John A. Sampson, "The Development of the Implantation Theory for the Origin of Peritoneal Endometriosis," *American Journal of Obstetrics & Gynecology* 40, no. 4 (1940): 549–57, https://doi.org/10.1016/S0002-9378 (40)91238-8.

166. J. Halme et al., "Retrograde menstruation in healthy women and in patients with endometriosis," *Obstetrics and Gynecology* 64, no. 2 (August 1984):151–4, https://pubmed.ncbi.nlm.nih.gov/6234483/.

167. Sampson, "Perforating Hemorrhagic (Chocolate) Cysts of the Ovary."

168. Ray Garry, "The Endometriosis Syndromes: A Clinical Classification in the Presence of Aetiological Confusion and Therapeutic Anarchy," *Human Reproduction* 19, no. 4 (April 1, 2004): 760–68, https://doi.org/10.1093 /humrep/deh147.

169. Dr. David Redwine, interview by Tracey Lindeman, July 27, 2021.

170. "David Redwine," Endopædia, accessed February 16, 2022, http://www .endopaedia.info/redwine.html.

171. Christina Rei, Thomas Williams, and Michael Feloney, "Endometriosis in a Man as a Rare Source of Abdominal Pain: A Case Report and Review of the Literature," *Case Reports in Obstetrics and Gynecology* 2018 (January 31, 2018), https://doi.org/10.1155/2018/2083121.

172. Suzanne White Junod and Lara Marks, "Women's Trials: The Approval of the First Oral Contraceptive Pill in the United States and Great Britain," *Journal of the History of Medicine and Allied Sciences* 57, no. 2 (April 1, 2002): 117–60, https://doi.org/10.1093/jhmas/57.2.117.

173. Robert W. Kistner, "The Use of Newer Progestins in the Treatment of Endometriosis," *American Journal of Obstetrics and Gynecology* 75, no. 2 (February 1, 1958): 264–78, https://doi.org/10.1016/0002-9378(58)90384-3.

174. "Management of Endometriosis," American College of Obstetricians and Gynecologists, July 2010, https://www.acog.org/en/clinical/clinical-guidance /practice-bulletin/articles/2010/07/management-of-endometriosis.

175. "Endometriosis—Treatment," National Health Service, December 4, 2017. https://www.nhs.uk/conditions/endometriosis/treatment/.

176. Parveen Parasar, Pinar Ozcan, and Kathryn L. Terry, "Endometriosis: Epidemiology, Diagnosis, and Clinical Management," *Current Obstetrics and Gynecology Reports* 6, no. 1 (March 1, 2017): 34–41, https://doi.org /10.1007/s13669-017-0187-1.

177. Parasar, Ozcan, and Terry, "Endometriosis."

178. ResearchAndMarkets, "$20+ Billion Hormonal Contraceptives Market by Product, Hormones, Age Group End User—Global Opportunity Analysis and Industry Forecast, 2021-2030," Yahoo! Finance, April 29, 2022, https://finance.yahoo.com/news/20-billion-hormonal-contraceptives-market-115700654.html.

179. Garry, "The Endometriosis Syndromes."

180. Antonio Simone Laganà et al., "The Pathogenesis of Endometriosis: Molecular and Cell Biology Insights," *International Journal of Molecular Sciences* 20, no. 22 (2019), https://doi.org/10.3390/ijms20225615.

181. Holly R. Harris et al., "Early Life Abuse and Risk of Endometriosis," *Human Reproduction* 33, no. 9 (September 1, 2018): 1657–68, https://doi.org/10.1093/humrep/dey248.

182. Shay M. Freger and Warren G. Foster, "The Link between Environmental Toxicant Exposure and Endometriosis Re-Examined," in *Endometriosis*, ed. Courtney Marsh (IntechOpen, 2021), https://www.intechopen.com/chapters/70843.

183. "Dioxins and Their Effects on Human Health," World Health Organization, accessed February 16, 2022, https://www.who.int/news-room/fact-sheets/detail/dioxins-and-their-effects-on-human-health.

184. "What Are Common Symptoms of Autoimmune Disease?" Johns Hopkins Medicine, accessed February 16, 2022, https://www.hopkinsmedicine.org/health/wellness-and-prevention/what-are-common-symptoms-of-autoimmune-disease.

185. "What Are Common Symptoms of Autoimmune Disease?" Johns Hopkins Medicine.

186. Emily C. Somers et al., "Are Individuals with an Autoimmune Disease at Higher Risk of a Second Autoimmune Disorder?" *American Journal of Epidemiology* 169, no. 6 (March 15, 2009): 749–55, https://doi.org/10.1093/aje/kwn408.

187. Adriana Rojas-Villarraga et al., "Introducing Polyautoimmunity: Secondary Autoimmune Diseases No Longer Exist," *Autoimmune Diseases* 2012 (February 20, 2012), https://doi.org/10.1155/2012/254319.

188. "What Are Common Symptoms of Autoimmune Disease?" Johns Hopkins Medicine.

189. Marine Peyneau et al., "Role of Thyroid Dysimmunity and Thyroid Hormones in Endometriosis," *Proceedings of the National Academy of Sciences* 116, no. 24 (June 11, 2019): 11894–99, https://doi.org/10.1073/pnas.1820469116.

190. Valeria Stella Vanni et al., "Concomitant Autoimmunity May Be a Predictor of More Severe Stages of Endometriosis," *Scientific Reports* 11, no. 1 (July 28, 2021): 15372, https://doi.org/10.1038/s41598-021-94877-z.

191. Warren B. Nothnick, "Treating Endometriosis as an Autoimmune Disease,"

Fertility and Sterility 76, no. 2 (August 1, 2001): 223–31, https://doi.org/10
.1016/S0015-0282(01)01878-7.

192. Dr. Jörg Keckstein, interview by Tracey Lindeman, July 1, 2021.

193. P. Vigano et al., "Time to Redefine Endometriosis Including Its Pro-Fibrotic Nature," *Human Reproduction* 33, no. 3 (March 1, 2018): 347–52, https://doi .org/10.1093/humrep/dex354.

194. Peyneau et al., "Role of Thyroid Dysimmunity."

195. Milena Králíčková and Václav Větvička, "Immunological Aspects of Endometriosis: A Review," *Annals of Translational Medicine* 3, no. 11 (July 2015): 153, https://doi.org/10.3978/j.issn.2305-5839.2015.06.08.

196. Vered H. Eisenberg, Mati Zolti, and David Soriano, "Is There an Association between Autoimmunity and Endometriosis?" *Autoimmunity Reviews* 11, no. 11 (September 1, 2012): 806–14, https://doi.org/10.1016/j.autrev.2012.01.005.

197. Vanni et al., "Concomitant Autoimmunity May Be a Predictor."

198. National Cancer Institute, "Macrophage," *NCI Dictionary of Cancer Terms*, February 2, 2011, https://www.cancer.gov/publications/dictionaries/cancer -terms/def/macrophage.

199. Chloe Hogg et al., "Macrophages Inhibit and Enhance Endometriosis Depending on Their Origin," *Proceedings of the National Academy of Sciences* 118, no. 6 (February 9, 2021), https://doi.org/10.1073/pnas.2013776118.

200. Chloe Hogg, Andrew W. Horne, and Erin Greaves, "Endometriosis-Associated Macrophages: Origin, Phenotype, and Function," *Frontiers in Endocrinology* 11 (January 23, 2020), https://doi.org/10.3389/fendo.2020.00007.

201. Dr. David Redwine, interview by Tracey Lindeman.

202. E. Pascoal et al., "Strengths and Limitations of Diagnostic Tools for Endometriosis and Relevance in Diagnostic Test Accuracy Research," *Ultrasound in Obstetrics & Gynecology*, accepted author manuscript, March 1, 2022, https://doi.org/10.1002/uog.24892.

203. "ESHRE Endometriosis Guidelines," European Society of Human Reproduction and Embryology (2022), https://www.eshre.eu /Guidelines-and-Legal/Guidelines/Endometriosis-guideline.aspx.

204. "Table B3. Number of Active Residents, by Type of Medical School, GME Specialty, and Sex," Association of American Medical Colleges, accessed March 9, 2022, https://www.aamc.org/data-reports/students-residents /interactive-data/report-residents/2021/table-b3-number-active-residents -type-medical-school-gme-specialty-and-sex.

205. "Table C1. Number of Graduates of U.S. MD-Granting and DO-Granting Schools, by Last Completed GME Specialty," Association of American Medical Colleges, accessed March 9, 2022, https://www.aamc.org/data -reports/students-residents/interactive-data/report-residents/2021/table-c1 -number-graduates-last-completed-gme-specialty.

206. "Match Results Statistics—Obstetrics and Gynecology 2021," National

Resident Matching Program, https://www.nrmp.org/fellowship-applicants
/participating-fellowships/obstetrics-gynecology-fellowship-match/;
"2021 MIGS Fellowship Match Results," American Association of
Gynecologic Laparoscopists, https://www.aagl.org/service/fellowships/.

207. "Table C1," Association of American Medical Colleges.

Chapter 3: Open Up and Bleed

208. "Starting Your Periods," National Health Service, April 9, 2018, https://www
.nhs.uk/conditions/periods/starting-periods/.

209. "Preventing Child Abuse & Neglect," Centers for Disease Control and
Prevention, March 23, 2021, https://www.cdc.gov/violenceprevention
/childabuseandneglect/fastfact.html.

210. Children's Bureau and the US Department of Health and Human Services,
"Child Maltreatment 2020" (U.S. Department of Health & Human Services
Administration for Children and Families Administration on Children,
Youth and Families Children's Bureau, 2022), https://www.acf.hhs.gov/cb
/data-research/child-maltreatment.

211. "Understanding the Effects of Maltreatment on Brain Development,"
Children's Bureau, Administration for Children and Families, April 2015,
https://www.childwelfare.gov/pubs/issue-briefs/brain-development/.

212. "Police-Reported Family Violence against Children and Youth in Canada,
2019," Government of Canada, Statistics Canada, December 5, 2018, https://
www150.statcan.gc.ca/n1/pub/85-002-x/2021001/article/00001/02-eng.htm.

213. June C. Paul and Emma Kahle Monahan, "Sexual Minority Status and
Child Maltreatment: How Do Health Outcomes among Sexual Minority
Young Adults Differ Due to Child Maltreatment Exposure?," *Child Abuse
& Neglect* 96 (October 1, 2019): 104099, https://doi.org/10.1016/j.chiabu
.2019.104099.

214. Holly R. Harris et al., "Early Life Abuse and Risk of Endometriosis," *Human
Reproduction* 33, no. 9 (September 1, 2018): 1657–68, https://doi.org/10.1093
/humrep/dey248.

215. Sarah M. Peitzmeier et al., "Intimate Partner Violence in Transgender
Populations: Systematic Review and Meta-Analysis of Prevalence and
Correlates," *American Journal of Public Health* 110, no. 9 (September 2020):
e1–14, https://doi.org/10.2105/AJPH.2020.305774.

216. A.A. Alonzo, "The Experience of Chronic Illness and Post-Traumatic Stress
Disorder: The Consequences of Cumulative Adversity," *Social Science &
Medicine* 50, no. 10 (May 2000): 1475–84, https://doi.org/10.1016/s0277-9536
(99)00399-8.

217. Tara (anonymous), interview by Tracey Lindeman, June 14, 2021.
218. "What Is Trauma Informed Care?," Trauma-Informed Care Implementation Resource Center, August 8, 2018, https://www.traumainformedcare.chcs.org /what-is-trauma-informed-care/.
219. Center for Substance Abuse Treatment (U.S.), *Understanding the Impact of Trauma, Trauma-Informed Care in Behavioral Health Services* (Substance Abuse and Mental Health Services Administration, U.S., 2014), http://www .ncbi.nlm.nih.gov/books/NBK207191/.
220. Paige L. Sweet, "The Sociology of Gaslighting," *American Sociological Review* 84, no. 5 (October 1, 2019): 851–75, https://doi.org/10.1177/0003122419874843.

Chapter 4: Typical Girls

221. Dr. Olga Bougie, interview by Tracey Lindeman, May 28, 2021.
222. Donna (anonymous), interview by Tracey Lindeman, June 16, 2021.
223. Committee Opinion, "Dysmenorrhea and Endometriosis in the Adolescent," American College of Obstetricians and Gynecologists, December 2018, https://www.acog.org/en/clinical/clinical-guidance/committee-opinion /articles/2018/12/dysmenorrhea-and-endometriosis-in-the-adolescent.
224. Nicholas Leyland, Robert Casper, and Philippe Laberge, "Endometriosis: Diagnosis and Management," *Society of Obstetricians and Gynecologists of Canada Clinical Practice Guideline* 32, no. 7, supplement 2 (July 2010): S1–S3, https://doi.org/10.1016/S1701-2163(16)34589-3.
225. Committee Opinion, "Dysmenorrhea and Endometriosis in the Adolescent."
226. "Rethinking Menstrual Hygiene as a Fundamental Human Right," United Nations Girls' Education Initiative, May 28, 2019, https://www.ungei.org /blog-post/rethinking-menstrual-hygiene-fundamental-human-right.
227. "More than One in Three UK Women Face Period Stigma," ActionAid UK, May 25, 2018, https://www.actionaid.org.uk/latest-news/more-one-three-uk -women-face-period-stigma.
228. Karla Kossler et al., "Perceived Racial, Socioeconomic, and Gender Discrimination and Its Impact on Contraceptive Choice," *Contraception* 84, no. 3 (September 2011): 273–79, https://doi.org/10.1016/j.contraception .2011.01.004.
229. "Obituary for Trinity Lillian Graves," Benson Family Funeral Home, August 23, 2021, https://www.bensonfamilyfuneralhome.com/obituary/Trinity-Graves.
230. "Adenomyosis," Jean Hailes for Women's Health, last updated June 29, 2021, https://www.jeanhailes.org.au/health-a-z/vulva-vagina-ovaries-uterus /adenomyosis.
231. Sarah Austin, "Sarah Austin, Whose Daughter Committed Suicide Due to

Endometriosis Pain, Speaks Out," Endometriosis Foundation of America, January 19, 2022, https://www.endofound.org/sarah-austin-whose-daughter -committed-suicide-due-to-endometriosis-pain-speaks-out.

232. Georgina Wren and Jenny Mercer, "Dismissal, Distrust, and Dismay: A Phenomenological Exploration of Young Women's Diagnostic Experiences with Endometriosis and Subsequent Support," *Journal of Health Psychology* (December 2, 2021), https://doi.org/10.1177/13591053211059387.

233. Howard Robinson, "Dualism," in *The Stanford Encyclopedia of Philosophy*, ed. Edward N. Zalta (Stanford, CA: Metaphysics Research Lab, Stanford University, 2020), https://plato.stanford.edu/archives/fall2020/entries/dualism/.

234. Robinson, "Dualism."

235. Mathew H. Gendle, "The Problem of Dualism in Modern Western Medicine," *Mens Sana Monographs* 14, no. 1 (2016): 141–51, https://doi.org /10.4103/0973-1229.193074.

236. Leen Aerts et al., "Psychosocial Impact of Endometriosis: From Co-morbidity to Intervention," *Best Practice & Research Clinical Obstetrics & Gynaecology* 50 (July 2018): 2–10, https://doi.org/10.1016/j.bpobgyn.2018.01.008.

237. R.B. Scott and R.W. TeLinde, "External Endometriosis: The Scourge of the Private Patient," *Annals of Surgery* 131, no. 5 (May 1950): 697–720, https:// doi.org/10.1097/00000658-195005000-00008.

238. Gladwin Hill, "Social Ill Is Laid to Endometriosis," *The New York Times*, October 21, 1948.

239. Hill, "Social Ill."

240. Olga Bougie, Jenna Healey, and Sukhbir S. Singh, "Behind the Times: Revisiting Endometriosis and Race," *American Journal of Obstetrics & Gynecology* 221, no. 1 (July 1, 2019): 35.e1–35.e5, https://doi.org/10.1016 /j.ajog.2019.01.238.

241. "The Jezebel Stereotype," Jim Crow Museum, accessed February 17, 2022, https://www.ferris.edu/HTMLS/news/jimcrow/jezebel/index.htm.

242. Donald L. Chatman, "Endometriosis in the Black Woman," *American Journal of Obstetrics and Gynecology* 125, no. 7 (August 1, 1976): 987–89, https://doi.org/10.1016/0002-9378(76)90502-0.

243. Dr. Melvin Thornton, interview by Tracey Lindeman, July 19, 2021.

244. Kimberlé Crenshaw, "Demarginalizing the Intersection of Race and Sex: A Black Feminist Critique of Antidiscrimination Doctrine, Feminist Theory and Antiracist Politics," *University of Chicago Legal Forum* 1989, no. 1, https://chicagounbound.uchicago.edu/uclf/vol1989/iss1/8.

245. Heather Guidone, interview by Tracey Lindeman, July 5, 2021.

246. Marcello Ceccaroni et al., "Pericardial, Pleural and Diaphragmatic Endometriosis in Association with Pelvic Peritoneal and Bowel Endometriosis: A Case Report and Review of the Literature," *Videosurgery*

and Other Miniinvasive Techniques 7, no. 2 (June 2012): 122–31, https://doi
.org/10.5114/wiitm.2011.26758.

247. Wendy Bingham, interview by Tracey Lindeman, July 14, 2021.

248. Kelly M. Hoffman et al., "Racial Bias in Pain Assessment and Treatment
Recommendations, and False Beliefs about Biological Differences between
Blacks and Whites," *Proceedings of the National Academy of Sciences of the
United States of America* 113, no. 16 (April 19, 2016): 4296–4301, https://doi
.org/10.1073/pnas.1516047113.

249. Hoffman et al., "Racial Bias."

250. Kiara M. Bridges, "Implicit Bias and Racial Disparities in Health Care,"
Human Rights 43, no. 3 (2018) https://www.americanbar.org/groups/crsj
/publications/human_rights_magazine_home/the-state-of-healthcare-in-the
-united-states/racial-disparities-in-health-care/.

251. Nancy E. Morden et al., "Racial Inequality in Prescription Opioid Receipt—
Role of Individual Health Systems," *New England Journal of Medicine* 385,
no. 4 (July 22, 2021): 342–51, https://doi.org/10.1056/NEJMsa2034159.

252. "White People Get Opioids," *Wanda Sykes: Not Normal,* directed by Linda
Mendoza (Netflix, 2019).

253. Samantha Artiga et al., "Health Coverage by Race and Ethnicity, 2010–
2019," KFF, July 16, 2021, https://www.kff.org/racial-equity-and-health
-policy/issue-brief/health-coverage-by-race-and-ethnicity/.

254. Keturah James and Ayana Jordan, "The Opioid Crisis in Black
Communities," *Journal of Law, Medicine & Ethics* 46, no. 2 (2018): 404–21,
https://doi.org/10.1177/1073110518782949.

255. "Health Insurance Coverage in the United States: 2018," United States
Census Bureau, https://www.census.gov/content/dam/Census/library
/publications/2019/demo/p60-267.pdf.

256. Lisa M. Pollack et al., "Racial/Ethnic Disparities/Differences in
Hysterectomy Route in Women Likely Eligible for Minimally Invasive
Surgery," *Journal of Minimally Invasive Gynecology* 27, no. 5 (July 1, 2020):
1167–1177.e2, https://doi.org/10.1016/j.jmig.2019.09.003.

257. Alessandra Spagnolia, James Beal, and Abe Sahmoun, "Differences in
Clinical Management and Outcomes of American Indian and White
Women Diagnosed With Endometriosis," *Journal of Family and Reproductive
Health* 14, no. 2 (October 18, 2020), https://doi.org/10.18502/jfrh.v14i2.4348.

258. Lloy Wylie and Stephanie McConkey, "Insiders' Insight: Discrimination
against Indigenous Peoples through the Eyes of Health Care Professionals,"
Journal of Racial and Ethnic Health Disparities 6, no. 1 (February 1, 2019):
37–45, https://doi.org/10.1007/s40615-018-0495-9.

259. Vikas Gampa, Kenneth Bernard, and Michael J. Oldani, "Racialization as a
Barrier to Achieving Health Equity for Native Americans," *AMA Journal of*

Ethics 22, no. 10 (October 2020): 874–81, https://doi.org/10.1001/amajethics .2020.874.

260. Morten Fibieger Byskov, "What Makes Epistemic Injustice an 'Injustice'?" *Journal of Social Philosophy* 52, no. 1 (March 1, 2021): 114–31, https://doi.org /10.1111/josp.12348.

261. "Research Identifies Gender Bias in Estimation of Patients' Pain," April 6, 2021, University of Miami News@TheU (blog), https://news.miami.edu/stories/2021 /04/research-identifies-gender-bias-in-estimation-of-patients-pain.html.

262. Lanlan Zhang et al., "Gender Biases in Estimation of Others' Pain," *The Journal of Pain* 22, no. 9 (September 2021): 1048–59, https://doi.org/10.1016 /j.jpain.2021.03.001.

263. Miranda Fricker and Katharine Jenkins, "Epistemic Injustice, Ignorance and Trans Experiences," in *The Routledge Companion to Feminist Philosophy* (Routledge, 2017), 268–78, https://doi.org/10.4324/9781315758152-23.

264. Fricker and Jenkins, "Epistemic Injustice, Ignorance and Trans Experiences."

265. Gráinne Schäfer et al., "Health Care Providers' Judgments in Chronic Pain: The Influence of Gender and Trustworthiness," *Pain* 157, no. 8 (August 2016): 1618–25, https://doi.org/10.1097/j.pain.0000000000000536.

266. Thomas Hadjistavropoulos, Bruce McMurtry, and Kenneth D. Craig, "Beautiful Faces in Pain: Biases and Accuracy in the Perception of Pain," *Psychology & Health* 11, no. 3 (March 1, 1996): 411–20, https://doi.org /10.1080/08870449608400268.

267. Heather D. Hadjistavropoulos, Michael A. Ross, and Carl L. Von Baeyer, "Are Physicians' Ratings of Pain Affected by Patients' Physical Attractiveness?" *Social Science & Medicine* 31, no. 1 (January 1, 1990): 69–72, https://doi.org/10.1016/0277-9536(90)90011-G.

268. Diane LaChapelle et al., "Attractiveness, Diagnostic Ambiguity, and Disability Cues Impact Perceptions of Women with Pain," *Rehabilitation Psychology* 59, no. 2 (May 2014): 162–70, https://doi.org/10.1037/a0035894.

269. Jing Meng et al., "The Interaction between Pain and Attractiveness Perception in Others," *Scientific Reports* 10, no. 1 (March 26, 2020): 5528, https://doi.org/10.1038/s41598-020-62478-x.

270. Daniel Z. Buchman, Anita Ho, and Judy Illes, "You Present like a Drug Addict: Patient and Clinician Perspectives on Trust and Trustworthiness in Chronic Pain Management," *Pain Medicine* 17, no. 8 (August 1, 2016): 1394–1406, https://doi.org/10.1093/pm/pnv083.

271. Daniel Z. Buchman, Anita Ho, and Daniel S. Goldberg, "Investigating Trust, Expertise, and Epistemic Injustice in Chronic Pain," *Journal of Bioethical Inquiry* 14, no. 1 (March 2017): 31–42, https://doi.org/10.1007/s11673-016-9761-x.

272. Kari Ann Phillips and Naykky Singh Ospina, "Physicians Interrupting Patients," *JAMA* 318, no. 1 (July 4, 2017): 93–94, https://doi.org/10.1001 /jama.2017.6493.

273. Gabrielle Jackson, "'Disgusting' Study Rating Attractiveness of Women with Endometriosis Retracted by Medical Journal," *The Guardian*, August 5, 2020, https://www.theguardian.com/society/2020/aug/05/disgusting-study-rating-attractiveness-of-women-with-endometriosis-retracted-by-medical-journal.

274. Anke Samulowitz et al., "'Brave Men' and 'Emotional Women': A Theory-Guided Literature Review on Gender Bias in Health Care and Gendered Norms towards Patients with Chronic Pain," *Pain Research & Management* 2018 (2018): 6358624, https://doi.org/10.1155/2018/6358624.

275. Larissa J. Strath et al., "Sex and Gender Are Not the Same: Why Identity Is Important for People Living with HIV and Chronic Pain," *Journal of Pain Research* 13 (April 24, 2020): 829–35, https://doi.org/10.2147/JPR.S248424.

276. Samulowitz et al., "Brave Men."

277. Strath et al., "Sex and Gender Are Not the Same."

278. Rich Schapiro, "'An Ongoing Nightmare': People with Obesity Face Major Healthcare Obstacles," NBC News, June 27, 2021, https://www.nbcnews.com/health/health-news/ongoing-nightmare-obese-people-face-major-obstacles-when-seeking-medical-n1272019.

279. Rita Rubin, "Addressing Medicine's Bias Against Patients Who Are Overweight," *JAMA* 321, no. 10 (March 12, 2019): 925–27, https://doi.org/10.1001/jama.2019.0048.

280. Beth Allan, interview by Tracey Lindeman, June 11, 2021.

281. Ted Combs, interview by Tracey Lindeman, May 29, 2021.

282. Anderson Sanches Melo, Rui Alberto Ferriani, and Paula Andrea Navarro, "Treatment of Infertility in Women with Polycystic Ovary Syndrome: Approach to Clinical Practice," *Clinics* 70, no. 11 (November 2015): 765–69, https://doi.org/10.6061/clinics/2015(11)09.

283. "The Trump Administration's Final Rule on Section 1557 Non-Discrimination Regulations Under the ACA and Current Status," KFF (blog), September 18, 2020, https://www.kff.org/racial-equity-and-health-policy/issue-brief/the-trump-administrations-final-rule-on-section-1557-non-discrimination-regulations-under-the-aca-and-current-status/.

284. Michael D. Shear and Margot Sanger-Katz, "Biden Administration Restores Rights for Transgender Patients," *The New York Times*, May 10, 2021, sec. U.S., https://www.nytimes.com/2021/05/10/us/politics/biden-transgender-patient-protections.html.

285. Julie Landry, "Trans, Gender-Diverse People with Endometriosis Fight 'Double Battle' against Pain and Lack of Recognition," CBC News, March 31, 2021, https://www.cbc.ca/news/canada/british-columbia/endometriosis-transgender-gender-diverse-non-binary-double-battle-1.5970374.

286. Rose Eveleth, "What Makes the Speculum Awful," *The Atlantic*, November 17, 2014, https://www.theatlantic.com/health/archive/2014/11/why-no-one-can-design-a-better-speculum/382534/.

287. Madeleine Freeman et al., "Acceptability of Non-Speculum Clinician Sampling for Cervical Screening in Older Women: A Qualitative Study," *Journal of Medical Screening* 25, no. 4 (December 2018): 205–10, https://doi .org/10.1177/0969141318756452.

288. Karen Canfell and Megan Smith, "Never Had a Pap Smear? Now There's a DIY Option for You," *The Conversation*, November 30, 2017, http:// theconversation.com/never-had-a-pap-smear-now-theres-a-diy-option-for -you-70706.

289. "A Self-Test Is Making Cervical Screening Even Easier," Healthdirect Australia, November 28, 2021, https://www.healthdirect.gov.au/blog /self-test-makes-cervical-screening-pap-smear-even-easier.

290. Marvellous Akinlotan et al., "Cervical Cancer Screening Barriers and Risk Factor Knowledge Among Uninsured Women," *Journal of Community Health* 42, no. 4 (2017): 770–78, https://doi.org/10.1007/s10900-017-0316-9.

291. Centers for Disease Control and Prevention, "Leading Cancers by Age, Sex, Race, and Ethnicity," United States Cancer Statistics: Data Visualizations, accessed March 10, 2022, https://gis.cdc.gov.

292. Kimberly D. Miller et al., "Cancer Statistics for the US Hispanic/Latino Population, 2021," *CA: A Cancer Journal for Clinicians* 71, no. 6 (2021): 466–87, https://doi.org/10.3322/caac.21695.

293. Rebekah Rollston, "Promoting Cervical Cancer Screening Among Female-to-Male Transmasculine Patients" (Fenway Institute, 2019).

294. Editorial, "Henrietta Lacks: Science Must Right a Historical Wrong," *Nature* 585, no. 7823 (September 1, 2020): 7, https://doi.org/10.1038/d41586-020 -02494-z.

295. Leah Samuel, "5 Important Ways Henrietta Lacks Changed Medical Science," *STAT* (blog), April 14, 2017, https://www.statnews.com/2017/04/14 /henrietta-lacks-hela-cells-science/.

296. "HeLa Cells (1951)," British Society for Immunology, accessed March 11, 2022, https://www.immunology.org/hela-cells-1951.

297. National Institutes of Health, "Significant Research Advances Enabled by HeLa Cells," Office of Science Policy (blog), accessed March 11, 2022, https:// osp.od.nih.gov/scientific-sharing/hela-cells-timeline/.

298. Art Caplan, "NIH Finally Makes Good with Henrietta Lacks' Family—and It's about Time, Ethicist Says," NBC News, August 7, 2013, http://www .nbcnews.com/healthmain/nih-finally-makes-good-henrietta-lacks-family-its -about-time-6C10867941.

299. "The U.S. Public Health Service Syphilis Study at Tuskegee," Centers for Disease Control and Prevention, May 3, 2021, https://www.cdc.gov/tuskegee /timeline.htm.

300. Heather Dron and Gianna May Sanchez, email to author, "Response to

Sterilization and Social Justice Lab Inquiry about Sterilization Statistics," April 12, 2022.

301. Victoria Bekiempis, "More Immigrant Women Say They Were Abused by Ice Gynecologist," *The Guardian*, December 22, 2020, https://www.theguardian.com/us-news/2020/dec/22/ice-gynecologist-hysterectomies-georgia.

302. Samantha Allen, "It's Not Just Japan. Many U.S. States Require Transgender People Get Sterilized," The Daily Beast, March 22, 2019, https://www.thedailybeast.com/its-not-just-japan-many-us-states-require-transgender-people-get-sterilized.

303. *Belly of the Beast*, directed by Erika Cohn, aired November 23, 2020, on PBS, https://www.pbs.org/independentlens/documentaries/belly-of-the-beast/.

304. Shilpa Jindia, "Belly of the Beast: California's Dark History of Forced Sterilizations," *The Guardian*, June 30, 2020, https://www.theguardian.com/us-news/2020/jun/30/california-prisons-forced-sterilizations-belly-beast.

305. Corey G. Johnson, "California Bans Coerced Sterilization of Female Inmates," *Reveal*, September 26, 2014, http://revealnews.org/article-legacy/california-bans-coerced-sterilization-of-female-inmates/.

306. UN Committee on the Rights of Persons with Disabilities, *Concluding Observations on the Initial Report of Canada* (Geneva: United Nations, May 8, 2017), https://digitallibrary.un.org/record/1310657.

307. National Women's Law Center, *Forced Sterilization of Disabled People in the United States* (Washington, DC: National Women's Law Center, January 2022), https://nwlc.org/resource/forced-sterilization-of-disabled-people-in-the-united-states/.

308. Bougie, Healey, and Singh, "Behind the Times."

309. Kellyn Pollard, interview by Tracey Lindeman, July 6, 2021.

310. Erika DuBose, "Black Wall Street Memorial March Led by Massacre Survivors on Horse-Drawn Carriage," *The Black Wall Street Times*, May 28, 2021, https://theblackwallsttimes.com/2021/05/28/black-wall-street-memorial-march-led-by-massacre-survivors-in-horse-drawn-carriage/.

311. Kellyn Pollard, "'Am I Crazy?': A Black Woman's Journey with Endometriosis," *The Black Wall Street Times*, March 17, 2021, https://theblackwallsttimes.com/2021/03/17/am-i-crazy-a-black-womans-journey-with-endometriosis/.

Chapter 5: Nervous Breakdown

312. *Competitive Problems in the Drug Industry: Hearings before the Subcomm. on Monopoly of the Select Comm. on Small Business, 2nd session, on the Present Status of Competition in the Pharmaceutical Industry, Part 16*, 91st Cong. 6451

(1970) (statement of Dr. Francis J. Kane), https://babel.hathitrust.org/cgi
/pt?id=msu.31293011705971&view=1up&seq=3&skin=2021.

313. *Competitive Problems in the Drug Industry*, 6451 (statement of Dr. Francis J. Kane).

314. Leanne R. McCloskey et al., "Contraception for Women with Psychiatric Disorders," *American Journal of Psychiatry* 178, no. 3 (March 2021): 247–55, https://doi.org/10.1176/appi.ajp.2020.20020154.

315. "No, Your Birth Control Won't Cause Depression," accessed February 5, 2022, https://news.northwestern.edu/stories/2020/11/birth-control-does-not-cause-depression/.

316. C. Lundin et al., "There Is No Association between Combined Oral Hormonal Contraceptives and Depression: A Swedish Register-Based Cohort Study," *BJOG: An International Journal of Obstetrics & Gynaecology* 129, no. 6 (May 2022), https://doi.org/10.1111/1471-0528.17028.

317. Charlotte Wessel Skovlund et al., "Association of Hormonal Contraception with Depression," *JAMA Psychiatry* 73, no. 11 (November 1, 2016): 1154–62, https://doi.org/10.1001/jamapsychiatry.2016.2387.

318. Skovlund et al., "Depression."

319. Heather Guidone, interview by Tracey Lindeman.

320. "Conversion Disorder," *Encyclopedia Britannica*, accessed February 17, 2022, https://www.britannica.com/science/conversion-disorder.

321. Sander Gilman et al., *Hysteria beyond Freud* (Berkeley, CA: University of California Press, 1993), 41.

322. Sabine Arnaud, *On Hysteria: The Invention of a Medical Category between 1670 and 1820* (Chicago: The University of Chicago Press, 2015).

323. Arnaud, *On Hysteria*, 1–8.

324. Gilman et al., *Hysteria beyond Freud*, 107–8.

325. Augustin Fabre, *L'hystérie viscérale: Les dilatations du coeur droit* (Paris: Adrien Delahaye et Emile Legrosnier, Place de l'école-de-médecine, 1883), 3.

326. Gilman et al., *Hysteria beyond Freud*, 294.

327. Arthur George Tansley, "Sigmund Freud 1856–1939," *Obituary Notices of Fellows of the Royal Society* 3, no. 9 (January 1941): 247–75, https://doi.org/10.1098/rsbm.1941.0002.

328. Sigmund Freud, *Fragment of an Analysis of a Case of Hysteria* (1905), 7–8.

329. Katrien Libbrecht and Julien Quackelbeen, "On the Early History of Male Hysteria and Psychic Trauma," *Journal of the History of the Behavioral Sciences* 31, no. 4 (October 1, 1995): 370–84, https://doi.org/10.1002/1520-6696(199510)31:4<370::AID-JHBS2300310404>3.0.CO;2-6.

330. Mark S. Micale, "The Salpêtrière in the Age of Charcot: An Institutional Perspective on Medical History in the Late Nineteenth Century," *Journal of Contemporary History* 20, no. 4 (October 1, 1985): 703–31, https://doi.org/10.1177/002200948502000411.

331. Micale, "The Salpêtrière."
332. Dana Haugh, "Salpêtrière Photographs," Text, Harvey Cushing/ John Hay Whitney Medical Library, August 27, 2021, https://library.medicine.yale.edu/historical/digitized-collections/salp%C3 %AAtri%C3%A8re-photographs.
333. Gilman et al., *Hysteria beyond Freud*, 345–46.
334. James C. Harris, "A Clinical Lesson at the Salpêtrière," *Archives of General Psychiatry* 62, no. 5 (May 1, 2005): 470–72, https://doi.org/10.1001/archpsyc .62.5.470.
335. Eva Figes, *Patriarchal Attitudes: Women in Society* (London: Faber & Faber, 1970), 146.
336. Andrea Tone, *The Age of Anxiety: A History of America's Turbulent Affair with Tranquilizers* (New York: Basic Books, 2008), 26.
337. Jack Drescher, "Out of DSM: Depathologizing Homosexuality," *Behavioral Sciences* 5, no. 4 (December 4, 2015): 565–75, https://doi.org/10.3390/bs5040565.
338. "Dr. Sandor Rado Dies at 82; An Original Disciple of Freud," *The New York Times*, May 16, 1972, sec. Archives, https://www.nytimes.com/1972 /05/16/archives/dr-sandor-rado-dies-at-82-an-original-disciple-of-freud -founder-of.html.
339. Jonathan M. Metzl, "'Mother's Little Helper': The Crisis of Psychoanalysis and the Miltown Resolution," *Gender & History* 15, no. 2 (August 1, 2003): 228–55, https://doi.org/10.1111/1468-0424.00300.
340. Jonathan Michel Metzl, *Prozac on the Couch: Prescribing Gender in the Era of Wonder Drugs* (Duke University Press, 2003), 80–81.
341. Metzl, *Prozac on the Couch*, 80–81.
342. Metzl, *Prozac on the Couch*, 74.
343. Matt Savelli, "Mind and Matter," Science History Institute, June 2, 2013, https://www.sciencehistory.org/distillations/mind-and-matter.
344. Patrick Radden Keefe, *Empire of Pain: The Secret History of the Sackler Dynasty* (Toronto: Bond Street Books, 2021), 53–65.
345. Metzl, "'Mother's Little Helper.'"
346. Tone, *The Age of Anxiety*, 27.
347. Tone, *The Age of Anxiety*, 27.
348. Radden Keefe, *Empire of Pain*, 53–65.
349. "Valium," *Encyclopaedia Britannica*, accessed March 12, 2022, https://www .britannica.com/science/Valium.
350. Radden Keefe, *Empire of Pain*, 53–55.
351. Radden Keefe, *Empire of Pain*, 62–64.
352. Metzl, "'Mother's Little Helper.'"
353. Radden Keefe, *Empire of Pain*, 58.
354. Samulowitz et al., "Brave Men."
355. Lanlan Zhang et al., "Gender Biases in Estimation of Others' Pain," *The*

       Journal of Pain 22, no. 9 (September 2021): 1048–59, https://doi.org/10.1016/j.jpain.2021.03.001.

356. Lanlan Zhang et al., "Gender Biases in Estimation of Others' Pain."

357. D.E. Hoffmann and A.J. Tarzian, "The Girl Who Cried Pain: A Bias against Women in the Treatment of Pain," *The Journal of Law, Medicine & Ethics* 29, no. 1 (2001): 13–27, https://doi.org/10.1111/j.1748-720x.2001.tb00037.x.

358. Nancy Petersen, interview by Tracey Lindeman, July 5, 2021.

359. Kate Weinstein, *Living with Endometriosis: How to Cope with the Physical and Emotional Challenges* (Reading, MA: Addison-Wesley Pub. Co, 1987).

360. "Endometriosis," Johns Hopkins Medicine, accessed February 16, 2022, https://www.hopkinsmedicine.org/health/conditions-and-diseases/endometriosis.

361. Erika Gebel Berg, "The Chemistry of the Pill," *ACS Central Science* 1, no. 1 (March 25, 2015): 5–7, https://doi.org/10.1021/acscentsci.5b00066.

362. "Birth Control Pills," Planned Parenthood, accessed March 12, 2022, https://www.plannedparenthood.org/learn/birth-control/birth-control-pill.

363. Michael Edwards and Ahmet S. Can, "Progestin," StatPearls, last updated September 21, 2021, http://www.ncbi.nlm.nih.gov/books/NBK563211/.

364. "Spironolactone," American Chemical Society, October 5, 2020, https://www.acs.org/content/acs/en/molecule-of-the-week/archive/s/spironolactone.html.

365. Alex V. Green, "Spironolactone, a Standard Drug in Hormone Treatment for Trans Women, Has Controversial Side Effects," Slate, June 10, 2019, https://slate.com/technology/2019/06/spironolactone-hormone-trans-women-side-effects.html.

366. Susanne Hiller-Sturmhöfel and Andrzej Bartke, "The Endocrine System," *Alcohol Health and Research World* 22, no. 3 (1998): 153–64, https://www.ncbi.nlm.nih.gov/pmc/articles/PMC6761896/.

367. Sarah E. Hill, *This Is Your Brain on Birth Control: The Surprising Science of Women, Hormones and the Law of Unintended Consequences* (New York: Avery, 2019), 81–85.

368. Donita Africander, Nicolette Verhoog, and Janet P. Hapgood, "Molecular Mechanisms of Steroid Receptor-Mediated Actions by Synthetic Progestins Used in HRT and Contraception," *Steroids* 76, no. 7 (June 1, 2011): 636–52, https://doi.org/10.1016/j.steroids.2011.03.001.

369. Richard Jones and Kristin H. Lopez, *Human Reproductive Biology—4th Edition* (Cambridge, MA: Academic Press, 2014), 249.

370. "Birth Control: How to Skip Your Monthly Period," Mayo Clinic, accessed March 12, 2022, https://www.mayoclinic.org/healthy-lifestyle/birth-control/in-depth/womens-health/art-20044044.

371. Robert W. Kistner, "The Treatment of Endometriosis by Inducing Pseudopregnancy with Ovarian Hormones: A Report of Fifty-Eight Cases," *Fertility and Sterility* 10, no. 6 (1959): 539–56, https://doi.org/10.1016/S0015-0282(16)33602-0.

372. Rei Shimoda, Anne Campbell, and Robert A. Barton. "Women's Emotional and Sexual Attraction to Men across the Menstrual Cycle," *Behavioral Ecology* 29, no. 1 (January 13, 2018): 51–59, https://doi.org /10.1093/beheco/arx124.

373. Hill, *This Is Your Brain on Birth Control.*

374. Rupali Sharma et al., "Use of the Birth Control Pill Affects Stress Reactivity and Brain Structure and Function," *Hormones and Behavior* 124 (August 1, 2020): 104783, https://doi.org/10.1016/j.yhbeh.2020.104783.

375. Shawn E. Nielsen et al., "Hormonal Contraception Use Alters Stress Responses and Emotional Memory," *Biological Psychology* 92, no. 2 (February 1, 2013): 257–66, https://doi.org/10.1016/j.biopsycho.2012.10.007.

376. American Psychological Association, "Stress Effects on the Body," American Psychologial Association (blog), November 1, 2018, https://www.apa.org /topics/stress/body.

377. Radiological Society of North America, "Study Finds Key Brain Region Smaller in Birth Control Pill Users," ScienceDaily, December 4, 2019, https://www.sciencedaily.com/releases/2019/12/191204090819.htm.

378. Nielsen et al., "Hormonal Contraception Use."

379. Mary Ann C. Stephens and Gary Wand, "Stress and the HPA Axis," *Alcohol Research : Current Reviews* 34, no. 4 (2012): 468–83, https://www.ncbi.nlm .nih.gov/pmc/articles/PMC3860380/.

380. Carlo Faravelli et al., "Childhood Stressful Events, HPA Axis and Anxiety Disorders," *World Journal of Psychiatry* 2, no. 1 (February 22, 2012): 13–25, https://doi.org/10.5498/wjp.v2.i1.13.

381. Nielsen et al., "Hormonal Contraception Use."

382. Johannes Hertel et al., "Evidence for Stress-Like Alterations in the HPA-Axis in Women Taking Oral Contraceptives," *Scientific Reports* 7, no. 1 (October 26, 2017): 14111, https://doi.org/10.1038/s41598-017-13927-7.

383. Marni N. Silverman and Esther M. Sternberg, "Glucocorticoid Regulation of Inflammation and Its Behavioral and Metabolic Correlates: From HPA Axis to Glucocorticoid Receptor Dysfunction," *Annals of the New York Academy of Sciences* 1261 (July 2012): 55–63, https://doi.org/10.1111/j.1749-6632.2012.06633.x.

384. Silvia Vannuccini et al., "Hormonal Treatments for Endometriosis: The Endocrine Background," *Reviews in Endocrine and Metabolic Disorders,* August 17, 2021, https://doi.org/10.1007/s11154-021-09666-w.

385. Muye Zhu and Roberta Brinton, "How Progestin, a Synthetic Female Hormone, Could Affect the Brain," *The Atlantic,* January 14, 2012, https://www.theatlantic.com/health/archive/2012/01/how-progestin-a -synthetic-female-hormone-could-affect-the-brain/251299/.

386. Bruce S. McEwen and Stephen E. Alves, "Estrogen Actions in the Central Nervous System," *Endocrine Reviews* 20, no. 3 (June 1, 1999): 279–307, https://doi.org/10.1210/edrv.20.3.0365.

387. Hill, *This Is Your Brain on Birth Control*, 88–89.
388. Katherine M. Scarpin et al., "Progesterone Action in Human Tissues: Regulation by Progesterone Receptor (PR) Isoform Expression, Nuclear Positioning and Coregulator Expression," *Nuclear Receptor Signaling* 7 (December 31, 2009): e009, https://doi.org/10.1621/nrs.07009; Keri Stephens, "Breast MRI Shows IUDs Have Systemic Effects," *AXIS Imaging News*, November 22, 2021, http://www.proquest.com/docview/2600470030 /abstract/A543FAB13BAD462EPQ/1.
389. René Zeiss et al., "Depressive Disorder with Panic Attacks after Replacement of an Intrauterine Device Containing Levonorgestrel: A Case Report," *Frontiers in Psychiatry* 11 (August 28, 2020): 561685, https://doi.org/10.3389 /fpsyt.2020.561685.
390. Jurate Aleknaviciute et al., "The Levonorgestrel-Releasing Intrauterine Device Potentiates Stress Reactivity," *Psychoneuroendocrinology* 80 (June 1, 2017): 39–45, https://doi.org/10.1016/j.psyneuen.2017.02.025.
391. Bayer AG, "Mirena Prescribing Information," https://labeling.bayerhealthcare.com/html/products/pi/Mirena_PI.pdf.
392. Jurate Aleknaviciute et al., "The Levonorgestrel-Releasing Intrauterine Device Potentiates Stress Reactivity."
393. Charlotte Wessel Skovlund, interview by Tracey Lindeman, June 5, 2020.
394. Skovlund et al., "Association of Hormonal Contraception with Depression."
395. Charlotte Wessel Skovlund et al., "Association of Hormonal Contraception with Suicide Attempts and Suicides," *American Journal of Psychiatry* 175, no. 4 (April 2018): 336–42, https://doi.org/10.1176/appi.ajp.2017.17060616.
396. "Management of Endometriosis," American College of Obstetricians and Gynecologists, July 2010, https://www.acog.org/en/clinical/clinical-guidance /practice-bulletin/articles/2010/07/management-of-endometriosis.
397. Gayle Markovitz, "Why Are Women More Depressed Than Men?" World Economic Forum (blog), March 6, 2020, https://www.weforum.org /agenda/2020/03/are-women-less-happy-than-men/.
398. Jaimie F. Veale et al., "The Mental Health of Canadian Transgender Youth Compared with the Canadian Population," *The Journal of Adolescent Health: Official Publication of the Society for Adolescent Medicine* 60, no. 1 (January 2017): 44–49, https://doi.org/10.1016/j.jadohealth.2016.09.014.
399. Noah J. Adams and Ben Vincent, "Suicidal Thoughts and Behaviors Among Transgender Adults in Relation to Education, Ethnicity, and Income: A Systematic Review," *Transgender Health* 4, no. 1 (October 16, 2019): 226–46, https://doi.org/10.1089/trgh.2019.0009.
400. Allan John Pollack et al., "Why Women See Their GP More Than Men," *The Conversation*, February 7, 2016, http://theconversation.com/why-women-see -their-gp-more-than-men-49051.
401. "Men and Depression," National Institute of Mental Health (blog), accessed

March 13, 2022, https://www.nimh.nih.gov/health/publications/men-and depression.

402. Nicholas R. Eaton et al., "An Invariant Dimensional Liability Model of Gender Differences in Mental Disorder Prevalence: Evidence from a National Sample," *Journal of Abnormal Psychology* 121, no. 1 (February 2012): 282–88, https://doi.org/10.1037/a0024780.

403. David Hubacher et al., "Preventing Copper Intrauterine Device Removals Due to Side Effects among First-Time Users: Randomized Trial to Study the Effect of Prophylactic Ibuprofen," *Human Reproduction* 21, no. 6 (June 1, 2006): 1467–72, https://doi.org/10.1093/humrep/del029.

Chapter 6: We're Desperate

404. Stephanie Lepage, interview by Tracey Lindeman, June 11, 2021.

405. Robert W. Kistner, "The Treatment of Endometriosis by Inducing Pseudopregnancy with Ovarian Hormones: A Report of Fifty-Eight Cases," *Fertility and Sterility* 10, no. 6 (1959): 539–56, https://doi.org/10.1016/S0015 -0282(16)33602-0.

406. Kistner, "Infertility with Endometriosis."

407. Kistner, "Infertility with Endometriosis."

408. Donna Shoupe, "The Progestin Revolution," *Contraception and Reproductive Medicine* 6, no. 1 (January 7, 2021): 3, https://doi.org/10.1186/s40834-020 -00142-5.

409. U.S. Food and Drug Administration, "Drugs@FDA: FDA-Approved Drugs," accessed February 19, 2022, https://www.accessdata.fda.gov /scripts/cder/daf/index.cfm?event=overview.process&ApplNo\=010976.

410. "ALESSE (Levonorgestrel, Ethinyl Estradiol) Dosage Forms, Composition And Packaging," Pfizer, accessed February 19, 2022, https://www .pfizermedicalinformation.ca/en-ca/alesse/dosage-forms-composition-and -packaging.

411. "Yasmin, Yaz (Drospirenone/Ethinyl Estradiol) Dosing, Indications, Interactions, Adverse Effects, and More," Medscape, accessed February 19, 2022, https://reference.medscape.com/drug/yasmin-yaz-drospirenone-ethinyl -estradiol-342768.

412. *Interagency Coordination in Drug Research and Regulation: Hearings before the Subcomm. on Reorganization and International Organizations of the Comm. on Government Operations, Part 4*, 88th Cong. 1925–42 (1963) (exhibit 237), https://babel.hathitrust.org/cgi/pt?id=osu.32437122474246&view=1up &seq=7.

413. Kistner, "Infertility with Endometriosis."

414. Kistner, "The Use of Newer Progestins."

415. *Competitive Problems in the Drug Industry: Hearings before the Subcomm. on Monopoly of the Select Comm. on Small Business, 2nd session, on the Present Status of Competition in the Pharmaceutical Industry, Part 15,* 91st Cong. 6062 (1970) (statement of Dr. Robert W. Kistner), https://babel.hathitrust.org/cgi /pt?id=msu.31293011705963&view=1up&seq=3&skin=2021.

416. *Competitive Problems in the Drug Industry, Part 15,* 91st Cong. 6074 (statement of Dr. Robert W. Kistner).

417. Naomi Kresge and Cynthia Koons, "Better Birth Control Exists, But Big Pharma Isn't Interested," *Bloomberg,* August 8, 2019, https://www.bloomberg .com/news/articles/2019-08-08/better-birth-control-exists-but-big-pharma-isn -t-interested.

418. Fernando M. Reis et al., "Progesterone Receptor Ligands for the Treatment of Endometriosis: The Mechanisms behind Therapeutic Success and Failure," *Human Reproduction Update* 26, no. 4 (May 16, 2020): 565–85, https://doi.org /10.1093/humupd/dmaa009.

419. Elodie Chantalat et al. "Estrogen Receptors and Endometriosis," *International Journal of Molecular Sciences* 21, no. 8 (April 17, 2020): 2815, https://doi.org /10.3390/ijms21082815.

420. Taisuke Mori et al., "Local Estrogen Formation and Its Regulation in Endometriosis," *Reproductive Medicine and Biology* 18, no. 4 (2019): 305–11, https://doi.org/10.1002/rmb2.12285.

421. Suzanne White Junod, "FDA's Approval of the First Oral Contraceptive, Enovid," *Update* (Food and Drug Law Institute), July–August 1998, https:// www.fda.gov/media/110456/download.

422. Becky Little, "Delivering 'The Pill' Wasn't Easy," *National Geographic,* December 18, 2014, https://www.nationalgeographic.com/adventure/article /141218-birth-control-pill-contraception-science-medicine-ngbooktalk.

423. Aliya Buttar and Sheraden Seward, "Enovid: The First Hormonal Birth Control Pill," The Embryo Project Encyclopedia, January 20, 2009, https:// embryo.asu.edu/pages/enovid-first-hormonal-birth-control-pill.

424. Gardiner Harris, "The Pill Started More Than a Sexual Revolution," *The New York Times,* May 3, 2010, https://www.nytimes.com/2010/05/04/health /04pill.html.

425. Barbara Seaman, "Letter from Barbara Seaman to Senator Gaylord Nelson, September 23, 1969," Jewish Women's Archive, https://jwa.org/media/letter -from-barbara-seaman-to-senator-gaylord-nelson.

426. *Competitive Problems in the Drug Industry, Part 15,* 91st Cong.

427. *Competitive Problems in the Drug Industry: Hearings before the Subcomm. on Monopoly of the Select Comm. on Small Business, 2nd session, on the Present Status of Competition in the Pharmaceutical Industry, Part 16,* 91st Cong. (1970), https://babel.hathitrust.org/cgi/pt?id=msu.31293011705971&view =1up&seq=3&skin=2021.

428. *Competitive Problems in the Drug Industry: Hearings before the Subcomm. on Monopoly of the Select Comm. on Small Business, 2nd session, on the Present Status of Competition in the Pharmaceutical Industry, Part 17,* 91st Cong. (1970), https://babel.hathitrust.org/cgi/pt?id=msu.31293026739346&view =1up&seq=1&skin=2021.

429. *Competitive Problems in the Drug Industry, Part 16,* 91st Cong. 6693–94 (statement of Mrs. Phyllis Piotrow).

430. *Competitive Problems in the Drug Industry, Part 16,* 91st Cong. 6749 (statement of Dr. Herbert Ratner).

431. *Competitive Problems in the Drug Industry, Part 16,* 91st Cong. 6749 (statement of Dr. Herbert Ratner).

432. "Poll Finds Shift in Views on Pill," *The New York Times,* March 1, 1970, https://www.nytimes.com/1970/03/01/archives/poll-finds-shift-in-views-on -pill-more-women-see-a-danger-in-oral.html.

433. *Competitive Problems in the Drug Industry, Part 16,* 91st Cong. 6689–90 (statement of Senator Nelson).

434. James J. Nagle, "Merger News," *The New York Times,* March 19, 1971, https:// www.nytimes.com/1971/03/19/archives/searle-seeking-howmedica-inc-accord -in-principle-reached-for.html.

435. "Sen. Nelson Accused of Creating a Fear of Birth Control Pill," *The New York Times,* March 4, 1970, https://www.nytimes.com/1970/03/04/archives /sen-nelson-accused-of-creating-a-fear-of-birth-control-pill.html.

436. *Population Crisis: Hearings before the Subcomm. on Foreign Aid Expenditures of the Comm. on Government Operations, 2nd session,* 89th Cong. (1966), https://www.govinfo.gov/app/details/CHRG-89shrg67785p5A/summary.

437. *Competitive Problems in the Drug Industry, Part 16,* 91st Cong., 6741–42 (statement of Dr. Herbert Ratner).

438. Morton Mintz, *The Pill: An Alarming Report* (Boston: Beacon Press, 1970), 20, 24–25.

439. Mintz, *The Pill,* 23.

440. Stephanie Banchero, "Obituary: Dr. H. Ratner, Family-Life Advocate," *The Chicago Tribune,* December 17, 1997, https://www.chicagotribune.com/news /ct-xpm-1997-12-17-9712170220-story.html.

441. *Competitive Problems in the Drug Industry, Part 16,* 91st Cong., 6716, 6731, 6735, 6742.

442. Christel Meuleman et al., "High Prevalence of Endometriosis in Infertile Women with Normal Ovulation and Normospermic Partners," *Fertility and Sterility* 92, no. 1 (July 1, 2009): 68–74, https://doi.org/10.1016/j.fertnstert .2008.04.056.

443. Divya Kelath Shah, "Diminished Ovarian Reserve and Endometriosis: Insult upon Injury," *Seminars in Reproductive Medicine* 31, no. 2 (March 2013): 144–49, https://doi.org/10.1055/s-0032-1333479.

444. "Carl Djerassi," *Science History Institute* (blog), June 1, 2016, https://www
.sciencehistory.org/historical-profile/carl-djerassi.

445. Gaby Wood, "Father of the Pill," *The Observer*, April 14, 2007, https://www
.theguardian.com/lifeandstyle/2007/apr/15/healthandwellbeing.features1.

446. Margaret Sanger, "Voluntary Motherhood," *Teaching American History* (blog),
1917, https://teachingamericanhistory.org/document/voluntary-motherhood/.

447. Margaret Sanger and Carrie Chapman Catt, *The Pivot of Civilization* (New
York: Brentano's, 1922), https://www.gutenberg.org/files/1689/1689-h/1689
-h.htm.

448. *Competitive Problems in the Drug Industry, Part 16*, 91st Cong., 6748
(statement of Dr. Herbert Ratner).

449. Sanger and Catt, *The Pivot of Civilization*.

450. "The History & Impact of Planned Parenthood," Planned Parenthood,
accessed March 13, 2022, https://www.plannedparenthood.org/about-us/who
-we-are/our-history.

451. Sanger and Catt, *The Pivot of Civilization*.

452. Jonathan Eig, *The Birth of the Pill: How Four Crusaders Reinvented Sex and
Launched a Revolution* (New York: W. W. Norton & Company, 2014).

453. Jonathan Eig, "The Team That Invented the Birth-Control Pill," *The Atlantic*,
October 9, 2014, https://www.theatlantic.com/health/archive/2014/10/the
-team-that-invented-the-birth-control-pill/380684/.

454. "The Boston Pill Trials," *American Experience*, PBS, accessed March 13, 2022,
https://www.pbs.org/wgbh/americanexperience/features/pill-boston-pilltrials/.

455. Eig, *The Birth of the Pill*, 174–180.

456. Eig, *The Birth of the Pill*, 159–159.

457. John Rock, "Suitable Experimental Subjects," OnView: Digital Collections &
Exhibits, https://collections.countway.harvard.edu/onview/items/show/6466.

458. Eig, *The Birth of the Pill*, 232.

459. Suzanne White Junod and Lara Marks, "Women's Trials: The Approval of the
First Oral Contraceptive Pill in the United States and Great Britain," *Journal
of the History of Medicine and Allied Sciences* 57, no. 2 (April 1, 2002): 117–60,
https://doi.org/10.1093/jhmas/57.2.117.

460. N. Ordover, "The Eugenics Archive: Puerto Rico," *The Eugenics Archive*
(blog), February 24, 2014, http://eugenicsarchive.ca/discover/tree
/530ba18176f0db569b00001b.

461. "The Pill and Informed Consent," *American Experience*, PBS, accessed April
15, 2022, https://www.pbs.org/wgbh/americanexperience/features/pill-and
-informed-consent/.

462. "The Great Bluff That Led to a 'Magical' Pill and a Sexual Revolution," *Fresh
Air*, NPR, October 7, 2014, https://www.npr.org/2015/10/02/445089125
/the-great-bluff-that-led-to-a-magical-pill-and-a-sexual-revolution.

463. Joanna Schoen, *Choice and Coercion: Birth Control, Sterilization, and Abortion*

in *Public Health and Welfare* (Chapel Hill, NC: University of North Carolina Press, 2005), 3.

464. William Green, *Contraceptive Risk: The FDA, Depo-Provera, and the Politics of Experimental Medicine* (New York: New York University Press, 2017), 1–14, 134.

465. William Green, "The Odyssey of Depo-Provera: Contraceptives, Carcinogenic Drugs, and Risk-Management Analyses," *Food, Drug, Cosmetic Law Journal* 42, no. 4 (1987): 567–87, http://www.jstor.org/stable/26658687.

466. Green, *Contraceptive Risk*, 20.

467. Green, *Contraceptive Risk*, 16.

468. Douglas F. Scutchfield and W. Newton Long, "Parenteral Medroxyprogesterone as a Contraceptive Agent," *Public Health Reports (1896–1970)* 84, no. 12 (1969): 1059–62, https://doi.org/10.2307/4593755.

469. Wendy Kline, *Bodies of Knowledge: Sexuality, Reproduction, and Women's Health in the Second Wave* (Chicago, IL: University of Chicago Press, 2010), 113–19.

470. Nicholas H. Wright and Joseph R. Swartwout, "A Program in Mass Family Planning for the Urban Indigent in a Charity Hospital," *American Journal of Obstetrics and Gynecology* 97, no. 2 (January 15, 1967): 181–188, https://doi.org/10.1016/0002-9378(67)90538-8.

471. Kline, *Bodies of Knowledge*, 115.

472. *Use of the Drug, Depo Provera, by the Indian Health Service: Oversight Hearing before the Subcomm. on General Oversight and Investigations of the Comm. on Interior and Insular Affairs*, 100th Cong. 157 (1987) (statement of Sybil Shainwald), https://babel.hathitrust.org/cgi/pt?id=uc1.31210014741084&view=1up&seq=1&skin=2021.

473. *Use of the Drug, Depo Provera, by the Indian Health Service*, 100th Cong. 168 (1987) (testimony of Sybil Shainwald).

474. *Use of the Drug, Depo Provera, by the Indian Health Service*, 100th Cong. 170 (1987) (testimony of Sybil Shainwald).

475. U.S. Food and Drug Administration, "Drugs@FDA: FDA-Approved Drugs," accessed February 20, 2022, https://www.accessdata.fda.gov/scripts/cder/daf/index.cfm?event=overview.process&ApplNo=020246.

476. David B. Thomas, Elizabeth A. Noonan, and WHO Collaborative Study of Neoplasia and Steroid Contraceptives, "Risk of Breast Cancer in Relation to Use of Combined Oral Contraceptives near the Age of Menopause," *Cancer Causes & Control* 2, no. 6 (November 1, 1991): 389–94, https://doi.org/10.1007/BF00054299.

477. U.S. Food and Drug Administration, "Depo-Provera Black Box Warning," 2004, https://www.pfizermedicalinformation.com/en-us/depo-provera/boxed-warning.

478. "Model List of Essential Medicines (2019)," World Health Organization, 42, https://www.who.int/publications/i/item/WHOMVPEMPIAU2019.06.

479. Interagency Coordination in Drug Research and Regulation: Hearings before the Subcomm. on Reorganization and International Organizations of the Comm. on Government Operations, 89th Cong. 1860 (1963) (official reply of George P. Larrick), https://babel.hathitrust.org/cgi/pt?id=osu.32437122474246&view=1up&seq=7&skin=2021.

480. Competitive Problems in the Drug Industry: Hearings before the Subcomm. on Monopoly of the Select Comm. on Small Business, 2nd session, on the Present Status of Competition in the Pharmaceutical Industry, Part 15, 91st Cong. 5925 (1970) (statement of Dr. Hugh J. Davis), https://babel.hathitrust.org/cgi/pt?id=msu.31293011705963&view=1up&seq=3&skin=2021.

481. Competitive Problems in the Drug Industry, Part 15, 91st Cong. 5941 (1970) (statement of Dr. Hugh J. Davis).

482. Rainey Horwitz, "The Dalkon Shield," The Embryo Project Encyclopedia (blog), January 10, 2018, https://embryo.asu.edu/pages/dalkon-shield.

483. Horwitz, "The Dalkon Shield."

484. Morton Mintz, At Any Cost: Corporate Greed, Women, and the Dalkon Shield (New York: Pantheon Books, 1985), 86.

485. Mintz, At Any Cost.

486. "Papers of the Dalkon Shield Claimants Trust, [1970–1998]," Arthur J. Morris Library, University of Virginia, accessed February 20, 2022, https://archives.law.virginia.edu/records/mss/00-4.

487. "All Dalkon Shields Taken off the Market," The New York Times, January 21, 1975, https://www.nytimes.com/1975/01/21/archives/all-dalkon-shields-taken-off-market.html.

488. James A. Miller, "Money for Mischief: USAID and Pathfinder Tag-Team Women in the Developing World," Population Research Institute (blog), September 1, 1996, https://www.pop.org/money-for-mischief-usaid-and-pathfinder-tag-team-women-in-the-developing-world/.

489. Mark Dowie, Barbara Ehrenreich, and Stephen Minkin, "The Charge: Gynocide; the Accused: The US Government," Mother Jones, November 1979, https://www.motherjones.com/politics/1979/11/charge-gynocide/.

490. "Contraceptive Use by Method 2019," United Nations, Population Division, https://digitallibrary.un.org/record/3849735.

491. Kresge and Koons, "Better Birth Control Exists."

492. "Health Facts: Hormonal Birth Control and Blood Clot Risk," National Women's Health Network, February 22, 2017, https://nwhn.org/hormonal-birth-control-blood-clot-risk/.

493. Adam Taylor, "Blood Clot Risks: Comparing the AstraZeneca Vaccine and the Contraceptive Pill," The Conversation, April 12, 2021, http://theconversation.com/blood-clot-risks-comparing-the-astrazeneca-vaccine-and-the-contraceptive-pill-158652.

494. Pushkala Aripaka, "Very Small Blood Clot Risk after First AstraZeneca

COVID Shot—UK Studies," Reuters, February 22, 2022, sec. Healthcare & Pharmaceuticals, https://www.reuters.com/business/healthcare-pharmaceuticals/very-small-blood-clot-risk-after-first-astrazeneca-covid-shot-uk-studies-2022-02-22/.

495. "Yaz, Yasmin Birth Control Pills Suspected in 23 Deaths," CBC News, June 11, 2013, https://www.cbc.ca/news/canada/british-columbia/yaz-yasmin-birth-control-pills-suspected-in-23-deaths-1.1302473.

496. "FDA Drug Safety Communication: Safety Review Update on the Possible Increased Risk of Blood Clots with Birth Control Pills Containing Drospirenone," U.S. Food and Drug Administration, June 28, 2019, https://www.fda.gov/drugs/drug-safety-and-availability/fda-drug-safety-communication-safety-review-update-possible-increased-risk-blood-clots-birth-control.

497. "Yasmin and Yaz (Drospirenone): Updated Information on Increased Risk of Blood Clots," Health Canada, December 5, 2011, https://recalls-rappels.canada.ca/en/alert-recall/yasmin-and-yaz-drospirenone-updated-information-increased-risk-blood-clots.

498. "Yaz Lawsuits," Drugwatch.com, accessed February 20, 2022, https://www.drugwatch.com/yaz/lawsuits/.

499. "Merck to Pay $100 Million in NuvaRing Contraceptive Settlement," Reuters, February 7, 2014, https://www.reuters.com/article/us-merck-nuvaring-idUSBREA1615F20140207.

500. "Bayer AG: Annual Report 2020," Bayer AG, 82, https://www.bayer.com/sites/default/files/2021-02/Bayer-Annual-Report-2020.pdf.

501. Janice Tibbetts, "Reproductive Health Experts Warn Women Not to Abandon Birth Control," *CMAJ : Canadian Medical Association Journal* 185, no. 11 (August 6, 2013): E517–18, https://doi.org/10.1503/cmaj.109-4529.

502. Stephanie Lepage, interview by Tracey Lindeman.

503. "Determination That LUPRON (Leuprolide Acetate) Injection, 1 Milligram/0.2 Milliliter, Was Not Withdrawn from Sale for Reasons of Safety or Effectiveness," Federal Register, May 30, 2019, https://www.federalregister.gov/documents/2019/05/30/2019-11243/determination-that-lupron-leuprolide-acetate-injection-1-milligram02-milliliter-was-not-withdrawn.

504. "ART Medications," Society for Assisted Reproductive Technology, accessed February 19, 2022, https://www.sart.org/patients/a-patients-guide-to-assisted-reproductive-technology/general-information/art-medications/.

505. Jong Hyuk Choi et al., "Therapeutic Effects of Leuprorelin (Leuprolide Acetate) in Sexual Offenders with Paraphilia," *Journal of Korean Medical Science* 33, no. 37 (July 23, 2018): e231, https://doi.org/10.3346/jkms.2018.33.e231.

506. "Puberty Blockers for Youth," Trans Care BC: Provincial Health Services Authority, accessed February 19, 2022, http://www.phsa.ca/transcarebc/child-youth/affirmation-transition/medical-affirmation-transition/puberty-blockers-for-youth.

507. April Grant, press officer at FDA, email to author, "Media Request Regarding Leuprolide Acetate and Elagolix," September 24, 2021.

508. "Management of Endometriosis," American College of Obstetricians and Gynecologists, July 2010, https://www.acog.org/en/clinical/clinical-guidance /practice-bulletin/articles/2010/07/management-of-endometriosis.

509. April Grant, email.

510. "FDA Adverse Events Reporting System (FAERS)," Food and Drug Administration, https://fis.fda.gov/sense/app/95239e26-e0be-42d9-a960 -9a5f7f1c25ee/sheet/7a47a261-d58b-4203-a8aa-6d3021737452/state/analysis.

511. Rodrigo de P. Sepulcri and Vivian F. do Amaral, "Depressive Symptoms, Anxiety, and Quality of Life in Women with Pelvic Endometriosis," *European Journal of Obstetrics and Gynecology and Reproductive Biology* 142, no. 1 (January 1, 2009): 53–56, https://doi.org/10.1016/j.ejogrb.2008.09.003.

512. D.J. Brody, L.A. Pratt, and J. Hughes, "Prevalence of Depression Among Adults Aged 20 and Over: United States, 2013–2016," National Center for Health Statistics, 2018, https://www.cdc.gov/nchs/products/databriefs /db303.htm.

513. Christina Jewett, "Women Fear Drug They Used to Halt Puberty Led to Health Problems," *Kaiser Health News*, February 2, 2017, https://khn.org /news/women-fear-drug-they-used-to-halt-puberty-led-to-health-problems/.

514. Kathryn Phillips, interview by Tracey Lindeman, June 23, 2021.

515. "ORILISSA® (Elagolix) 150 Mg or 200 Mg Tablets," AbbVie, accessed February 21, 2022, https://www.orilissa.com/about/what-is-orilissa.

516. "Discover ORIAHNN®," AbbVie, accessed February 21, 2022, https://www .oriahnn.com/.

517. Ivan Urits et al., "An Evidence-Based Review of Elagolix for the Treatment of Pain Secondary to Endometriosis," *Psychopharmacology Bulletin* 50, no. 4 suppl. 1 (October 15, 2020): 197–215, https://pubmed.ncbi.nlm.nih.gov /33633426/.

518. "Institute for Clinical and Economic Review Final Report Highlights Limitations in Evidence on Long-Term Safety and Effectiveness of Elagolix for Endometriosis, Discusses Options for Insurance Coverage Criteria," Institute for Clinical and Economic Review, August 3, 2018, https://icer.org /news-insights/press-releases/elagolix-final-report/.

519. "Elagolix for Treating Endometriosis—Final Evidence Report," Institute for Clinical and Economic Review, 36, https://icer.org/wp-content/uploads /2020/10/ICER_Elagolix_Final_Evidence_Report_080318.pdf.

520. "Orilissa Prices," GoodRx.com, accessed February 21, 2022, https://www .goodrx.com/orilissa.

521. "Institute for Clinical and Economic Review Final Report," Institute for Clinical and Economic Review.

522. "ORILISSA Prescribing Information," AbbVie, October 29, 2021, https://

www.abbvie.ca/content/dam/abbvie-dotcom/ca/en/documents/products /ORILISSA_PM_EN.PDF.

523. April Grant, email.

524. Dr. Jeff Arrington, interview by Tracey Lindeman, September 2, 2021.

525. Dr. Jeff Arrington, interview by Tracey Lindeman.

526. "Management of Endometriosis," American College of Obstetricians and Gynecologists, 2010, https://www.acog.org/clinical/clinical-guidance/practice -bulletin/articles/2010/07/management-of-endometriosis.

527. Dr. Jeff Arrington, interview by Tracey Lindeman.

528. Dr. Christopher Zahn (ACOG), interview by Tracey Lindeman, July 18, 2022.

529. "Missed Miscarriage," The Miscarriage Association, accessed February 16, 2022, https://www.miscarriageassociation.org.uk/information/miscarriage /missed-miscarriage/.

530. Stephanie Lepage, email to author, September 19, 2021.

531. Center for Drug Evaluation and Research: Approval Package for Application Number 020517/S002" (Food and Drug Administration, May 30, 1997).

532. Yun-Fei Zhu et al., Gonadotropin-releasing hormone receptor antagonists and methods relating thereto, U.S. Patent US6,346,534B1, filed May 12, 2000, and issued February 12, 2002.

533. "Neurocrine Wins $20M from Abbott Related to Elagolix for Endometriosis," *Genetic Engineering and Biotechnology News*, October 5, 2011, https://www.genengnews.com/topics/drug-discovery/neurocrine-wins -20m-from-abbott-related-to-elagolix-for-endometriosis/.

534. "Neurocrine Biosciences 10-K Filings: 2010–2021, Inclusively," United States Securities and Exchange Commission, https://www.sec.gov/edgar/browse /?CIK=914475&owner=exclude.

535. "AbbVie 10-K Filings: 2018–2021, Inclusively," United States Securities and Exchange Commission, https://www.sec.gov/edgar/browse/?CIK=1551152 &owner=exclude.

536. "Dollars for Docs: AbbVie: Orilissa 2018," ProPublica, https://projects .propublica.org/docdollars/products/11208.

537. Jessica Meiselman, "The Sneaky Way Pharmaceutical Companies Use Celebs to Market Their Drugs," *The Outline*, April 15, 2019, https://theoutline.com/ post/7290/julianne-hough-abbvie-endometriosis-orilissa.

538. "Neurocrine Biosciences 10-K Filings," United States Securities and Exchange Commission.

539. "Dollars for Docs: AbbVie: Lupron 2018," ProPublica, https://projects .propublica.org/docdollars/products/9191.

540. "AbbVie 10-K Filings," United States Securities and Exchange Commission.

541. "TAP Pharmaceutical Products Inc. and Seven Others Charged with Health Care Crimes Company Agrees to Pay $875 Million to Settle Charges," U.S.

Department of Justice, press release, October 3, 2001, https://www.justice
.gov/archive/opa/pr/2001/October/513civ.htm.

542. Melody Petersen, "2 Drug Makers to Pay $875 Million to Settle Fraud Case,"
The New York Times, October 4, 2001, https://www.nytimes.com/2001/10/04
/business/2-drug-makers-to-pay-875-million-to-settle-fraud-case.html.

543. "Takeda Pharmaceuticals and TAP Pharmaceutical Products Inc. Merge,"
Takeda Pharmaceuticals, press release, June 30, 2008, https://www.takeda
.com/en-us/newsroom/news-releases/2008/takeda-pharmaceuticals-and-tap
-pharmaceutical-products-inc.-merge/.

544. United States et al. vs. Takeda Pharmaceutical Company et al., Civil Action
1-11-cv-10343-FDS (District Court of Massachusetts 2012), 35.

545. "Open Payments Data Overview, Centers for Medicare & Medicaid
Services," Open Payments, accessed February 19, 2022, https://www.cms.gov
/OpenPayments/Data.

546. "Open Payments Data Overview," Open Payments.

547. Charles Ornstein, Mike Tigas, and Ryann Grochowski Jones, "Now There's
Proof: Docs Who Get Company Cash Tend to Prescribe More Brand-
Name Meds." ProPublica, March 17, 2016, https://www.propublica.org
/article/doctors-who-take-company-cash-tend-to-prescribe-more-brand
-name-drugs?token=9YmWuD9Dnei8kq4XpeZOIjXk4eC-4NHL.

548. "Voluntary Disclosure of Payments," Innovative Medicines Canada, accessed
February 19, 2022, http://innovativemedicines.ca/ethics/voluntary-disclosure
-of-payments/.

549. "Responsibility: Voluntary Disclosure of Payments," AbbVie, accessed
February 19, 2022, https://www.abbvie.ca/content/dam/abbvie-dotcom
/ca/en/documents/Voluntary-Disclosure-PaymentsHealthcareProfessionals
-HealthcareOrganization-EN_2019.pdf.

550. Aaron P. Mitchell et al., "Are Financial Payments from the Pharmaceutical
Industry Associated with Physician Prescribing? A Systematic Review,"
Annals of Internal Medicine 174, no. 3 (March 2021): 353–61, https://doi.org
/10.7326/M20-5665.

551. Committee Opinion, "Professional Relationships with Industry," American
College of Obstetricians and Gynecologists, November 2012, https://www
.acog.org/en/clinical/clinical-guidance/committee-opinion/articles/2012/11
/professional-relationships-with-industry.

552. Micah R. Wright et al., "Evaluating Financial Conflicts of Interest Among
Contributors to Clinical Practice Guidelines of the American College of
Obstetricians and Gynecologists," *Journal of Osteopathic Medicine* 120, no. 7
(July 1, 2020): 462–70, https://doi.org/10.7556/jaoa.2020.059.

553. Kate Connors, senior media relations manager at ACOG, email to author,
June 29, 2022.

554. Micah R. Wright et al., "Evaluating Financial Conflicts."

555. "Clinical Consensus Methodology," ACOG, https://www.acog.org/clinical /clinical guidance/clinical-consensus/articles/2021/09/clinical-consensus -methodology.

556. Heather Guidone, interview by Tracey Lindeman.

557. Dr. Christopher Zahn (ACOG), interview by Tracey Lindeman.

558. Dr. Jeff Arrington, interview by Tracey Lindeman.

559. Dr. Christopher Zahn (ACOG), interview by Tracey Lindeman.

560. "Global Endometriosis Drug Forecast and Market Analysis Report 2021-2030: Current Therapies Leave Significant Unmet Needs & Pipeline Therapies Present Promise in Closing Treatment Gaps," Yahoo! Finance, January 31, 2022, https://finance.yahoo.com/news/global-endometriosis -drug-forecast-market-163500890.html?guccounter=1.

Chapter 7: I Wanna Be Well

561. Richard E. Allen and Karl A. Kirby, "Nocturnal Leg Cramps," *American Family Physician* 86, no. 4 (August 15, 2012): 350–55, https://www.aafp.org /afp/2012/0815/p350.html.

562. "When Sex Is Painful," *American College of Obstetricians and Gynecologists* (blog), accessed February 17, 2022, https://www.acog.org/en/womens-health /faqs/when-sex-is-painful.

563. Giussy Barbara et al., "What Is Known and Unknown About the Association Between Endometriosis and Sexual Functioning: A Systematic Review of the Literature," *Reproductive Sciences* 24, no. 12 (December 1, 2017): 1566–76, https://doi.org/10.1177/1933719117707054.

564. Leona K. Shum et al., "Deep Dyspareunia and Sexual Quality of Life in Women With Endometriosis," *Sexual Medicine* 6, no. 3 (May 22, 2018): 224–33, https://doi.org/10.1016/j.esxm.2018.04.006.

565. Shaoli Yin et al., "Diagnosis of Deep Infiltrating Endometriosis Using Transvaginal Ultrasonography," *Frontiers in Medicine* 7 (November 23, 2020), https://www.frontiersin.org/article/10.3389/fmed.2020.567929.

566. Philip J. Quartana, Claudia M. Campbell, and Robert R. Edwards, "Pain Catastrophizing: A Critical Review," *Expert Review of Neurotherapeutics* 9, no. 5 (May 2009): 745–58, https://doi.org/10.1586/ERN.09.34.

567. Rodrigo de P. Sepulcri and Vivian F. do Amaral, "Depressive Symptoms, Anxiety, and Quality of Life in Women with Pelvic Endometriosis," *European Journal of Obstetrics and Gynecology and Reproductive Biology* 142, no. 1 (January 1, 2009): 53–56, https://doi.org/10.1016/j.ejogrb.2008.09.003.

568. "Endometriosis: Women 'Taking Their Own Lives' Due to Lack of Support," BBC News, October 7, 2019, https://www.bbc.com/news/uk -wales-49933866.

569. Togas Tulandi, "Endometriosis and Pelvic Pain Awareness: Infertility, Suicidal Ideation, and Cancer," *Journal of Obstetrics and Gynaecology Canada* 43, no. 5 (May 1, 2021): 543–44, https://doi.org/10.1016/j.jogc.2021.03.001.

570. Thomas George, "Woman, 26, Suffering Agonising Endometriosis Pain Died after Accidental Painkillers Overdose," *Manchester Evening News*, June 24, 2021, https://www.manchestereveningnews.co.uk/news/greater-manchester -news/woman-26-suffering-agonising-endometriosis-20876642.

571. Tian Li et al., "Endometriosis Alters Brain Electrophysiology, Gene Expression and Increases Pain Sensitization, Anxiety, and Depression in Female Mice," *Biology of Reproduction* 99, no. 2 (August 1, 2018): 349–59, https://doi.org/10.1093/biolre/ioy035.

572. Jiyao Sheng et al., "The Link between Depression and Chronic Pain: Neural Mechanisms in the Brain," *Neural Plasticity* 2017 (June 19, 2017), https://doi .org/10.1155/2017/9724371.

573. Sawsan As-Sanie et al., "Changes in Regional Gray Matter Volume in Women with Chronic Pelvic Pain—a Voxel Based Morphometry Study," *Pain* 153, no. 5 (May 2012): 1006–14, https://doi.org/10.1016/j.pain.2012.01.032.

574. Abhijeet Gummadavelli and Hal Blumenfeld, "Thalamus," *Encyclopaedia Britannica*, accessed February 17, 2022. https://www.britannica.com/science /thalamus.

575. Antonio Simone Laganà et al., "Anxiety and Depression in Patients with Endometriosis: Impact and Management Challenges," *International Journal of Women's Health* 9 (May 16, 2017): 323–30, https://doi.org/10.2147/IJWH .S119729.

576. D.J. Brody, L.A. Pratt, and J. Hughes, "Prevalence of Depression Among Adults Aged 20 and Over: United States, 2013–2016," National Center for Health Statistics, 2018, https://www.cdc.gov/nchs/products/databriefs /db303.htm.

577. Gabrielle Jackson, "Why Don't Doctors Trust Women? Because They Don't Know Much About Us," *The Guardian*, September 1, 2019, https://www .theguardian.com/books/2019/sep/02/why-dont-doctors-trust-women -because-they-dont-know-much-about-us.

578. Lara Wellman, interview by Tracey Lindeman, June 9, 2021.

579. Patrick Radden Keefe, *Empire of Pain*, 210.

580. Chris McGreal, "US Medical Group That Pushed Doctors to Prescribe Painkillers Forced to Close," *The Guardian*, May 25, 2019, https://www .theguardian.com/us-news/2019/may/25/american-pain-society-doctors -painkillers.

581. William Heisel, "Journalists Bag a Big One: The American Pain Foundation," *Center for Health Journalism* (blog), May 14, 2012, https:// centerforhealthjournalism.org/blogs/2012/05/14/journalists-bag-big-one -american-pain-foundation.

582. Clara Scher et al., "Moving beyond Pain as the Fifth Vital Sign and Patient Satisfaction Scores to Improve Pain Care in the 21st Century," *Pain Management Nursing: Official Journal of the American Society of Pain Management Nurses* 19, no. 2 (April 2018): 125–29, https://doi.org/10.1016/j.pmn.2017.10.010.

583. N. Levy, J. Sturgess, and P. Mills, "'Pain as the Fifth Vital Sign' and Dependence on the 'Numerical Pain Scale' Is Being Abandoned in the US: Why?," *British Journal of Anaesthesia* 120, no. 3 (March 1, 2018): 435–38, https://doi.org/10.1016/j.bja.2017.11.098.

584. Jackson, "Why Don't Doctors Trust Women?"

585. Juno Obedin-Maliver, "Pelvic Pain and Persistent Menses in Transgender Men | University of California, San Francisco—Gender Affirming Health Program," June 17, 2016, https://transcare.ucsf.edu/guidelines/pain-transmen.

586. Frances W. Grimstad, Elizabeth Boskey, and Meredith Grey, "New-Onset Abdominopelvic Pain After Initiation of Testosterone Therapy Among Trans-Masculine Persons: A Community-Based Exploratory Survey," *LGBT Health* 7, no. 5 (July 2020): 248–53, https://doi.org/10.1089/lgbt.2019.0258.

587. Hillary D. White and Thomas D. Robinson, "A Novel Use for Testosterone to Treat Central Sensitization of Chronic Pain in Fibromyalgia Patients," *International Immunopharmacology* 27, no. 2 (August 1, 2015): 244–48, https://doi.org/10.1016/j.intimp.2015.05.020.

588. Susan F. Evans et al., "Androgens, Endometriosis and Pain," *Frontiers in Reproductive Health* 3 (2021), https://www.frontiersin.org/article/10.3389/frph.2021.792920.

589. Amelia M. Stanton et al., "Differences in Mental Health Symptom Severity and Care Engagement among Transgender and Gender Diverse Individuals: Findings from a Large Community Health Center," *PLOS ONE* 16, no. 1 (January 25, 2021): e0245872, https://doi.org/10.1371/journal.pone.0245872.

590. Agustín Fuentes, "Biological Science Rejects the Sex Binary, and That's Good for Humanity," SAPIENS, May 11, 2022, https://www.sapiens.org/biology/biological-science-rejects-the-sex-binary-and-thats-good-for-humanity/.

591. Dr. Jeffrey S. Mogil, interview by Tracey Lindeman, June 2, 2021.

592. Jeffrey S. Mogil, "Qualitative Sex Differences in Pain Processing: Emerging Evidence of a Biased Literature," *Nature Reviews Neuroscience* 21, no. 7 (July 2020): 353–65, https://doi.org/10.1038/s41583-020-0310-6.

593. Margaret Waltz et al., "Evaluating the National Institutes of Health's Sex as a Biological Variable Policy: Conflicting Accounts from the Front Lines of Animal Research," *Journal of Women's Health* 30, no. 3 (March 2021): 348–54, https://doi.org/10.1089/jwh.2020.8674.

594. Theresa M. Wizemann and Mary-Lou Pardue, eds., *Exploring the Biological Contributions to Human Health: Does Sex Matter?* (Washington, DC: National Academies Press, 2001), https://www.ncbi.nlm.nih.gov/books/NBK222292/.

595. Wizemann and Pardue, *Exploring the Biological Contributions.*

596. Jamie White et al., "The Integration of Sex and Gender Considerations into Biomedical Research: Lessons from International Funding Agencies," *The Journal of Clinical Endocrinology & Metabolism* 106, no. 10 (October 1, 2021): 3034–48, https://doi.org/10.1210/clinem/dgab434.

597. "NIH Policy and Guidelines on the Inclusion of Women and Minorities as Subjects in Clinical Research," National Institutes of Health, accessed February 17, 2022, https://grants.nih.gov/grants/guide/notice-files/NOT -OD-18-014.html.

598. White et al., "The Integration of Sex and Gender."

599. Maayan Sudai et al., "Law, Policy, Biology, and Sex: Critical Issues for Researchers," *Science* 376, no. 6595 (May 20, 2022): 802–4, https://doi.org /10.1126/science.abo1102.

600. Mogil, "Qualitative Sex Differences."

601. Zoë Slote Morris, Steven Wooding, and Jonathan Grant, "The Answer Is 17 Years, What Is the Question," *Journal of the Royal Society of Medicine* 104, no. 12 (December 2011): 510–20, https://doi.org/10.1258/jrsm.2011.110180.

602. Stephen R. Hanney et al., "How Long Does Biomedical Research Take? Studying the Time Taken between Biomedical and Health Research and Its Translation into Products, Policy, and Practice," *Health Research Policy and Systems* 13, no. 1 (January 1, 2015): 1, https://doi.org/10.1186/1478-4505-13-1.

603. Beata Smolarz, Krzysztof Szyłło, and Hanna Romanowicz, "Endometriosis: Epidemiology, Classification, Pathogenesis, Treatment, and Genetics (Review of Literature)," *International Journal of Molecular Sciences* 22, no. 19 (January 2021): 10554, https://doi.org/10.3390/ijms221910554.

604. Amy E. Lacroix, Hurria Gondal, and Michelle D. Langaker, "Physiology, Menarche," StatPearls, last update March 17, 2022, http://www.ncbi.nlm.nih. gov/books/NBK470216/.

605. "How Do I Know When I'm in Menopause?," The North American Menopause Society, https://www.menopause.org/for-women /menopauseflashes/menopause-symptoms-and-treatments/how-do-i-know -when-i%27m-in-menopause-.

606. Meike Schuster and Dhanya A. Mackeen, "Fetal Endometriosis," *Fertility and Sterility* 103, no. 1 (January 1, 2015): 160–62, https://doi.org/10.1016 /j.fertnstert.2014.09.045.

607. Fernanda de Almeida Asencio et al., "Symptomatic Endometriosis Developing Several Years after Menopause in the Absence of Increased Circulating Estrogen Concentrations: A Systematic Review and Seven Case Reports," *Gynecological Surgery* 16, no. 1 (February 15, 2019): 3, https://doi.org /10.1186/s10397-019-1056-x.

608. Dr. Jeff Arrington, interview by Tracey Lindeman.

609. "Excision of Endometriosis," The Center for Endometriosis Care, accessed

February 16, 2022, https://centerforendo.com/lapex-laparoscopic-excision -of-endometriosis.

610. Rui Li et al., "Prevalence and Time of Diagnosis of Endometriosis across Racial and Ethnic Groups in the US," medRxiv preprint, July 31, 2021, https://doi.org/10.1101/2021.07.28.21261303.

611. Tobin Siebers, *Disability Theory* (University of Michigan Press, 2008), 46–48.

612. Jax (anonymous), interview by Tracey Lindeman, June 28, 2021.

613. Marit Stiles, interview by Tracey Lindeman, June 29, 2021.

614. Catherine Reisch, interview by Tracey Lindeman, June 18, 2021.

615. Sally Zori, interview by Tracey Lindeman, June 20, 2021.

616. Celia (anonymous), interview by Tracey Lindeman, June 27, 2021.

617. Jasmine Galang, interview by Tracey Lindeman, June 18, 2021.

618. Donna (anonymous), interview by Tracey Lindeman.

619. Ted Combs, interview by Tracey Lindeman.

620. Lana Krupey, interview by Tracey Lindeman, June 10, 2021.

621. Nancy Petersen, interview by Tracey Lindeman.

622. Eileen Mary Holowka, interview by Tracey Lindeman, June 14, 2021.

623. Shelia Ivany, interview by Tracey Lindeman, June 17, 2021.

624. Brandi LaPerle, interview by Tracey Lindeman, August 10, 2021.

625. US Congresswoman Jenniffer González-Colón, "House Approves Push by Finkenauer and Endometriosis Caucus to Double Research Funding," press release, July 30, 2020, https://gonzalez-colon.house.gov/media/press-releases /house-approves-push-finkenauer-and-endometriosis-caucus-double-research -funding.

626. "Budget," National Institutes of Health, 2020, https://www.nih.gov/about -nih/what-we-do/budget.

627. "Estimates of Funding for Various Research, Condition, and Disease Categories," National Institutes of Health RePORT, June 25, 2021, https:// report.nih.gov/funding/categorical-spending#/.

628. Esther Eisenberg, "Pre-IVF Treatment with a GnRH Antagonist in Women with Endometriosis—A Prospective Double-Blind Placebo-Controlled Trial," clinical trial registration (February 1, 2022), https://clinicaltrials.gov/ct2/show /NCT04173169.

629. Hugh Taylor, "Pre-IVF Treatment with a GnRH Antagonist in Women with Endometriosis—A Prospective Double Blind Placebo Controlled Trial (Pregnant)," NIH RePORTER, accessed March 14, 2022, https://reporter .nih.gov/project-details/10025594.

630. "HUGH S TAYLOR," Open Payments, 2018, https://openpaymentsdata.cms .gov/physician/331812.

631. Emily Ritter, public affairs specialist at National Institutes of Health, emails to author, "Media Info Request on Endometriosis Funding," April 14, 2022.

632. "Endometriosis Research Funding Bill Passed in Congress," *Endometriosis*

Foundation of America (blog), March 17, 2022, https://www.endofound.org /press-release-endometriosis-research-funding-bill-passed-in-congress.

633. Jeanne Rebillard, director of communications and government relations at Endometriosis Foundation of America, emails to author, "Media Request for End of Day—Endo Funding," April 6, 2022.·

634. "IRS Form 990 for Endometriosis Foundation of America, EIN 20-4904437. 2006–2020," Internal Revenue Service, https://apps.irs.gov/app/eos/, https:// projects.propublica.org/nonprofits/organizations/204904437.

635. "U.S. Census Bureau QuickFacts: Percent of Female Persons," United States Census Bureau, 2021, https://www.census.gov/quickfacts/fact/dashboard/US /SEX255219.

636. Jessica Glenza, "Endometriosis Often Ignored as Millions of American Women Suffer," *The Guardian*, September 28, 2015, https://www.theguardian.com /us-news/2015/sep/27/endometriosis-ignored-federal-research-funding.

637. "20 Painful Health Conditions," National Health Service, May 28, 2018, https://web.archive.org/web/20180528122513/https://www.nhs.uk/live-well /healthy-body/20-painful-health-conditions/.

638. National Institutes of Health, "Estimates of Funding for Various Research, Condition, and Disease Categories," NIH RePORT, July 2, 2022, https:// report.nih.gov/funding/categorical-spending#/.

639. Suneel D. Kamath, Sheetal M. Kircher, and Al B. Benson, "Comparison of Cancer Burden and Nonprofit Organization Funding Reveals Disparities in Funding Across Cancer Types," *Journal of the National Comprehensive Cancer Network* 17, no. 7 (July 1, 2019): 849–54, https://doi.org/10.6004/jnccn .2018.7280.

640. "Ductal Carcinoma in Situ (DCIS)," American Cancer Society, accessed March 14, 2022, https://www.cancer.org/cancer/breast-cancer/about/types -of-breast-cancer/dcis.html.

641. "Breast Cancer Statistics," American Cancer Society, 2021, https://www .cancer.org/cancer/breast-cancer/about/how-common-is-breast-cancer.html.

642. "Breast Cancer Statistics," American Cancer Society.

643. "Breast Cancer—Statistics," American Society of Clinical Oncology, 2022, https://www.cancer.net/cancer-types/breast-cancer/statistics.

644. Arthur A. Mirin, "Gender Disparity in the Funding of Diseases by the U.S. National Institutes of Health," *Journal of Women's Health (2002)* 30, no. 7 (July 2021): 956–63, https://doi.org/10.1089/jwh.2020.8682.

645. Kamath, Kircher, and Benson, "Comparison of Cancer Burden."

646. Mirin, "Gender Disparity."

647. Mirin, "Gender Disparity."

648. Rachel E. Gross, "They Call It a 'Women's Disease.' She Wants to Redefine It," *The New York Times*, April 27, 2021, https://www.nytimes.com/2021/04 /27/health/endometriosis-griffith-uterus.html.

Chapter 8: Notice of Eviction

649. N. Senn, "The Early History of Vaginal Hysterectomy," *JAMA* XXV, no. 12 (September 21, 1895): 476–482, https://doi.org/10.1001/jama.1895 .02430380006002.

650. Senn, "The Early History of Vaginal Hysterectomy."

651. Senn, "The Early History of Vaginal Hysterectomy."

652. Senn, "The Early History of Vaginal Hysterectomy."

653. Senn, "The Early History of Vaginal Hysterectomy."

654. Ludwig Emil Grimm, *Portrait of Konrad Johann Martin Langenbeck (1776–1851), Professor of Anatomy and Surgery at Göttingen*, etching, 1826, https://www.philamuseum.org/collection/object/12427.

655. Innie Chen, Abdul Jamil Choudhry, and Togas Tulandi, "Hysterectomy Trends: A Canadian Perspective on the Past, Present, and Future," *Journal of Obstetrics and Gynaecology Canada* 41 (December 1, 2019): S340–42, https://doi.org/10.1016/j.jogc.2019.09.002.

656. "Hysterectomy," Office on Women's Health, accessed March 14, 2022, https://www.womenshealth.gov/a-z-topics/hysterectomy#references.

657. Elodie Chantalat et al. "Estrogen Receptors and Endometriosis," *International Journal of Molecular Sciences* 21, no. 8 (April 17, 2020): 2815, https://doi.org/10 .3390/ijms21082815.

658. B. Rizk et al., "Recurrence of Endometriosis after Hysterectomy," *Facts, Views & Vision in ObGyn* 6, no. 4 (2014): 219–27, https://www.ncbi.nlm.nih.gov/pmc /articles/PMC4286861/.

659. Rizk et al., "Recurrence."

660. Dr. Jeff Arrington, interview by Tracey Lindeman.

661. "Management of Endometriosis," American College of Obstetricians and Gynecologists.

662. Dr. Christopher Zahn (ACOG), interview by Tracey Lindeman.

663. The Committee on Clinical Practice Guidelines–Gynecology," ACOG, https://www.acog.org/about/leadership-and-governance/committees.

664. Nancy Petersen, interview by Tracey Lindeman.

665. Zoë Pugsley and Karen Ballard, "Management of Endometriosis in General Practice: The Pathway to Diagnosis," *The British Journal of General Practice* 57, no. 539 (June 1, 2007): 470–76, https://www.ncbi.nlm.nih.gov/pmc/articles /PMC2078174/.

666. Sally Zori, interview by Tracey Lindeman.

667. Sunshine, interview by Tracey Lindeman, June 28, 2021.

Chapter 9: Bad Reputation

668. *Girl, Interrupted*, directed by James Mangold (Columbia Pictures, 1999).
669. Alan E. Fruzzetti, "Why Borderline Personality Disorder Is Misdiagnosed," *National Alliance on Mental Illness* (blog), October 3, 2017, https://www.nami.org/Blogs/NAMI-Blog/October-2017/Why-Borderline-Personality-Disorder-is-Misdiagnose.
670. Clare Shaw and Gillian Proctor, "Women at the Margins: A Critique of the Diagnosis of Borderline Personality Disorder," *Feminism & Psychology* 15, no. 4 (November 1, 2005): 483–90, https://doi.org/10.1177/0959-353505057620.
671. Dr. Jessica Taylor, *Sexy but Psycho* (New York: Little, Brown, and Company, 2022), xiii.
672. Sally King, "Premenstrual Syndrome (PMS) and the Myth of the Irrational Female," in *The Palgrave Handbook of Critical Menstruation Studies*, edited by Chris Bobel et al. (Singapore: Springer, 2020), 287, https://doi.org/10.1007/978-981-15-0614-7_23.
673. Beth Allan, interview by Tracey Lindeman.
674. "Data Shows Women, People of Color Affected Most by 'Medical Gaslighting,'" *Good Morning America* (ABC News), April 5, 2022, https://www.youtube.com/watch?v=Ec5wq9oDWTY.
675. Stephen Humphreys, "The Unethical Use of BMI in Contemporary General Practice," *The British Journal of General Practice* 60, no. 578 (September 1, 2010): 696–97, https://doi.org/10.3399/bjgp10X515548.
676. Carly Stern, "Why BMI Is a Flawed Health Standard, Especially for People of Color," *Washington Post*, May 5, 2021, https://www.washingtonpost.com/lifestyle/wellness/healthy-bmi-obesity-race-/2021/05/04/655390f0-ad0d-11eb-acd3-24b44a57093a_story.html.
677. Giles Yeo, "BMI: We Know It's Flawed, so Why Do We Still Use It?," *BBC Science Focus Magazine*, July 6, 2021, https://www.sciencefocus.com/comment/bmi-we-know-its-flawed-so-why-do-we-still-use-it/.
678. Nancy Petersen, interview by Tracey Lindeman.
679. American Association of Gynecologic Laparoscopists, "AAGL Fellowship Program," *AAGL* (blog), accessed July 2, 2022, https://www.aagl.org/service/fellowships/.
680. Dr. Antonio Simone Laganà, emails to author, questions and answers sent between May 27–June 16, 2021.
681. Dr. Jörg Keckstein, interview by Tracey Lindeman.
682. "National Action Plan for Endometriosis," Australian Government Department of Health, last updated August 31, 2021, https://www.health.gov.au/resources/publications/national-action-plan-for-endometriosis.
683. "Premier comité de pilotage de la Stratégie nationale contre l'endométriose,"

Gouvernement français, accessed February 21, 2022, https://www.gouvernement.fr/premier-comite-de-pilotage-de-la-strategie-nationale-contre-l-endometriose.

684. Audre Lorde, "The Master's Tools Will Never Dismantle the Master's House," *Sister Outsider: Essays and Speeches* (Berkeley, CA: Crossing Press, 1984), 110–114.

For every book sold, 1% of the cover price will be donated to Moon Time Sisters, a collective of people who want to help menstruators in northern, remote communities across Canada access menstrual products that they otherwise could not afford.

This book is also available as a Global Certified Accessible™ (GCA) ebook. ECW Press's ebooks are screen reader friendly and are built to meet the needs of those who are unable to read standard print due to blindness, low vision, dyslexia, or a physical disability.

At ECW Press, we want you to enjoy our books in whatever format you like. If you've bought a print copy just send an email to ebook@ecwpress.com and include:

Get the ebook free!*
*proof of purchase required

- the book title
- the name of the store where you purchased it
- a screenshot or picture of your order/receipt number and your name
- your preference of file type: PDF (for desktop reading), ePub (for a phone/tablet, Kobo, or Nook), mobi (for Kindle)

A real person will respond to your email with your ebook attached. Please note this offer is only for copies bought for personal use and does not apply to school or library copies.

Thank you for supporting an independently owned Canadian publisher with your purchase!